# SUPER
# BETTER

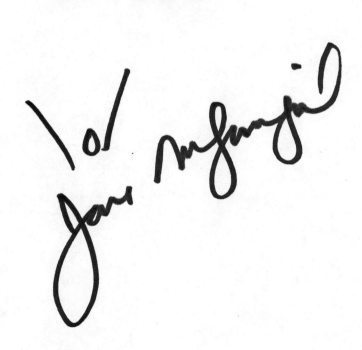

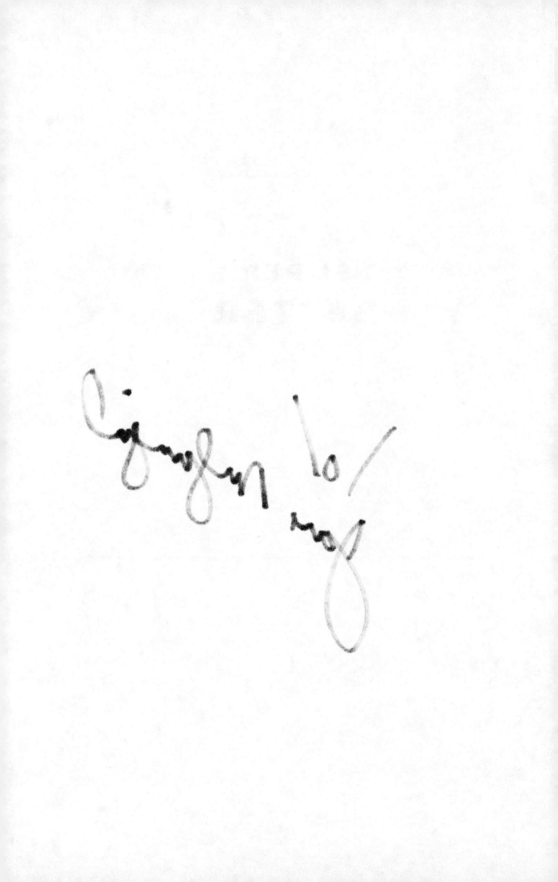

# SUPER
# BETTER

A Revolutionary
Approach to Getting
Stronger, Happier,
Braver, *and*
More Resilient*

## Jane McGonigal

*POWERED BY THE SCIENCE OF GAMES

VIKING

VIKING
an imprint of Penguin Canada Books Inc., a Penguin Random House Company

Published by the Penguin Group
Penguin Canada Books Inc.,
320 Front Street West, Suite 1400, Toronto, Ontario M5V 3B6, Canada

Penguin Group (USA) LLC, 375 Hudson Street, New York, New York 10014,
U.S.A. • Penguin Books Ltd, 80 Strand, London WC2R 0RL, England •
Penguin Ireland, 25 St Stephen's Green, Dublin 2, Ireland (a division of Penguin
Books Ltd) • Penguin Group (Australia), 707 Collins Street, Melbourne, Victoria
3008, Australia (a division of Pearson Australia Group Pty Ltd) • Penguin Books
India Pvt Ltd, 11 Community Centre, Panchsheel Park, New Delhi – 110 017,
India • Penguin Group (NZ), 67 Apollo Drive, Rosedale, Auckland 0632,
New Zealand (a division of Pearson New Zealand Ltd) • Penguin Books (South
Africa) (Pty) Ltd, 24 Sturdee Avenue, Rosebank, Johannesburg 2196, South Africa

Penguin Books Ltd, Registered Offices:
80 Strand, London WC2R 0RL, England

Published in Viking hardcover by Penguin Canada Books Inc., 2015
Simultaneously published in the United States by The Penguin Press

1   2   3   4   5   6   7   8   9   10   (RRD)

Manufactured in the U.S.A.

LIBRARY AND ARCHIVES CANADA CATALOGUING IN PUBLICATION

McGonigal, Jane, author
SuperBetter : a revolutionary approach to getting
stronger, happier, braver and more resilient--powered by the
science of games / Jane McGonigal.
Includes bibliographical references and index.
ISBN 978-0-670-06954-5 (bound)
1. Computer games--Social aspects.   2. Computer games--Health
aspects.   3. Computer games--Psychological aspects.   I. Title.   II. Title: Super
better.
GV1469.17.S63M34 2015           306.4'87           C2015-902065-4

eBook ISBN 978-0-14-319466-8

DESIGN BY AMANDA DEWEY
ICONS BY LAUREN KOLM

Visit the Penguin Canada website at www.penguin.ca

Special and corporate bulk purchase rates available; please see
www.penguin.ca/corporatesales or call 1-800-810-3104.

*To Tilden and Sibley—*
*May you grow up to be the heroes of your own stories*

# Contents

**PART 3**

•────────•

# Adventures

# Before You Play,
# Here's What You Need to Know

The SuperBetter method is designed to make you stronger, happier, braver, and more resilient.

It's based on the science of games—and there's *a lot* of evidence that it works.

A **randomized, controlled study conducted by the University of Pennsylvania** found that playing SuperBetter for thirty days significantly reduces symptoms of depression and anxiety and increases optimism, social support, and players' belief in their own ability to succeed and achieve their goals. The study also found that people who followed the SuperBetter rules for one month were significantly happier and more satisfied with their lives.

A **clinical trial funded by the National Institutes of Health** and conducted at Ohio State University Wexner Medical Center and Cincinnati Children's Hospital found that the SuperBetter method improves mood, decreases anxiety and suffering, and strengthens family relationships during rehabilitation and recovery.

Meanwhile, **data collected from more than 400,000 SuperBetter players** has helped me improve the method, to make it easier to learn and more fun to use in everyday life.

Every single day for the past five years I've heard from someone who says that the SuperBetter method has changed their life. It is my greatest hope that SuperBetter will help *you* tackle your toughest challenges, and pursue your biggest dreams, with more courage, creativity, optimism, and support.

Please remember, the SuperBetter method is *not* a substitute for medical advice or treatment. Many successful SuperBetter players—including a majority of participants in the University of Pennsylvania study and all the participants in the clinical trial—followed the SuperBetter method alongside some form of continuing counseling, medication, or rehabilitation, or with a doctor's supervision. *The SuperBetter method is NOT an alternative to therapy, counseling, ongoing medical treatment, or medication—nor is any game recommended or discussed in this book.*

Now that you know—let's play!

# SUPER
# BETTER

# Introduction

*You are stronger than you know.*

*You are surrounded by potential allies.*

*You are the hero of your own story.*

These three qualities are all it takes to become happier, braver, and more resilient in the face of any challenge.

Here's the good news: You already have these qualities within you. You don't have to change a thing. You are *already* more powerful than you realize.

You have the ability to control your attention—and therefore your thoughts and feelings.

You have the strength to find support in the most unexpected places, and deepen your existing relationships.

You have a natural capacity to motivate yourself and supercharge your heroic qualities, like willpower, compassion, and determination.

This book will help you understand the powers you already have—and show you that accessing these powers is *as easy as playing a game.*

◄►

And yet this book is not about playing games—at least, not exactly. It's about learning *how to be gameful* in the face of extreme stress and personal challenge.

Being gameful means bringing the psychological strengths you naturally display when you play games—such as optimism, creativity, courage, and determination—to your real life. It means having the curiosity and openness to play with different strategies to discover what works best. It means building up the resilience to tackle tougher and tougher challenges with greater and greater success.

The best way I know to explain what it means to be gameful—and how being gameful can make you stronger, happier, and braver—is to tell you a story. It's the story of how I invented the SuperBetter method—and the life-threatening challenge I had to overcome to be able to write this book.

◄►

In the summer of 2009, I hit my head and got a concussion. It didn't heal properly, and after thirty days I still had constant headaches, nausea, and vertigo. I couldn't read or write for more than a few minutes at a time. I had trouble remembering things. Most days I felt too sick to get out of bed. I was in a total mental fog. These symptoms left me more anxious and depressed than I had ever been in my life.

I had trouble communicating clearly to friends and family exactly what I was going through. I thought if I could write something down, it would help. I struggled and struggled to put together words that made sense, and this is what I came up with:

*Everything is hard.*

*The iron fist is pushing against
my thoughts.*

*My whole brain feels vacuum
pressurized.*

*If I can't think who am I?*

Unfortunately, there is no real treatment for postconcussion syndrome. You just rest as much as you can and hope for the best. I was told I might not feel better for months or even a year or longer.

There was one thing I could do to try to heal faster. My doctor told me I should avoid everything that triggered my symptoms. That meant no reading, no writing, no running, no video games, no work, no email, no alcohol, and no caffeine. I joked to my doctor at the time: "In other words, no reason to live."

There was quite a bit of truth in that joke. I didn't know it then, but suicidal ideation is very common with traumatic brain injuries—even mild ones like mine.[1] It happens to one in three, and it happened to me. My brain started telling me: *Jane, you want to die.* It said, *You're never going to get better. The pain will never end. You'll be a burden to your husband.*

These voices became so persistent and so persuasive that I started to legitimately fear for my life.

And then something happened. I had one crystal-clear thought that changed everything. Thirty-four days after I hit my head—and I will never forget this moment—I said to myself, *I am either going to kill myself, or I'm going to turn this into a game.*

Why a game? By the time I hit my head in 2009, I'd been researching the psychology of games for nearly a decade. In fact, I was the first person in the world to earn a Ph.D. studying the psychological strengths of gamers and how those strengths can translate to real-world problem solving. I knew from my years of research at the University of California at Berkeley that when we play a game, we tackle tough challenges with more creativity, more determination, and more optimism. We're also more likely to reach out to others for help. And I wanted to bring these gameful traits to my real-life challenge.

So I created a simple recovery game called "Jane the Concussion Slayer." This became my new *secret identity*, a way to start feeling heroic and determined instead of hopeless.

The first thing I did as the concussion slayer was to call my twin sister, Kelly, and tell her, "I'm playing a game to heal my brain, and I want you to play with me." This was an easy way to ask for help. She became my first *ally* in the game. My husband, Kiyash, joined next.

Together we identified and battled the *bad guys*. These were anything that could trigger my symptoms and therefore slow down the healing process—things like bright lights and crowded spaces.

We also collected and activated *power-ups*. These were anything I could do on even my worst day to feel just a little bit good or happy or powerful. Some of my favorite power-ups were cuddling my Shetland sheepdog for five minutes, eating walnuts (good for my brain), and walking around the block twice with my husband.

The game was that simple: adopt a secret identity, recruit allies, battle the bad guys, and activate power-ups. But even with a game so simple, within just a couple days of starting to play, that fog of depression and anxiety went away. It just vanished. It felt like a miracle to me. It *wasn't* a miracle cure for the headaches or the cognitive symptoms—they lasted more than a year, and it was the hardest year of my life by far. But even when I still had the symptoms, even while I was still in pain, *I stopped suffering*. I felt more in control of my own destiny. My friends and family knew exactly how to help and support me. And I started to see myself as a much stronger person.

What happened next with the game surprised me. After a few months, I put up a blog post and a short video online explaining how to play. Not everybody has a concussion, and not everyone wants to be "the slayer," so I renamed the game *SuperBetter*.

Why SuperBetter? Everyone had told me to "get better soon" while I was recovering from the concussion, but I didn't want just to get better, as in back to normal. I wanted to get *super*better: happier and healthier than I'd been before the injury.

Soon I started hearing from people all over the world who were adopting their own secret identities, recruiting their own allies, and fighting their own bad guys. They were getting "superbetter" at facing challenges like depression and anxiety, surgery and chronic pain, migraines and Crohn's disease, healing a broken heart and finding a job after years of unemployment. People were even playing it for extremely serious, even terminal diagnoses, like stage-five cancer and Lou Gehrig's disease (ALS). And I could tell from their messages and their videos that the game was helping them in the same ways that it helped me.

These players talked about feeling stronger and braver. They talked about feeling better understood by their friends and family. And they talked about feeling happier, even though they were in pain, even though they were tackling the toughest challenges of their lives.

At the time, I thought to myself, *What on earth is going on here?* How could a game so seemingly trivial, so admittedly simple, intervene so powerfully in such serious, in some cases life-and-death, circumstances? To be frank, if it hadn't already worked for me, there's no way I would have believed it was possible.

When I was recovered enough to do research, I dove into the scientific literature. And here's what I learned: some people get stronger and happier after a traumatic event. And that's what was happening to us. The game was helping us experience what scientists call *post-traumatic growth,* which is not something we usually hear about. More commonly, we hear about *post-traumatic stress disorder,* in which individuals experience ongoing anxiety and depression.

But research has shown that traumatic events don't always lead to long-term difficulty. Instead, some individuals find that struggling with highly challenging life circumstances helps them unleash their best qualities and eventually lead happier lives.[2]

To give you a better idea of what post-traumatic growth looks like, here are the top five things that people with post-traumatic growth say:

1. My priorities have changed. I'm not afraid to do what makes me happy.
2. I feel closer to my friends and family.
3. I understand myself better. I know who I really am now.
4. I have a new sense of meaning and purpose in my life.
5. I'm better able to focus on my goals and dreams.[3]

Taken together, these five traits represent a powerful positive transformation. But it's more than that. There's actually something quite astonishing about the benefits of post-traumatic growth, something I noticed in the course of my research.

A few years ago an Australian hospice worker named Bronnie Ware published an article called "Regrets of the Dying."[4] Ware would know—she had spent a decade caring for patients at the end of their lives. She wrote that the same regrets were repeated again and again by her patients, year after year—and after she published her article, she heard from hundreds of hospice workers and caretakers all over the world who confirmed her findings. They had heard the same five regrets over the years. Apparently they are nearly universal. Not everyone has regrets on their deathbed—but if they do, they are likely to be one or more of the following:

1. I wish I hadn't worked so hard.
2. I wish I had stayed in touch with my friends.
3. I wish I had let myself be happier.
4. I wish I'd had the courage to express my true self.
5. I wish I'd lived a life true to my dreams, instead of what others expected of me.

Think about this list for a moment. Are you having the same "aha!" moment that I had, two years ago, when I first encountered it?

Remarkably, the top five regrets of the dying are essentially the *exact opposite* of the top five experiences of post-traumatic growth. With post-traumatic growth, we find the strength and courage to do the things that make us happy, and to understand and express our true selves. We prioritize relationships and meaningful work that inspires us.

Post-traumatic growth is not the opposite of post-traumatic stress disorder, by the way. Many people who suffer post-traumatic stress disorder *also* go on to experience post-traumatic growth. The two are not mutually exclusive by any means. In fact, one study found that symptoms of post-traumatic stress were actually predictive of eventual post-traumatic growth—possibly because transformative growth requires wrestling in a deep and sustained way with something very difficult. If we bounce back too quickly, we miss the growth.[5]

Extreme personal challenge—if we respond in the right way—unlocks our ability to lead a life truer to our dreams and free of regrets. Looked at this way, post-traumatic growth—or getting superbetter—seems like a pretty strong candidate for the single most desirable personal transformation anyone could hope to undertake.

But how do you get from extreme stress or trauma to these five benefits? Research shows that not everyone who experiences a trauma goes on to have post-traumatic growth. So what exactly is the right process?

More important, is there any way to experience these benefits *without having a trauma*? I'm pretty sure no one would ever choose to suffer a terrible loss, an injury, an illness, or any other kind of trauma just to get these benefits. But at the same time, who wouldn't want to lead a life truer to their dreams and free of regret?

And so I set off on another two years of research. And here's what I discovered: you *can* experience the benefits of post-traumatic growth without the trauma, if you are willing to undertake an extreme challenge in your life—such as running a marathon, writing a book, starting a business, becoming a parent, quitting smoking, or making a spiritual journey. Researchers call this *post-ecstatic growth*. Ann Marie Roepke, a practicing clinical psychologist who first identified the phenomenon as a University of Pennsylvania doctoral candidate, describes it as "gains without pains"— or at least, far fewer pains.[6] It works the same way post-traumatic growth docs, except you get to choose your own challenge. Instead of waiting for life to throw a terrible trauma at you, you can cultivate post-ecstatic growth at any time by intentionally undertaking a meaningful project or mission that creates significant stress and challenge for you. This stressful adventure you've chosen for yourself creates the necessary conditions for you to struggle and grow as much as someone who is battling a trauma.

So if post-traumatic growth and post-ecstatic growth work the same way, what exactly is that process? What makes the difference between buckling under extreme stress and flourishing because of it? What determines whether you'll be weakened by adversity or strengthened by it?

This is where the research gets really exciting—at least for a game designer like me.

It turns out that there are seven ways of thinking and acting that contribute to post-traumatic and post-ecstatic growth. *And they are all ways that we commonly think and act when we play games.*

1. **Adopt a challenge mindset.** You need to be willing to engage with obstacles and look at stressful life events as a challenge, not a threat. In games, we call this simply "accepting the challenge to play."

2. **Seek out whatever makes you stronger and happier.** When you are facing a tough challenge, you need constant access to positive emotions, and you must look after your physical health. In games, we practice this rule by seeking out "power-ups," items that make us stronger, faster, and more powerful.

3. **Strive for psychological flexibility.** Be open to negative experiences, such as pain or failure, if they help you learn or get closer to your larger goal. Be driven by courage, curiosity, and the desire to improve. In games, we follow this rule whenever we battle a tough opponent or "bad guys," knowing we may fail many times before we become clever or skillful enough to defeat them.

4. **Take committed action.** Make small steps toward your biggest goal, every single day. Taking committed action means trying to take a step forward, even if it is difficult for you. It means always keeping your eyes on the larger goal. In games, we have a structure to do this. It's called a "quest," and it helps us stay focused on making progress toward the goal that matters most to us.

5. **Cultivate connectedness.** Try to find at least two people you feel you can ask for help, and who you can speak to honestly about your stress and challenges. In multiplayer games, we practice the art of making "allies"—people who understand the obstacles we're facing and who have our back.

6. **Find the heroic story.** Look at your life and find the heroic moments. Focus on the strength you've shown and the meaning and purpose to your struggles. In games, heroic stories abound. We often take on the "secret identity" of heroic characters as part of the journey; their stories inspire and motivate us to try harder and become better versions of ourselves.

**7. Learn the skill of benefit finding.** Be aware of good outcomes that can come even from stress or challenge. In games, we have the notion of "epic wins," or extremely positive outcomes that can arise when you least expect them, from the most unlikely or daunting circumstances.

No wonder SuperBetter works so well for so many people! Once you understand the science, it makes perfect sense. Of course a game designer like me would create a system that taps into these naturally gameful ways of thinking and acting. I didn't know it at the time, but SuperBetter was essentially a perfect road map to post-traumatic and post-ecstatic growth. Not because I was a genius but because I was a good game designer, and *all* good games train us in the seven ways of thinking and acting that help us turn extreme stress and challenge into positive transformation.

These seven rules to live by make up the SuperBetter method, and they are the heart of this book:

*1. Challenge yourself.*

*2. Collect and activate power-ups.*

*3. Find and battle the bad guys.*

*4. Seek out and complete quests.*

*5. Recruit your allies.*

*6. Adopt a secret identity.*

*7. Go for an epic win.*

If you're already facing a tough challenge—an illness, an injury, a loss, a personal struggle—following these rules will not only help you be more successful in dealing with the challenge; you'll also be more likely to experience the benefits of post-traumatic growth.

If you're *not* facing an extremely stressful challenge at the moment, but you still want to become stronger, happier, braver, and more resilient, just pick a meaningful and challenging goal for yourself—and then follow these rules as you try to achieve it. You will have the satisfaction of doing something extraordinary *and* start to unlock the benefits of post-ecstatic growth.

◀▶

If I sound quite confident that you can transform your life for the better with a gameful mindset and the SuperBetter method, it's because I am.

Since I invented SuperBetter, more than 400,000 people have played an online version of the game. We've recorded every power-up they've activated, every bad guy they've battled, and every quest they've completed—so we know what works and what doesn't. I've joined forces with data scientists to analyze all the information we've collected from these 400,000 players over the past two years. I wanted answers to some of the same questions you might have: Who can the SuperBetter method work for? (Virtually anyone—young or old, male or female, avid game player or someone who has never played a video game in their life.) How long do you have to play by the seven rules before you start to feel stronger, happier, and braver? (Our studies show measurable improvements within two weeks and even bigger improvements at four weeks and six weeks.) And most important, do these benefits last? (As far as we know, yes. This method has existed for only a few years, but we've followed up with successful players at six months, a year, and when possible two years later. We found that gameful ways of thinking and acting are a skill set that, once learned, you are likely to keep practicing and benefiting from.)

I've waited five years to write this book because I wanted to be absolutely sure that the gameful method works. I waited for early research on the positive benefits of games to be confirmed in larger, more robust studies. I waited for scientists from a wider range of fields, including neuroscience and behavioral psychology, to weigh in with their theories on how a gameful mindset can help. Most important, I waited until I could team up with doctors and psychology researchers myself to test the SuperBetter method in rigorous studies—and I have, with a randomized, controlled trial with the University of Pennsylvania *and* with a clinical trial with the Ohio State University Wexner Medical Center and Cincinnati Children's Hospital. (You'll read about that research in "About the Science," at the end of this book.)

Not a day has gone by in these five years that I haven't received an email or Facebook message from someone telling me how much SuperBetter has inspired them or helped their family. I hear from people from all walks of life, like Norman J. Cannon, a commander in the air force.

> I was taking command of a 2,000-person squadron in the air force and wanted to talk to them about resilience. Meanwhile, my wife had just fallen down the stairs in September 2012 and had a severe concussion. She had all the same thoughts and experiences you mentioned. I showed my wife your SuperBetter video. She cried while watching, realizing that somebody understands. I then showed the video to all 2,000 of my military and civilian employees in a commander's call that I had. It hit home with a lot of people.

I hear from parents like Michelle T., a mom in West Virginia, who says:

> My thirteen-year-old son has juvenile diabetes, and this is EXACTLY what I've been praying for. Our family has formed our own superhero team, and the emotional change I see in my son is glorious! I'm getting my son back! Thank you!

And I hear from patients like Jessica MacDonald, then a thirty-year-old administrative assistant from Denver who played SuperBetter while she battled multiple surgeries and hospitalization for a severe staph infection.

> When you're ill or injured, the world becomes one of can'ts. I can't lift that because of the antibiotics IV in my arm; I can't attend that event because I'm too tired; I can't go to work because I'm on enough medications to kill a horse and barely know my own name. A million times a day the word *can't* goes through your mind, and it murders your soul by inches. If I boil all the benefits of this game down to one thing, it is this: SuperBetter turns *can't* into *can*. Sure, there are still things you aren't allowed to or shouldn't do, but you stop focusing so much on the limitations. You begin to see and celebrate your achievements.

Jessica invited her doctors and nurses to be allies, and they had a lot to say about the game, too.

> The question everyone asks is "Did it help speed your recovery?" I can't say unequivocally that I got better faster because of this game, but I will tell you what my infectious disease doctor told me. In nearly fifty years of medical practice, he said he's come to one conclusion: patients' attitudes overwhelmingly influence the recovery process. He told me, "I don't know if you got better faster, but you got better *better*."

It doesn't matter if you're a lifelong game player or you've never played a video game. It doesn't matter if you prefer sports, card games, or board games to digital games. Whatever your history with games, you have the capacity to tap into your natural strengths by playing games—and you can learn to bring these gameful strengths to your real life challenges and goals.

Most people see games as nothing more than a pleasant distraction—or worse, as an addicting waste of time. But I see them differently—and not just because of my personal experience with SuperBetter. I've been researching the psychology of games for nearly fifteen years. I've studied games that decrease anxiety, alleviate depression, prevent pain, and treat posttraumatic stress disorder. I've analyzed games that increase willpower, boost self-esteem, improve attention skills, and strengthen family relationships. The mounting scientific evidence about games from the fields of psychology, medicine, and neuroscience has changed my mind about what games are—and what they can teach us. Games are not just a source of entertainment. They are a model for how to become the best version of ourselves.

I want you to look at games differently, too. I want you to discover the connection between the strengths you naturally express when you play games and the strengths you need to be happy, healthy, and successful in real life. To be more specific, I want you to see games as an opportunity to practice the seven life-changing skills that will make you a stronger person in every way: mentally, emotionally, physically, and socially.

You don't have to be an avid game player to activate your gameful strengths in everyday life, but if you love or play any game regularly—golf, bridge, Scrabble, soccer, poker, *Candy Crush Saga,* solitaire, sudoku—you're probably a bit more in touch with your gameful strengths already.

To lead a more gameful life, you simply have to be open to learning about the psychology of games—and be willing to experiment with new ways of thinking and acting that can help you increase your natural resilience.

The *fastest* way I know to get you to see games—and your own capabilities—differently is to play a game with you.

So let's play a game together—right now.

◄►

*I challenge you to complete four life-changing quests in the next five minutes.*

Don't worry, it's easier than it sounds. I've watched some amazing people complete the same four quests you're about to undertake—including Oprah Winfrey, legendary skateboarder and entrepreneur Tony Hawk, and Colonel Bat Masterson, the surgeon general for the U.S. Armed Forces. If they can do it, you can do it, too.

These are the first four quests that every SuperBetter player completes. I guarantee that if you successfully complete them all, roughly five minutes from now you will already be a stronger person—mentally, emotionally, physically, and socially. (You'll also have a much better idea of how this book can help you unleash your gameful qualities.)

Ready to play? Let's go!

# THE GAME STARTS NOW

Here's your first life-changing quest. I want you to complete it, right now, before you read any further.

Do not skip this first quest. I repeat: DO NOT SKIP THIS QUEST. If you skip it, you'll be tempted to skip others—and then the game will be over before you've even started playing. So here we go. Your first quest—I know you can do it!

**QUEST 1: Physical Resilience**

*Pick one:*

Stand up and take three steps.

*or*

Make your hands into fists and hold them over your head

as high as you can for five seconds.

*Go!*

Did you do it? Well done!

By completing this quest, you've just boosted your physical resilience.

*Physical resilience* is your body's ability to withstand stress and heal itself. And research shows that the number-one thing people can do to boost their physical resilience is to not sit still. Whenever you sit still for more than a few minutes, your body starts to shut down at the metabolic level. This shutdown negatively impacts every aspect of your health, from your immune system to your ability to handle stress.[7]

Every single second you're *not* sitting still, however, you're actively improving the health of your heart, your lungs, and your brain.[8] You'll have more energy and sleep better, too—which is crucial when you're facing a hard challenge, even if it isn't primarily physical in nature.

So stand up for just one second. Take three steps. Throw your arms in the air. That's all it takes. You are now physically stronger than you were thirty seconds ago.

Ready for your next quest?

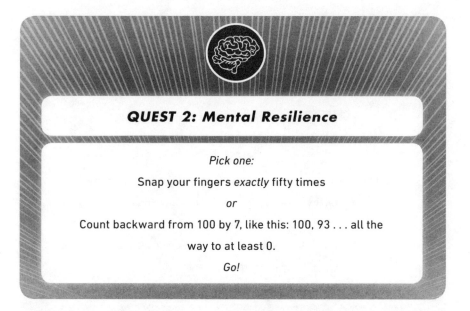

**QUEST 2: Mental Resilience**

*Pick one:*

Snap your fingers *exactly* fifty times

*or*

Count backward from 100 by 7, like this: 100, 93 . . . all the

way to at least 0.

*Go!*

All done? Good work.

By completing this quest, you've just increased your mental resilience.

*Mental resilience* is motivation, focus, and willpower—strengths that are essential to achieving any goal.

Researchers have figured out that willpower is like a muscle. It gets stronger the more you exercise it—as long as you don't exhaust it.[9] Accomplishing tiny challenges—even ones as absurd as snapping your fingers exactly fifty times or counting backward by seven—helps you exercise this muscle without wearing it out. That means you're more likely to have the motivation and determination you need when it's time to tackle tougher obstacles. So congratulations: you are now mentally stronger than you were a minute ago.

Let's keep playing!

### QUEST 3: Emotional Resilience

*Pick one:*

If you're inside, find a window and look outside for thirty
seconds. If you're outside, find a window and look in.

*or*

Do a Google Image or YouTube video search for
"baby [your favorite animal]."

*Go!*

Mission accomplished? Great!

By completing this quest, you've just strengthened your emotional resilience.

*Emotional resilience* is the ability to access positive emotions at will. It doesn't matter if you're stressed, or bored, or angry, or in pain—when you have emotional resilience, you can choose to feel something good instead.

Emotional resilience is a particularly important strength. Research has shown that if, on average, people experience more positive emotions than negative ones, they gain a huge range of benefits. They're more creative at solving problems. They're more ambitious and successful at school and at work. They're less likely to give up when things are hard. People around them are more likely to offer help and support them in their goals.[10]

To achieve emotional resilience, you don't need to eliminate negative emotions—that's obviously impossible. You just need enough positive emotions, over the course of a day, to beat out the negative ones.

Both options in this quest are scientifically validated methods for provoking a specific positive emotion. Looking through a window provokes *curiosity*—the positive emotion that psychologists define as "a desire to gratify the mind with new information or objects of interest."[11] (Hopefully you saw something interesting through the window!) Meanwhile, researchers have demonstrated that looking at photos or videos of baby animals is all it takes to make virtually anyone feel the emotion of *love*. (Baby animal cuteness brings out our nurturing instinct!) Better yet, this quick burst of love from looking at baby animals doesn't just feel good, it also improves attention and productivity.[12]

Even if you felt the curiosity or the love for only a few seconds, you just got emotionally stronger. Enjoy it.

Let's try one more quest.

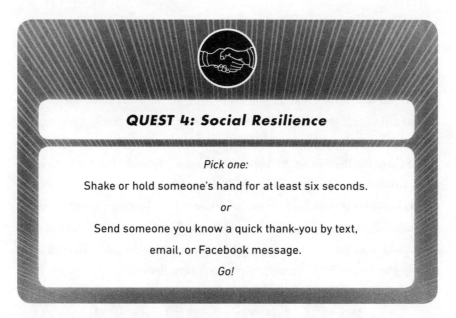

**QUEST 4: Social Resilience**

*Pick one:*

Shake or hold someone's hand for at least six seconds.

*or*

Send someone you know a quick thank-you by text,

email, or Facebook message.

*Go!*

All done? Awesome.

By completing this quest, you've boosted your social resilience.

*Social resilience* is the ability to get support from friends, family members, neighbors, and co-workers. You're able to ask for the help you need—and you're more likely to receive it. Social support is crucial to tackling challenges successfully. You can try to go it alone, but your odds of success are vastly improved when someone else has your back.

There are lots of ways to increase your social resilience. Touch and gratitude are two of the most effective.

Studies show that shaking or holding someone's hand for at least six seconds increases the level of the "trust hormone," oxytocin, in both of your bloodstreams.[13] Boosted oxytocin levels make you want to help and protect each other. The more oxytocin you release together, the deeper your bond.[14]

Meanwhile, expressing thanks is one of the most reliable ways to cultivate good feelings and a closer connection. Gratitude is the single most important relationship-strengthening emotion because, as researchers explain, "it requires us to see how we've been supported and affirmed by other people."[15]

So whether you just touched or thanked someone, you are now socially stronger than you were a page ago. Success!

◄►

I knew you could do it: you've completed four simple quests, and you're already building up life-changing skills and abilities. You're discovering that you are, in fact, stronger than you know; you are indeed surrounded by potential allies; and you really can become a hero to others just by tapping into your natural resilience.

Are you having fun yet? I hope so. Because my goal is to make this the most fun book you've ever read. You'll complete nearly one hundred more quests before this book is through. Each one is based on a different scientific breakthrough about what makes you more resilient. And at the start of each quest, you'll see one of these four icons to let you know if you're building primarily physical, mental, emotional, or social resilience:

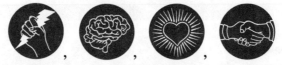

I promise you these quests will make you feel more confident, more in control, and more optimistic about all your real-life challenges. (As with any good game, these quests will get a little bit trickier the further you go!)

Seeking out and completing quests is just one of the seven gameful skills that will help you become stronger, happier, and braver in everyday life. Now that you've gotten a taste of what it feels like to adopt a gameful mindset, let me tell you a little bit more about what you can expect from this book.

I won't ask you to start leading a more gameful life until you're absolutely convinced of the ability of games to solve real problems and change real lives. So in Part 1, "Why Games Make Us Superbetter," we'll start with an overview of the evidence on games. What strengths do they tap into, and what psychological benefits do they bring? We'll look at games that increase motivation and willpower, that block the feeling of physical pain more powerfully than morphine, that help you overcome anxiety and depression, that can change your eating habits, develop your compassion for others, and help you forge stronger, happier relationships with friends and family. Most of the games we discuss in Part 1 are readily available for you to play on your phone or your computer as a way to practice and understand your gameful strengths better. However, even if you decide never to play any of these games, Part 1 will give you a solid foundation to understand what it means to be gameful. You will know exactly what it takes to tap into your three most important challenge-facing, problem-solving powers: your abilities to control your attention, to make allies and get support, and to motivate yourself to do what's important, even when it's difficult for you. We'll finish by exploring the research on why some game players are better able than others to bring these powers from their favorite games into their real lives.

Part 1 is full of gameful quests for you to complete, just like the ones in this introduction—so you'll have plenty of opportunity to play and get stronger with every page.

In Part 2, "How to Be Gameful," we'll talk about your life. Now that you understand your strengths, what is the best way to harness them in everyday life? We'll go in depth with each of the seven gameful skills that can help you tackle real-life challenges with more courage, creativity, and determination. I'll give you seven simple rules to follow to practice each of these skills in daily life. This is the SuperBetter method, and it's designed to make it easy for you to lead a more gameful life—*whether or not you have the time to play games.*

In Part 2, you'll meet people who have used the SuperBetter method to grow stronger, healthier, and happier in the face of challenges like anxiety, depression, chronic pain, and PTSD. You will hear stories from people who have adopted a gameful mindset to find a better job, have a more satisfying love life, run a marathon, start their own company, and simply enjoy life more. And because everything in this book is grounded in research, you will discover the science behind these success stories—more than two hundred studies from the fields of psychology, medicine, and neuroscience that explain exactly why living by these seven gameful rules builds mental, emotional, physical, and social strengths.

**If you're facing a major challenge in your life, and you want to start using the SuperBetter method *right now*, you can skip directly to Part 2.** Come back to Part 1 whenever you want. (I think that once you see for yourself how well SuperBetter works, you'll be even more curious to understand the science behind it!)

Part 3, "Adventures," brings it all together with three SuperBetter journeys I've created so that you can continue practicing your new gameful skills. Each journey is full of targeted power-ups, bad guys, and quests to help you achieve a major resilience breakthrough. On the "Love Connection" adventure, you'll build your social resilience with ten quests designed to help you find love in the most surprising ways and places. In "Ninja Body Transformation," you'll learn twenty-one sneaky ways to increase your physical resilience. And on your final adventure, you'll discover what it means to be "Time Rich"—the feeling that you have abundant free time to spend on all the things that matter most to you. Getting time rich is an excellent way to build your emotional and mental resilience.

Taken together, these three adventures contain *just* enough quests for you to keep playing SuperBetter for six weeks. That's an important number— because six weeks is exactly how long participants followed the SuperBetter rules in our clinical trial and randomized controlled study. In those cases, playing SuperBetter for six weeks resulted in significantly better mood, stronger social support, more optimism, less depression and anxiety, and higher self-confidence. If *you* complete all three of these adventures—by tackling just one quest a day—you'll have achieved a full, life-changing dose of the game.

Together, the stories and the science in this book will reveal how adopting a gameful mindset can change your life for the better. They will not only change what you think games are capable of. They will change what you think *you* are capable of.

Let's go get superbetter.

# PART 1

## Why Games Make Us Superbetter

The evidence that games can make us stronger is all around us. Over the past decade, thousands of scientists and researchers working at hospitals and universities across the globe have documented an astonishing range of real-life positive impacts of video games and virtual worlds.

In this part of the book, you will discover games that:

- increase your motivation and willpower
- block the feeling of physical pain more powerfully than morphine
- help you overcome anxiety and depression
- make you a better learner
- inspire you to exercise more
- help prevent post-traumatic stress disorder
- make you more likely to come to a stranger's rescue
- forge stronger, happier relationships with friends and family

Chances are, you've already played one or more of these potentially life-changing games—from *Tetris* to *Words with Friends* to *Call of Duty* to *Candy Crush Saga*. But even if you play games regularly, you're probably not getting all the benefits. That's because when it comes to unlocking the benefits of games, it's not just *what* you play or *how much* you play—it's why you play, when you play, and who you play with that really matter. In other words, you need to *play with purpose*.

As you'll learn in Part 1, when you play games with purpose, you tap into three core psychological strengths:

- *Your ability to control your attention* and therefore your thoughts and feelings
- *Your power to turn anyone into a potential ally* and to strengthen your existing relationships
- *Your natural capacity to motivate yourself* and supercharge your heroic qualities, like willpower, compassion, and determination

These strengths exist inside you already. Games are just an incredibly reliable and efficient way to discover and practice them—so you're better able to access them in everyday life.

Playing games isn't the only way to tap into these strengths. But the scientific research on *why* games make it so much easier to do so will help you understand these strengths more clearly.

Let me be clear: the point of Part 1 is *not* to persuade you to spend more time playing video games. You *do not* have to become an ardent game player to benefit from games research. Instead, I want to help you learn from the science of games how to be stronger, happier, braver, and more resilient—*whether you ever play any of these games or not.*

One important thing to note: although *all* kinds of games develop these gameful strengths, including sports, puzzles, board games, and card games, Part 1 focuses primarily on digital games, for several reasons.

More than one billion people on this planet currently play digital games for, on average, at least one hour a day.[1] This number will undoubtedly rise in the future; according to a Pew Internet Life study, in the United States, 99 percent of boys under eighteen and 92 percent of girls under eighteen report playing video games regularly (on average thirteen hours a week for boys and eight hours a week for girls).[2] The sheer time and energy poured into digital games by such a vast and growing number of people make it crucial to understand how digital games in particular impact us psychologically. The science of games can help us minimize the potential harms and maximize the potential benefits.

Equally important is the fact that over the past two decades, scientific research on the psychology of games has focused almost exclusively on digital games, largely for the reasons stated above. This book is grounded in the science of games, which means it necessarily focuses on the kinds of games that scientists have dedicated the most time and energy to understanding.

Finally, as you will see in the next four chapters, digital technology can actually heighten and accelerate many of the psychological benefits we experience from all games. For example, all games teach us to be comfortable with failure, because loss is always a possibility. However, digital games tend to have a higher and more rapid rate of failure. In digital games, we fail as much as 80 percent of the time, on average twelve to twenty times an hour.[3] This extremely high and rapid rate of failure helps players more quickly cultivate the strengths of grit and perseverance, as well as the ability to learn effectively from mistakes. You can build these same strengths by failing at basketball or Scrabble or chess, but the capability of digital games to automatically adjust the difficulty level upward so you are constantly playing at the edge of your ability helps you develop them faster.

This is just one example of the kind of research you'll read about in this part of the book. But before we dive deeper into the science of games, you have a special quest to complete.

Chapter 1 has some of the most surprising and eye-opening information in the entire book. It contains some *very* unexpected scientific findings.

I want you to be fully prepared to absorb these findings and act on them in your own life, no matter how surprised you are by them! So here's a quest to help you get ready.

## QUEST 5: Palms Up!

Trying to solve a problem? Want to learn something new? You can prime your brain to be more open to creative solutions and more receptive to surprising ideas. Here's how.

**What to do:** Turn your palms up, and leave them that way. You should start to notice a more open mindset in as little as fifteen seconds.

**Why it works:** Turning our palms up triggers a powerful mind-body response. With our palms up, we adopt an "approach and consider" mindset. We're less likely to reject or dismiss new information or ideas, and we're better able to spot new opportunities and solutions. With palms down, however, we adopt a "refuse and resist" mindset. We're more likely to reject new information and overlook creative ideas.

It sounds like a simple action to have such a big effect, but the evidence is compelling: peer-reviewed research published by the American Psychological Association shows that out of seven different experiments on the palms-up phenomenon, all seven showed the same mind-opening effect.[4]

Researchers theorize that this mind-body link stems from physical behaviors we exhibited thousands of years ago before we invented language.[5] When we offer someone a helping hand, our palm is upturned. When we ask for help ourselves, or when we prepare to receive something, we also turn our hands up. And when we welcome someone into our arms, our palms are facing up. But when we want to reject something, we slap it away with our hands turned downward. When we push someone away, the palms are turned away from us as well.

Through thousands of years of these gestures, we are biologically primed to associate *upward palms* with receptiveness and openness, *downward palms* with rejection and closing ourselves off.

So before you read the next chapter, **turn your palms upward for at least fifteen seconds.** Do this right now. 15 . . . 14 . . . 13 . . .

**Quest complete:** All done? Good job. You're ready for some surprising science! And in the future, whenever you're brainstorming, problem solving, or trying to wrap your head around some new information, remember the power you have to open your mind with a simple palms up.

# 1

## You Are Stronger Than You Know

### Your Mission

Unlock the ability to control what you think
and feel, even during extreme stress or pain

G ames are famously, perhaps even notoriously, attention grabbing. Players frequently become so immersed, they lose track of time and seem to ignore everything and everyone around them. Parents and spouses of gamers often complain that it's nearly impossible to tear their loved ones away from their favorite games. But could the highly immersive quality of good games actually be a clue to how our attention works—and how we can better control it?

In this chapter, we'll look at video game research that reveals the power we have to prevent anxiety, depression, trauma, and physical pain, by learning to *control our attention*. Whether you struggle with any of these challenges currently, or you just want to increase your mental and emotional resilience, games provide the perfect platform for mastering life-changing attention skills. This chapter will show you the science behind attention control and teach you the practical, gameful techniques you can use to discover and develop your attention superpowers.

.  .  .

Nothing hurts more than a severe burn injury. Doctors describe it as the most intense and prolonged pain a human being can experience. Naturally, burn patients receive powerful drugs during wound care, most commonly morphine. But the drugs aren't very effective at alleviating this uniquely excruciating pain. Medical researchers have spent decades searching for something better. Is there anything that can treat the most severe pain in the world more effectively than the traditional morphine approach?

Yes. And it's a video game.

*Snow World* is a 3-D virtual environment created by University of Washington researchers to help patients undergoing treatment for severe burns. Patients are given a virtual reality (VR) headset to wear and a joystick for navigating a virtual frozen ice world. There are ice caves to explore, snowballs to throw, and a whole landscape of winter delights to encounter. Patients wear their VR headset and play this game during the most painful part of burn treatment, while their wounds are being cleaned and redressed.

Medical researchers have tested *Snow World* in clinical trials. Here's what they learned: this VR game reduced pain by a whopping *30 to 50 percent*. For the most severe burn patients, the game proved to have a bigger impact on their pain and overall suffering than the morphine they also received.[1]

Better yet, *Snow World* players were able to almost entirely ignore whatever pain did remain. They reported being consciously aware of pain only 8 percent of the time. Compare this with traditional burn treatment: even with the highest doses of opiates that can be safely administered, patients typically report spending *100 percent* of treatment time thinking about their excruciating pain.

Simply by playing *Snow World*, patients discovered they were able to control what they were thinking and feeling *an extraordinary 92 percent of the time*. As a result, doctors have found that with the game, they can reduce the level of medication and dramatically improve pain management at the same time. And the benefits are more than psychological. When patients feel less pain, doctors are able to pursue more aggressive wound care and physical therapy—two factors that can speed up recovery and reduce medical costs. Most important, the patients feel more in control and suffer far less.[2]

How exactly did a video game create such a powerful change? In scientific papers describing the game's positive impacts, *Snow World*'s inventors, Dr. Hunter Hoffman and Dr. David Patterson, attribute its success to a well-established psychological phenomenon: the *spotlight theory of attention*.[3]

According to this theory, human attention is like a spotlight. Your brain can process and absorb only a limited amount of new information at any given moment. So you focus on one source of information at a time, ignoring everything else. As a result, information everywhere competes constantly for your brain's attention—sights, sounds, tastes, smells, thoughts, and physical sensations.

What does this have to do with pain? The signals from your nerves that cause pain are just one of many competing streams of information. It's a particularly compelling stream. Your nerves are sending signals to your brain to let you know that you're injured—which is pretty important information! It makes perfect sense that without conscious intervention, you'd be more likely to focus your attention spotlight on these pain signals than just about any other source of information.

But you're not powerless against pain signals. In fact, if you learn to control your attention spotlight, you can actually stop your brain from spending its limited processing resources on pain signals from your nerves.

For burn patients, that's where *Snow World* comes in. In order to prevent pain *signals* from turning into a *conscious awareness* of pain, patients need to swing their spotlight of attention somewhere else—and keep it there. How? By deliberately monopolizing all their brain's processing power with as challenging and information-rich a target as possible. Games, and particularly virtual worlds rich in 3-D imagery, serve this purpose perfectly. They require so much active attention, the patient runs out of cognitive resources to process the pain.

This is exactly what scientists observed when they decided to study the brain activity of *Snow World* players using functional magnetic resonance imaging (fMRI). This technology allows researchers to see where blood is flowing in the brain—the more blood flow, the more active that region of the brain. In *Snow World* studies, fMRI footage showed reduced blood flow to all five regions of the brain associated with processing pain. This data revealed that players weren't just doing a better job of dealing with the pain they felt—they were actively blocking the brain from dedicating resources to processing the pain signals.[4] No cognitive resources, no pain.

This is the real breakthrough at the heart of the *Snow World* technique: the game isn't merely a distraction from feelings of pain; it actively *prevents* conscious feelings of pain in the first place. And you can learn to use this technique in your own life.

You may never be in as much physical pain as a burn patient. But if and when you do find yourself in pain, you now know: *You don't have to pay attention to the signals from your nerves. You can choose to pay attention to anything you want.* Even when you're in pain, even when you're suffering, you can control your attention spotlight and change your experience for the better.

And you don't necessarily need a fancy 3-D VR headset to do it. Although advanced game technology makes it easier to commandeer cognitive resources, other studies on pain and gaming show that in less extreme cases, a simple handheld game—the kind you can play on your mobile phone or iPad—can also block pain signals effectively.[5]

Or if you prefer a nongaming solution, you can choose any challenging activity that successfully captures your full attention. Research suggests, for example, that knitting and crafting both require enough brain-processing resources to successfully reduce chronic pain.[6] The key is simply to realize that *you* are in charge of your cognitive resources. If you don't want your brain to pay attention to pain signals, give it something else to pay attention to instead.

*Snow World* is an important health care innovation—but it's also much more than that. It's a clear lesson in how much untapped power we all have over what we physically feel. Even when we're in pain, even when we're suffering, we can control our attention spotlight and change our experience for the better.

As you'll see in the coming pages, this finding is repeated again and again in video game research: we have more power, more mental control, over what we feel, moment to moment, than we realize.

*You* have this power—and it comes from your ability to control your attention spotlight, and in doing so, to change what is happening in your body and your brain.

Let's start practicing that power now, with your next quest.

## QUEST 6: Stop the Pink Elephant!

Don't think of a pink elephant. Whatever you do, do *not* think of a pink elephant.

Stop reading this book for the next ten seconds, and in that time, be absolutely sure you do not *once* think about a pink elephant. Go!

10 . . . 9 . . . 8 . . .

Did you think of a pink elephant? Of course you did, even though I told you not to. Fortunately, that's not your quest. At least not yet—not until you have a concrete strategy for controlling your attention spotlight.

The command "Don't think of an elephant" (or sometimes "Don't think of a bear") is one of the most widely employed exercises in cognitive psychology. Devised by Harvard University professor Daniel Wegner and later made popular by University of California at Berkeley professor George Lakoff, the idea is simple: once you evoke a concept in someone's mind, they are essentially powerless to block it. Despite the instructions to *not* picture a large gray (or pink) mammal with a trunk and floppy ears, the brain is incapable of obeying. The word *elephant* calls up the idea of an elephant, and you're stuck with it, for better or for worse.[7]

We're going to try a different experiment here. I want you to keep trying to not think about a pink elephant, but I'm going to give you a strategy for doing just that.

**What to do:** This time you're going to control your attention spotlight by focusing your cognitive resources on a challenging, high-attention task.

To stop the pink elephant from commanding your attention, I want you picture a giant letter P and E (short for *pink elephant*, naturally). P and E. Got it?

Now I'm going to give you sixty seconds—set a timer, or just estimate it—to list as many words that contain *both* the letter P and the letter E, in any order. Here are a few to get you started: *help, hope, pickle, peanut.*

Write the words down, or if it's easier, just think of them and tick them off on your fingers, or keep a mental tally.

If you can think of at least ten more words with a P and an E in sixty seconds, that's very good. If you can think of twenty or more, that's amazing. If you can think of thirty or more, you're a rock star at this, one of the best in the world. Try to aim for at least ten—and remember, while you're doing it, don't think about a pink elephant.

*Go!*

Okay, now I want you to notice two things.

1. Were you better able to stop thinking about a pink elephant while you were engaged in this high-attention, challenging task? I hope so. The higher your word score, the more likely you are to have completely blocked that silly animal out of your mind. (If you don't like your score or you couldn't stop the pink elephant from occupying your thoughts, give it another try with these two letters: S and B, for *SuperBetter*!)

2. As you go back to reading this book or go about the rest of your day, see which is more likely to occur: you keep picturing a pink elephant *or* you randomly think of or spot another word with the letters P and E in them. If you are like most people, you're more likely to flash back to the word game than to the mental image of an ele-

phant. That's because your attention spotlight is more likely to drift back to something that engaged more cognitive resources. Be sure to notice what happens in the next few minutes or hours to see if this is true for you!

**Quest complete:** If you found this word game an effective technique to control your attention spotlight, congratulations. You now have a new tool in your toolkit for blocking unwanted thoughts, feelings, or physical sensations. Try it anytime, with any two letters, to practice swinging that spotlight of attention quickly and more effectively.

**Just for fun:** Check out the following footnote for twenty P and E words you could have thought of!*

---

* People, preach, happen, pamphlet, prairie, prayer, apple, yelp, rope, dampen, patent, prehistoric, petal, penumbra, pennant, sniper, eclipse, epicenter, spine, rapture, empty, prince, poke.

As you're hopefully starting to see, researchers have figured out all kinds of ways people can get better at controlling their attention spotlight. Let's take a look at other types of mental and emotional resilience you can develop by mastering this important skill—such as the power to prevent trauma, fight cravings, block anxiety, and heal from depression.

◄►

You've almost certainly seen *Tetris*, the falling blocks puzzle game, even if you've never played it. It's estimated to be one of the most widely played video games of all time, with nearly half a billion players to date.

Despite having been around since 1984, it wasn't until recently that researchers realized that *Tetris* can do more than entertain us. It can, remarkably, help us recover more quickly from traumatic events.

Post-traumatic stress disorder, or PTSD, is a psychological condition that can develop after an individual witnesses or experiences a terrifying or tragic event. The hallmark symptom of PTSD is recurring flashbacks. Unwanted, intrusive memories can haunt individuals for months or even years after a traumatic event, disrupting sleep, triggering panic attacks, and causing severe emotional distress. Typically, these flashbacks have a strong visual component. Someone repeatedly "sees" a traumatic event in their mind's eye, as vividly as if it were really happening all over again. Psychologists consider these flashbacks to be the single most stressful and difficult-to-treat symptom of PTSD.

But what if, instead of trying to treat flashbacks as an unavoidable symptom of trauma, we could prevent them in the first place? Cognitive scientists have shown that memories change and take shape for up to six hours after a traumatic event. That has led some researchers to wonder: Is there anything we can do in the first six hours after trauma to inhibit our brains from forming the kinds of visual memories that lead to flashbacks?

Yes, there is. You can play *Tetris*.

In 2009 and 2010 a team of psychiatrists at Oxford University completed two studies showing that playing *Tetris* within six hours of viewing traumatic imagery helped reduce flashbacks of the traumatic events. It worked so well, in fact, that the Oxford researchers proposed that a single ten-minute session of *Tetris* could effectively serve as a "cognitive vaccine" against PTSD. Play the game as soon as possible after a traumatic event, and you may significantly reduce your likelihood of experiencing severe post-traumatic stress.[8]

How did the Oxford researchers figure this out? It's not easy to study trauma in a laboratory, as you can imagine. It's simply not ethical for researchers to do horrible things to study participants just to measure their traumatic response. So the Oxford team used an experimental method that has been tested and validated in hundreds of other trauma studies: they gathered together test subjects in a laboratory and showed them a series of extremely graphic, gory images of death and injury. (Trust me, these are the kind of images you truly hope you will never see.) Then they measured the subjects' emotional response to the images to ensure that they were truly disturbed.

In the hours that followed, half of the test subjects played *Tetris* for ten minutes while the other group did nothing special. Here's what the researchers found: most of the group that did nothing special reported a high number of disturbing visual flashbacks from the images over the next week. The group that played *Tetris*, however, had just half as many flashbacks. And when both groups completed a psychological survey one week later, the *Tetris* players had significantly fewer symptoms of PTSD than the group that did not play.

So how did ten minutes of game play prevent flashbacks and PTSD symptoms? The Oxford researchers explain that *Tetris* occupies the visual processing circuitry of the brain with something *other* than what it's usually preoccupied with after a trauma—involuntarily remembering and replaying the trauma over and over again. It's similar to how *Snow World* works to prevent pain, but it's a more targeted approach. To interfere with involuntary visual memories of the trauma, you have to swing the attention spotlight to something that specifically demands a huge amount of *visual attention*.

Crucially, the Oxford researchers found that not every video game can successfully hijack the visual processing centers. It must be a game that requires a massive amount of constant, visual processing—ideally, a pattern-matching game like *Tetris* or *Candy Crush Saga*, in which your goal is to move and connect game pieces according to a visual pattern. These kinds of games are so visually engaging, players notoriously report seeing game play flashbacks—typically, colored blocks falling, or matching candies swapping places—whenever they close their eyes, even hours after they've stopped playing. But if you play a less visual game, like Scrabble or a trivia quiz, this technique doesn't work. Your brain will have too many visual processing resources still available to replay traumatic images.[9]

One more important detail from the Oxford study: playing *Tetris* did *not* prevent individuals from voluntarily remembering details of what they saw. A week later, when they were asked questions like "What color was the hair of the man who drowned?" or "About how old was the woman on the stretcher?" the *Tetris* players accurately recalled as many details as the group that did not play. Their memories were intact—they just weren't as haunted by them.

This is extremely important, so I'll say it again: the *Tetris* technique does not erase memories; it simply stops the cognitive process of *involuntary* memory. It gives you control over the memory. You won't think about it when you don't want to.

The Oxford researchers have not followed up their initial study with research on how well this technique works in real-world contexts. However, since they publicly shared this work five years ago at scientific conferences and in the media, many individuals have had the chance to learn and try it outside formal scientific studies. As part of my ongoing work to understand how people use games to become stronger and heal faster, I've heard from many people who have conducted successful *Tetris*-style interventions in their own lives: a runner who, after the 2013 Boston marathon bombings, found herself worried about whether she would ever be able to participate in road races again; a high school student in Norway who lost a friend in the 2011 mass shooting and kept replaying media images of the scene in his mind; a woman who did not want to suffer flashbacks of her elderly father's final moments, which were not peaceful. What I have heard from individuals like these is that a short period of game play in the hours, days, and even weeks after the trauma gave them control over what they were thinking and seeing in their mind's eye—and that this level of control not only helped limit flashbacks but also gave them a sense of comfort and strength.

Let's put this *Tetris* research into a bigger perspective. The power to prevent flashbacks can potentially help anyone, even someone not directly involved with a traumatic event. We often see traumatic images of violence or accidents in the media. Children can be especially disturbed by these images. But a quick session of visually absorbing game play can help them avoid nightmares or intrusive memories.

The *Tetris* technique also has potential to change how you respond to ordinary negative events. When you have a particularly upsetting day, or if you can't stop thinking about something that went wrong, you can activate this gameful ability.

You can put a stop to involuntary thoughts quickly and simply. This power to control what you're remembering *in the moment*, right now, ensures that you can choose to truly leave difficult moments in the past when you need to.

There's one more surprising—and potentially life-changing—way to apply the *Tetris* technique in everyday life.

To find out what it is, try this quick quest!

## QUEST 7: Control the Mind's Eye

**What to do:** Think of something you often crave—something that, once you start thinking about it, it usually feels impossible to resist. Imagine it in detail. Picture yourself enjoying it, as vividly as you can. Do you have a specific craving in mind? Good.

The next time this craving kicks in—including right now, if you're already feeling it!—I want you to **play a pattern-matching game like *Tetris* for three minutes**. Do this, and you will be much better able to successfully resist your craving.

**Why it works:** Multiple studies have shown that playing *Tetris* for three minutes while feeling an intense craving cuts the intensity of the craving by 25 percent.[10]

This may not sound like a lot, but a 25 percent reduction in craving intensity is enough to change behavior. It's just enough of a boost to give your willpower a fighting chance. (Keep in mind that if you're hungry when you play *Tetris*, you'll still be hungry afterward—but you'll be less likely to give in to a specific, unhealthy craving, and more likely to make a smarter choice about what to eat.)

This anticraving strategy works on exactly the same scientific principle as the strategy of using a pattern-matching game to prevent flashbacks and PTSD. Research has shown that cravings have a very strong visual component. The more you mentally imagine yourself enjoying what you crave, the more likely you are to give in. To resist a craving, you simply need to give your brain's visual-processing centers something else to visualize—and you'll find the craving significantly reduced.[11]

**What to play:** You can find countless pattern-matching games for free online and on your mobile phone or tablet. The easiest ones to pick up from scratch if you've never played them are *Tetris*, *Bejeweled*, and *Candy Crush Saga*. (This last is the first video game my sixty-seven-year-old mom played in her entire life—and she taught herself how to play it in less than a minute.)

If you don't want to play a digital game, a wonderful pattern-matching card game called *SET* offers the same powerful flashback effects. You can find it on Amazon or at Setgame.com. Finally, some SuperBetter players report that solving jigsaw puzzles is another way to control visual attention and stave off cravings effectively.

## A SuperBetter Story: The Bride- and Groom-to-Be

When Joe and Elisa decided to get married, they promised each other that they would both successfully quit smoking by their wedding day.

In the months before the big day, the Michigan-based couple both wore nicotine patches, which helped them fight their cravings at work. But when they came home in the evening, Joe told me, it was harder to avoid reverting back to old habits.

"There was so much going on at work, the patch was enough—we didn't need anything else. But at home, with less going on, we were really tempted. We thought about lighting up constantly."

Thanks to the nicotine-replacement therapy, their physical cravings were in check. But they hadn't yet gotten control over their *mental* cravings. They kept picturing themselves smoking and imagining how good it would feel. Those mental images were the real problem.

The gameful solution? Joe and Elisa decided to start a new tradition: puzzle nights. Every evening after dinner they sat down at the kitchen table to work on a giant jigsaw puzzle together.

"It totally worked for us," Joe told me. "Zero cigarettes on puzzle nights." It worked so well, in fact, that they worked on puzzles every night all the way up to their wedding. Two years later the happily married couple are still smoke-free.

Puzzle nights had one additional surprise benefit for the bride- and groom-to-be: working cooperatively on the puzzles together for so many hours, night after night, boosted their communication and problem-solving skills. "We got really good at working together and solving the puzzles as a team." Not a bad way to prepare for marriage!

Joe and Elisa were, as it turns out, ahead of the curve with their creative solution. In 2014 a team of researchers from the American Cancer Society, Brown University, and Stony Brook University found that nicotine-deprived smokers were able to reduce their cravings by playing two-player cooperative games with their relationship partners. Functional magnetic resonance imaging (fMRI) scans showed that cooperative game play and puzzle solving lit up the same reward centers of the brain that nicotine does. The scientists believe this is evidence that social games and puzzles could provide smokers with an alternative neurological pathway to feeling a reward when they crave it most.[12]

In other words, game play provides a powerful one-two punch for changing behavior. First, it gives you control over your thoughts and mental cravings by fully absorbing the visual-processing center of the brain. Second, it gives you a pleasurable neurochemical reward—the same kind you would get from a cigarette or a cookie or whatever else you might crave. Who needs a

cigarette or cookie when you already feel deeply satisfied by the
game?

Sweethearts Joe and Elisa might not be surprised to hear about
one final scientific discovery from the same team of fMRI-scanning
researchers: falling in love also dampens cravings for food, alcohol, and drugs, by activating the same reward pathways.[13] "Intense,
passionate love," as the researchers put it, is like kryptonite to
cravings—they just can't stand up to it.

The moral of the story: if you want to quit something, anything,
just solve a puzzle—or fall in love. Or if you're really lucky, like Joe
and Elisa, do both at the same time.

By now, you're catching on: purposefully controlling your attention has
all sorts of real-life benefits. By why are games such an effective means of
attention control, compared with other activities? Let's explore this question by taking a look at another strength you can develop through game
play: the ability to block anxiety, even in extremely stressful situations.

Surgery is scary—especially for kids. Over the past twenty-five years,
doctors have tested every idea imaginable to reduce kids' anxiety in the
operating room. They've tested powerful medications. They've allowed parents to hold their kids' hands while they go under and wake up from anesthesia. They've even tested *clowns* in the operating room.

What works best? Not surprisingly, it's not clowns. But it's not parents or
medication either. Kids who are allowed to play handheld video games—
such as *Super Mario* on the Nintendo DS—experience virtually *no* anxiety
before surgery. And after surgery, they wake up from anesthesia with less
than half the anxiety of children given drugs—and with zero medication
side effects.[14]

It's another headline-worthy scientific result: "Ordinary video games
prevent anxiety more effectively than the most powerful antianxiety medications." But what makes it work? The research team at the department of

anesthesiology at New Jersey Medical School argues that—as with the *Snow World* and *Tetris* techniques—*cognitive absorption* is the key. By focusing intensely on something *other* than the impending surgery, young patients avoid becoming upset or panicked.

This hypothesis makes perfect sense, given what we already know about the spotlight theory of attention. Anxiety—just like pain, traumatic memory, and cravings—requires conscious attention in order to develop and unfold. It's fueled by active thoughts about what could possibly go wrong. Fear is a response to something actually going wrong right now. Anxiety, on the other hand, is the anticipation that something *might* go wrong in the future. The more vividly we imagine something bad happening, the more anxious we get.

Physiological sensations can contribute to anxiety—for example, caffeine can cause rapid heartbeats and sweaty palms, and a sudden surprise can trigger a jolt of adrenaline. If we notice these physical sensations, we may start to rack our brains for something specific to be nervous about, which can lead to a full-blown case of anxiety or even a panic attack. But without a conscious story about what might go wrong next, these symptoms are just physical sensations. They become an *emotional feeling* of anxiety only when we actively start to imagine terrible things happening in the future. Such imaginings can trigger more physiological changes—more adrenaline, an even faster heart rate—that we interpret as more reason to worry, and so the vicious cycle of anxiety goes.

Game play, the research shows, helps us stop imagining what might go wrong. The game breaks the cycle of attention. Even if we feel physical symptoms of anxiety while we're playing, we're too preoccupied with the game to actively imagine the worst. And without a nervous imagination, there is no anxiety.

In some situations, anxiety can be a helpful emotion—if it alerts you to a potential problem in the future, and if you have the time and ability to take steps now to prevent that problem. For example, if you're anxious about an upcoming exam or presentation, anxiety can be a useful cue to study or practice more. For this reason, you should not *always* seek to block anxiety. However, for most people, in most situations, anxiety does not lead to productive action. Instead, it merely creates needless suffering and can prevent us from taking helpful action. Here's a good rule of thumb for when to safely use a gameful technique to block anxiety: if the anxiety is *not* helping you identify concrete positive steps you can take, but rather is simply creating distress, play a game. Likewise, if the anxiety is trying to talk you out of doing something you truly want or need to do (like getting on a plane, giving a presentation, or going to a social event), go ahead and block it with a few minutes of play.

I s *any* form of pleasurable distraction a viable tool for disrupting the anxiety cycle? It turns out, no. Studies have shown that other similar attempts to prevent presurgery anxiety in kids have limited or no impact. Comic books, music, cartoons—none of these distractions tested nearly as well as games in the operating room.[15] The problem? They just don't offer the same level of cognitive absorption.

When we play games, we're not just paying attention to the game—we're paying a special *quality* of attention. That quality is called flow.

*Flow* is the state of being completely cognitively absorbed in an activity. It's not mere distraction or engagement; it's *full* engagement. It's being totally immersed in, motivated by, and energized from the challenge at hand. In a state of flow, you not only lose track of time, you lose a sense of self-awareness. You experience a "deep focus" on the activity and no conscious awareness of competing thoughts or emotions.[16]

First identified by American psychology researcher Mihaly Csikszentmihalyi in the 1970s, flow is considered an extremely positive psychological state—indeed, perhaps the most optimal psychological state.[17] A flow state can be achieved in many different ways, as long as the right conditions are met. It emerges when we have a clear goal, a challenging task to perform, and sufficient skills to meet the challenge—or at least to come close enough that we are energized to try again and do better. People find flow playing guitar, cooking, running, gardening, doing complex mathematics, and dancing—to name just a few ways. However, compared with a quick video game, these activities aren't always as easy to perform in stressful contexts and everyday environments (and definitely not in an operating room before surgery). Moreover, when Csikszentmihalyi first wrote about the phenomenon of flow, he identified games and play as the quintessential flow activity.

Perhaps surprisingly, many leisure activities that we commonly think of as a good source of distraction do *not* typically lead to a flow state: watching television or movies, listening to music, or even reading.[18] While these may be pleasurable and can indeed take our mind off our problems, they are not usually challenging and interactive in the way that flow-inducing activities must be. This is an important insight, because many people naturally turn to relaxing activities as a way to deal with stress, anxiety, or pain. But flow research shows that a challenging interactive task actually gives us more control over what we think and feel than a passive relaxing activity.

Flow is the reason that games, more than any other activity, are uniquely able to help us exert more control over anxiety and many other emotions as well. Games give us a clear goal. They require focus and effort to succeed. And digital games provide near-constant feedback so we can improve our performance. As soon as we improve our skills, the game gets harder, ensuring that we are always sufficiently challenged. Video games are such a reliable and efficient way to reach a flow state, in fact, that when scientists want to study the phenomenon of flow in the laboratory, they typically have participants play them.[19] No activity that we know of creates flow more quickly, for so many people, as digital game play. And when we are in flow, we are in full control of our attention spotlight.

If you can create flow for yourself, you're not just blocking negative feelings like pain and anxiety. You're also actively creating better psychological and physical health.

Scientists at the Psychophysiology Lab and Biofeedback Clinic at East Carolina University recently completed a series of three studies to measure the mind-and-body impacts of video game play. They were interested in one particular genre: casual video games, the simple single-player ones like

*Angry Birds*, solitaire, and *Bejeweled*. They can be learned quickly and are easy to stop and start again. They are highly correlated with flow states.[20] And unlike more complex games, such as *World of Warcraft* and *Madden NFL Football*, they require no special video game skills, expertise, or regular time commitment.

The scientists' interest in casual video games was sparked when a senior executive at PopCap Games, one of the largest casual game makers in the world, shared findings from a formal survey of its players. It turned out that 77 percent of players were seeking some form of mental or emotional health benefit from playing, not merely entertainment.[21] These players reported using casual video games to improve their mood, stop anxiety, and relieve stress, and in some cases even as a kind of "self-medication."

Were the players' mental health benefits real or imagined? That's what PopCap wanted to find out. So it created a research program with East Carolina University (ECU), known for its leading biofeedback research. The goal was to measure changes in brain waves, heart rate, and breathing patterns in game players to see if they aligned with physiological signs of improved mood, decreased depression, and resilience to stress.

The scientists at ECU attached monitoring devices to game players in order to track two specific measures of emotional and physical resilience: electroencephalographic (EEG) changes in alpha brain waves, which can indicate whether you're distressed, depressed, or in an overall good mood; and heart rate variability, which reflects how quickly your body can recover from emotional or physical stress.

The group's first randomized, controlled trial found that a twenty-minute session of casual game play *decreased* left frontal alpha brain waves, which typically indicates improved mood. Indeed, on a survey, the players with decreased alpha brain waves reported feeling in a better mood. They had significantly less anger, depression, and tension and more energy. A comparison group that simply surfed the Internet for twenty minutes had no significant EEG changes and no reported improvements in mood or energy level. The game players, meanwhile, also experienced significant improvements in heart rate variability. After just twenty minutes of play, their hearts were able to withstand more stress and recover more quickly.[22]

These initial findings were so promising that the team decided to conduct a longer-term study of casual video games. In their next trial, they studied the impact of thirty minutes of game play, three times a week, on reported mood, as well as on the same EEG and heart rate variability measures. Participants were all suffering from anxiety, depression, or both at the start of the study. After one month of this game play routine, they saw significant reductions in depression, anxiety, and general stress levels across the board. Their EEG and heart rate variability measures—both significantly improved—confirmed these perceived emotional changes at a physiological level.[23] As a result of these significant findings, the researchers have called for the development of prescriptive interventions.

Someday soon it's quite likely that psychologists or doctors will commonly write prescriptions for *Angry Birds* to reduce anxiety, or *Peggle* to treat depression, or *Call of Duty* for anger management. Indeed, I already frequently hear from therapists and counselors who do just that! And the science is increasingly on their side. A 2012 meta-analysis of thirty-eight randomized, controlled trials of video games published in the *American Journal of Preventive Medicine* found significant promise for video games to improve psychological health outcomes. (The article also encouraged researchers and the game industry to conduct trials of longer duration as a necessary next step for this emerging field of research.)[24]

Keep in mind that gameful prescriptions are not necessarily an alternative to traditional forms of therapy or medication. Indeed, 23 percent of participants in the ECU casual games trial continued to take antidepressants during the study. We are still at the beginning of understanding the full range and depth of the positive impact that games can have on our health and well-being. For now, and perhaps for the long term, these tools should be seen as a complement, and not necessarily as an alternative, to other forms of support and treatment.

G ame play isn't the only flow activity that can lead to these positive mind-and-body results. As you start to practice the gameful techniques in this chapter, you'll become better and better at spotting a wide range of activities that help you tap in to your natural ability to control your attention.

Mindfulness meditation, for example, has been measured to have quite similar physiological benefits as casual game play. During mindfulness meditation, participants are challenged to focus on their breath above all other thoughts, emotions, or physical sensations. This is actually quite a difficult task that requires a tremendous amount of attention! If you'd like to try it, set aside a few minutes where you can sit quietly and simply count your breaths. Each inhalation and exhalation counts as one breath. See how high you can count before you realize that you've been distracted by a thought or sound or feeling and lost count. Start over from zero and try again. Continue trying to increase the number of breaths you can count without distraction until five or ten minutes have passed. (As you can see, you can take a gameful approach to meditation simply by setting a high score!)

This activity, it turns out, is nearly identical to playing a casual video game in terms of its physiological benefits.[25] Two decades' worth of research shows that mindfulness meditation leads to significant heart rate variability improvement and EEG changes consistent with improved mood and decreased stress.[26] More recently, researchers have proposed that precisely the concept of flow explains these physiological changes during and after meditation.[27] They describe the benefits of mindfulness meditation as stemming directly from "a state of positive and full immersion in an effortful activity." Meditation, it turns out, is a form of play!

I have to admit, I am heartened by this scientific link between the benefits of meditation, which many already accept as an important and valuable mental and physical health practice, and the benefits of casual game play, which is more typically dismissed as a trivial pastime or even a waste of time. Thanks to the efforts of researchers, we now know that even though games are fun, we can and should take them seriously as a tool for becoming stronger, happier, and healthier.

## A SuperBetter Story:
## The Game-Playing Monk

I met Vasily on the other side of the world, high in the mountains of Ganghwa Island, an hour outside of Seoul, South Korea. I had escaped the city for a weekend stay at the ancient Jeongdeungsa Temple, built in AD 381, where visitors are invited to learn about Buddhist cultures and traditions.

Vasily was our teacher for the weekend. Tall, handsome, and Russian, he was not quite the kind of monk I expected to meet at a temple in South Korea! I soon learned that while he had been ordained as a monk in Russia, he had chosen to make Jeongdeungsa his home, as he preferred the peace and beauty of the landscape.

After two days of practicing Buddhist methods of meditation and prayer and chanting with our group of twenty students, I had a chance to sit down for a chat with Vasily. I wanted to ask him his opinion about the role of play and games in a spiritual and happy life. I knew that the Buddha had famously rejected games, compiling a list of all the games he would not play—including those with balls or dice and even "guessing at letters traced with the finger in the air or on a friend's back."[28] Yet given everything contemporary science has said about game play as a way to learn to control our attention—which is one of the primary aims of Buddhist practice!—I wondered (perhaps a bit impudently) if there wasn't a place for games at a Buddhist temple after all.

Vasily first explained to me that the Buddha rejected games on the grounds that they were "a waste of time." (Worrying about games as a waste of time? Apparently, not much has changed in the past twenty-five hundred years!) The problem, according to the Buddha, was that games distracted players from the more important work of seeking enlightenment. Vasily shared this concern and discouraged me from using games to "escape reality" rather than be present in the moment.

But then Vasily lowered his voice and said something that rather shocked me: "Of course, I play *Angry Birds* every night." Looking a bit sheepish, he explained, "We meditate for hours. We pray for hours. There are still many hours in the day." He did not see his game play as an escape: "Especially in the evening when I am tired, one hour of *Angry Birds* is a way to focus and calm my thoughts. It is skillful practice, not escape."

Here was someone who had spent years training in the Buddhist practice, mastering some of the most powerful attention-control techniques ever devised. And even he, a master of highly complex forms of meditation, breathing, and prayer, had decided to integrate video games into his daily rituals!

It's been almost three years since I met Vasily, but whenever I pull out my phone for a quick session of *Angry Birds*, I find myself thinking about him. I picture him in his monastery robe, seated on a meditation cushion in the oldest temple in Korea, slinging the same adorable birds through the same virtual space, both of us enjoying the peaceful experience of controlling our spotlight of attention.

From *Snow World* and *Tetris* to *Super Mario* and *Bejeweled*, healing video games teach an important lesson that extends far beyond the virtual world: you are mentally and emotionally stronger than you realize, especially in the face of stress, trauma, or pain. You can control your attention spotlight. And therefore you can control your thoughts, emotions, and even physical sensations.

# MISSION COMPLETE

***Skills Unlocked: Why You Are Stronger Than You Know***

- Control over your attention spotlight is a hidden superpower you already have, one that can help you combat stress, anxiety, depression, and pain.
- Games help you discover and practice this power—and prepare you to wield it even under the most difficult real-world conditions.
- To prevent traumatic flashbacks or curb cravings, swing your attention spotlight toward something that is highly visually engaging, like *Tetris* or jigsaw puzzles.
- To block pain or anxiety, don't try to relax. Instead, focus your attention on any flow-inducing activity—something that challenges you and requires active effort.
- If you need to quickly pull your attention away from an unwanted thought or feeling, play the two-letter word game (in which you try to list as many words that contain both letters as possible).
- Thirty minutes of a "deep focus" activity—such as casual game play or meditation—three times a week can improve your mood, decrease stress, and help reduce symptoms of depression. It will also improve your heart rate variability, one of the best measures of physical resilience.
- Playing games is not a waste of time to feel guilty about. It's a skillful, purposeful activity that gives you direct control over your thoughts and feelings.

# 2

## You Are Surrounded by Potential Allies

### Your Mission

Discover just how many people are ready
to help you with any problem, at any time.

What if you were surrounded by people ready and willing to help you with any problem at any time? How much more could you accomplish? How much more ambitious could you be?

You already have this power. You can *turn almost anyone into an ally*—even a stranger, even someone who thinks they don't like you—just by playing a game with them.

In this chapter, we'll examine the unique properties of games that make them the perfect platform for learning how to strengthen real-life relationships and find more common ground with others. You'll see how the benefits of playing a game with others last long after the game is played. Plus, you'll learn practical strategies for bringing the positive ways we interact in games into the rest of your daily life.

. . .

H*edgewars* is a cute and funny video game, despite the word *wars* in its title. Players are invited to commandeer an army of pink hedgehogs for intergalactic space battle. (Think *Angry Birds* but a bit more challenging—and with flying spiny mammals instead of birds.) It's relatively simple to learn, playable on any computer or mobile phone—and as researchers at the University of Helsinki recently discovered, it has a powerful effect on our bodies and brains.

When two people play *Hedgewars* together in the same room, they experience what Dr. Michiel Sovijärvi-Spapé and Dr. Niklas Ravaja describe as "neurological and physiological linkage."[1] The two players start to make the same facial expressions, smiling and frowning in unison. Their heart rates adapt to the same rhythm. Their breathing patterns sync. Most astonishingly, their brain waves sync, as their neurons start to "mirror" each other—a process that helps each of them anticipate what the other will do next. All these changes happen almost immediately, within minutes of starting to play.

Surprisingly, this synchronization occurs whether the two players are cooperating *or* competing with each other. It doesn't matter whether you consider your fellow player a teammate or an opponent. When you play *Hedgewars* together, your minds and bodies start to operate in near-perfect harmony.

What makes these biological linkages so interesting to researchers? As psychologists have recently discovered, all four types of synchronization—facial expression, heart rate, respiration, and neural activity—are strongly correlated with increased empathy and social bonding. The more we sync up with someone, the more we like them—and the more likely we are to help them in the future.[2]

It's not surprising, then, that in surveys conducted afterward, *Hedgewars* players do indeed report feeling high levels of empathy and connection with each other—again, regardless of whether they played cooperatively or competitively.

*Hedgewars*, as it turns out, is not special in this regard. In fact, as an expanding field of research shows, *any* game played simultaneously by two people in the same physical location creates this same kind of "mind meld" and body synchronization—laying the foundation for a more powerful and positive relationship after the game is over.[3]

How do games trigger a mind-and-body connection so quickly and effectively—and is there anything else you can do to achieve a similar effect? Let's dig into the science of synchronization to find out.

Humans unconsciously mirror and imitate each other constantly. We fall into lockstep when walking together. We return someone's smile naturally, without thinking. We shift our body language to match the posture of people we like. And it's not just a one-on-one phenomenon. At sporting events and concerts, we make the same facial expressions and move in unison with other fans, creating entire crowds of biologically linked individuals.[4]

Not all synchronization is visibly obvious. Research shows, for example, that a mother's heartbeat synchronizes with her infant's when she holds her.[5] And when a close friend tells you a story about his day, you experience what scientists call *neural coupling*. Your brain activity mirrors your friend's as closely as if it were your own experience he was describing.[6] It's quite amazing when you think about it: your brain processes *your friend's* story as if what happened to him had actually happened to *you*.

Why are these spontaneous biological connections so common? Scientists argue that without them, survival—let alone successful social interaction—would be impossible.

In order to interact with other people, we have to be able to understand them. What are they thinking? What are they feeling? What action are they about to take? Do they want to hurt you or help you? But it's not easy to read someone else's mind or guess what they're feeling. In fact, the only way we can do it is by *re-creating their thoughts and feelings in our own minds and bodies*.

Consider this example: A stranger is smiling at you. Does he mean you well, or does he mean you harm? You involuntarily smile back—with the same kind of smile he just gave you. Your smile may be fleeting—maybe it lasts just for a microsecond, barely detectable. But now your brain understands the stranger's intentions. It knows whether the smile you just gave back is the kind of warm, genuine smile you typically give people you intend to be nice to, or a pained, insincere smile you give to people you don't like. Only by becoming a mirror for someone else are you able to accurately deduce his intentions.

Here's another example: You run to catch up to someone and start walking beside her. You naturally fall into lockstep, and in doing so, you get important information about her state of mind. Perhaps your stride feels slightly longer and faster than usual—you physically start to feel her sense of urgency. Or perhaps you notice yourself relaxing, walking more slowly than usual. You start to feel the same sense of calm as your partner. By unconsciously mimicking her physical movement, you suddenly have access to her emotions!

We synchronize like this hundreds of times every day without thinking about it. People who do it more tend to score higher on measures of empathy and social intelligence. That's because the more you mirror and mimic, the better you understand the people around you.

That just leaves one important question to answer: why do we *like* people better when we mimic and mirror them? It's not just a matter of better understanding. Countless studies have shown that we become closer to, more affectionate toward, and more likely to help the people we sync up with. Why?

Scientists theorize that syncing up creates an "upward spiral" of positive connection between two people.[7] It helps us understand each other better, which means we have smoother social interactions—and that makes us more willing to interact with each other again in the future. When we're biologically synced up, studies show, we also perform more effectively together, because we're better able to anticipate each other's actions. Experiencing success together makes us more likely to help each other in the future. Meanwhile we more naturally like people who we perceive to be like ourselves. So when we unconsciously notice someone else mirroring us, we start to feel more positively about them. And the more positively we feel about someone, the more time we tend to spend with them, giving us more opportunities to sync up and strengthen our bond.

Not all synchronization leads to positive feelings or stronger bonds. If you intuit through a quick neural connection that someone else means you harm, you're not going to befriend her. And synchronizing around an emotion like anger or frustration can create more stress, not more empathy. Research suggests, for example, that unhappily married couples actually go into *downward* spirals of synchronization when they argue.[8] The more they fight, the more their minds and bodies align—but with negative, rather than positive, emotions. (More happily married couples, on the other hand, are actually *less* biologically linked during fights. Researchers theorize that they are better able to quickly mirror and process their partner's negative feelings without having to fully embody them.)

However, syncing up around negative feelings may have at least one benefit. The increased biological connection when some couples fight may explain why so many attest that a good argument can lead to great sex. If you're synced up, you're much more in tune with each other's mind and body. Still, all things considered, the biggest benefits come from syncing up around positive emotions like interest, excitement, curiosity, and wonder—emotions that are extremely common during game play.

Will you notice the next time you're on a positive upward spiral with someone? Here's a quest to help you increase your social intelligence right now.

## QUEST 8: The Love Detector

When you understand how synchronization works, you spot it happening all around you. It's almost like developing a sixth sense—you see relationships sparking and connections strengthening right before your eyes.

I want you to think of your new sixth sense as a powerful *love detector.*

**What to do:** Look for the telltale sign of deep biological synchronization between two people.

What's the telltale sign? When two people are feeling positively connected, their **body language starts to mirror each other**. When one person leans forward, the other leans forward. When one rests her head thoughtfully on her right hand, the other follows suit. When one sits cross-legged, soon the other does as well.

This kind of spontaneous, unconscious mirroring happens in all kinds of situations: over coffee conversations with friends, during work meetings and job interviews, on first dates, and at parties. It's what happens whenever you feel like you're really "clicking" with someone.

**Why it works:** Dr. Barbara Fredrickson, one of the world's leading researchers of positive emotion, describes these mirror moments as "micro-moments of love." Whenever our brain activity and biochemistry align, she says, we lay the foundation for future friendship or even intimacy. While *love* might seem too strong a word to denote these everyday moments, Dr. Fredrickson's research shows that every time we sync up in a safe and positive context, we are actually feeling a miniburst of deep human connection. Every time we mirror, it's like we're practicing and strengthening our ability to love.[9]

Some people may advise you to purposefully mimic your boss's or your date's body language to help gently nudge the love along, but I don't recommend it. Instead, it's much more fun (and definitely less creepy!) to simply **become aware of mirroring** when it happens—and to delight in these micro-moments of love whenever you notice them.

So here's your quest to learn how to use your new love detector: for the next twenty-four hours, **pay special attention to the body language of people around you** (and to your own body language).

**Quest complete:** If you see body language being mirrored, congratulations—you've completed this quest by detecting a micro-moment of love!

If synchronization happens all the time, what makes the syncing that takes place during game play so special?

In some regards, there's nothing special about it—it works exactly as synchronization works during *any* kind of social interaction. Because you and your fellow player are focusing your attention on the same activity at the same time, your neurons start to mirror each other. And because emotions are contagious, you will pass your emotions back and forth—whether it's pride in a successful move, or frustration over a difficult obstacle, or surprise at an unexpected outcome. As your feelings align, so do your bodies—from the muscles in your face that express different feelings to the amount of sweat on your skin that reveals how excited or stressed out you are.

All shared activities—such as watching a movie, having a conversation, or listening to music—have a similar potential to create mind-and-body links. However, the *intensity* of game-based linkage is typically much stronger.

Remember from Chapter 1 the special kind of attention we give to games: when we play, we go into a state of deep focus, or *flow*. And when two people are in flow together, the synchronization is far greater (and far more enjoyable) than when they participate in less mentally absorbing activities.[10] Likewise, because we tend to feel heightened emotions like excitement and joy during game play, the quality of emotional linkage is heightened as well. The stronger our synchronized feelings, the deeper our mind-and-body connection.

But what's *really* special about syncing during game play is best explained by what psychologists call *theory of mind,* which is short for having an accurate theory of what's going on in someone else's mind. When you're playing a game with someone else, you spend a tremendous amount of time trying to anticipate what they're going to do next. This is true whether you're playing cooperatively or competitively: the more you can accurately model what your coplayer is thinking, the more successful you'll be in the game.

Game play requires a powerful theory of mind, much more so than ordinary social interactions.[11] Compared with taking a walk together or having a conversation, game play—with all its unpredictability and constant decision making—demands much tighter and more sustained synchronization. It's due to this high-demand social environment that neurological and physiological links happen so quickly and easily whenever we play. It's simply the nature of the game.

Because synchronization happens so rapidly, reliably, and deeply during game play, many gamers find it particularly useful for creating stronger social bonds. This is especially true for introverted individuals, who seem to benefit greatly from the easy and powerful social connections afforded by games.

Real-world studies offer even more insight into the benefits of syncing up through game play. Research from Brigham Young University's School of Family Life, for example, shows that playing video games together regularly in the same physical space increases the sense of connection between parent and child.[12] And for children with autism, multiplayer video games have been shown to increase cooperation, improve family social interactions, and increase social intelligence.[13] Children with autism communicate more directly and confidently with their peers and siblings after playing a game together. They also pay each other more compliments and engage more frequently in positive touching, such as giving each other high-fives.[14]

If you're not a frequent gamer but have a gamer in your life, consider taking the time to play together more often. It may be one of the most productive things you could do with your free time—if you want to enjoy a closer, happier relationship.

*A SuperBetter Story:*
*The Secret Language Between*
*Father and Daughter*

Antonio, a senior sales executive with a Fortune 500 company, doesn't seem like the kind of man with a lot of time to play video games. When I met him at his company's annual offsite leadership meeting in Chicago, he was juggling important calls and emails the whole time and flagging down colleagues to touch base about upcoming sales meetings around the country.

Although I was invited to the offsite to speak about how game psychology could improve motivation and productivity in the workplace, Antonio, like most of the executives I met that day, seemed more interested in talking to me about the role that games played in his family.

"I set aside a few hours every week to play games with my daughter," he told me. "It's very important to me, especially now that she's a teenager, that we keep playing together. It helps keep the lines of communication open."

Antonio's daughter Julia had just turned thirteen, and her new favorite game was *Minecraft*, the Lego-like building universe where players gather resources to architect whatever they can imagine. Monsters roam the *Minecraft* world, requiring players to build safe rooms and craft armor to protect themselves.

Apparently *Minecraft* was giving Julia a new way to think about real-life problems—and a way to talk to her dad about them. "Just last week I was dropping Julia off at school, and she really didn't want to go in. She's had some problems with bullying this year, nothing physical, just verbal. A few friends of hers decided they didn't want to be her friend anymore and have been giving her a really hard time. It's been rough on her.

"It's not something she usually talks to me about—she'd rather talk to her mom about that stuff. But when we pulled up at school last week, she turned to me and said, 'Dad, you know what I can do? I can put my armor on.' I knew what she meant immediately. When she puts on her armor in *Minecraft*, the monsters, the lava, all the bad stuff—it can't hurt her.

"I told her that was a great way to think about it. 'You're going to put on your diamond armor today, and it won't matter what anyone says to you. It'll bounce right off you.' And she said, 'Yep,' and smiled, and hopped out of the car. It was a little thing, but now we've got this conversation going. It's like a secret code, where I can ask her if she needs her armor today, and she knows what I mean, and she knows that I'm proud of her for being so resilient."

As we've seen, games are a particularly easy and efficient way to create mind-and-body synchrony. When you play a game with someone, you don't have to focus consciously on mirroring or imitating—it just happens naturally as a result of your mutual engagement with the game. But even without games, there are lots of other ways you can intentionally jump-start your biological linkage. Find out how in your next quest.

## QUEST 9: The Power of a Good Sync

If you want to strengthen your mind-and-body connection to friends and family, all it takes is a good sync.

**What to do**: Take one or two minutes out of your day to coordinate your actions as closely as possible with another person.

These simple methods work to stimulate mirror neurons and synchronize heart and breathing rates:

- Take a walk around the block together, and match your stride as closely as possible, in both rhythm and length.
- Listen to a song together—everyone taps their fingers or claps their hands to the beat.
- Learn a simple dance routine, and perform it together.
- Rock in rocking chairs, or swing in swings, next to each other, at the same pace, for at least ninety seconds.
- Work together to lift and carry a heavy piece of furniture.[15]

Walking, tapping, clapping, dancing, rocking, and swinging together all work in the same way—they create biological linkage through near-perfect physical mirroring and synchronization. Carrying a piece of heavy furniture together, however, is more like playing a video game: in order to avoid dropping it, bumping it, or hurting yourself, you have to successfully anticipate your partner's thoughts and movements. This kind of intense neurological linkage stimulates the same increase in connection, affection, and empathy as physical mirroring.

There are countless ways to get a good sync in, and it only takes a few minutes. Be creative and invent your own favorite traditions.

**Examples:** Here are some ideas from SuperBetter players:

- "My son and I walk in sync for one minute every day when I pick him up from school. He decides how fast or far to step, and I have to try to match him!"
- "My wife and I have been taking turns picking a song to listen to each night before we go to bed. We don't try to move together on purpose, because that feels forced and kind of awkward. But we somehow wind up tapping our feet or swaying together by the end of the song, without even consciously trying."

- "Whenever there's a big disagreement at the office, we have the people who are disagreeing move the conference room table into the hallway and back again. I'm sure the syncing helps, but it also breaks the tension and brings some humor to the situation. Everyone knows what it means when they see the table coming into the hall!"

*Tip:* Your partner doesn't need to know all the science for it to work. But if you're going to make it a habit, clue them in so they can share in this powerful knowledge with you.

Also, it helps if your go-to syncing activity is something you both enjoy doing for its own sake. Don't force it. Let the synchronizing happen naturally, while you're focusing on the fun or the challenge.

◄►

Being able to strengthen bonds with people you already know is a powerful ability. Starting to see the entire world around you as full of potential allies is another superpower altogether.

Sometimes, to get more support in our lives, we have to be willing to look in the most unlikely places. And games can help us do that—by opening up our minds to friendship with people we would ordinarily overlook. One of my favorite game studies in recent years explains how.

Social scientists at Nanyang Technological University (NTU) in Singapore have been studying the real-life impacts of video games for more than a decade—and recently they made a major breakthrough. They discovered that playing the Nintendo game *Wii Bowling* with a stranger not only makes you like that person more—something you'd expect from almost any enjoyable activity two people perform together—but also makes you like more *everyone else in the world who you perceive to be like your game partner.* Let me explain.

One of the biggest social problems in Singapore today is alienation between young people and senior citizens. According to national surveys, they don't like each other very much, and they avoid spending time together. The result is that seniors in Singapore are often socially isolated, which is terrible for their mental and physical health. Meanwhile, young people miss out on significant opportunities to be mentored and cared for by seniors.

Could games help solve this widespread social problem? The NTU researchers set up a pilot study to find out. They paired up college students and senior citizens for weekly video game dates lasting thirty minutes each. After six weeks of playing Nintendo *Wii Bowling* together, the seniors and the young people not only considered each other friends, they had dramatically revised their opinion of the entire other group.

The young people decided they liked senior citizens, in general, a whole lot more. Meanwhile the seniors were much less anxious about interacting with young people. Both groups said they were more likely to seek out social interaction with someone from the other group in the future. This represented a huge psychological shift. They didn't just make one new friend; they started to see *all* seniors or young people as potential friends.

Crucially, this powerful change did *not* occur in the study's control group, in which young people and seniors spent the same exact amount of time together making conversation, watching TV, or working on arts and crafts together. The individuals liked each other more after six weeks of hanging out, but they continued to *dislike* other seniors or young people in general. In short, they changed their mind about just one person, not the whole group. They remained, unfortunately, psychologically closed off from a whole world of potential allies.

By now, you can probably guess how the *Wii Bowling* video game accomplished what other common social interactions could not: deep synchronization was surely at play. And one particular outcome of synchronization—increased empathy—makes all the difference when it comes to reversing prejudice or healing social tension.

Empathy is the ability to imagine and relate to what someone else is feeling—and fortunately, a little bit of empathy goes a long way. Research shows that increasing our empathy for just *one person* in a group will improve our opinions about the *entire group* in general.[16] However, if we simply *like* one person in a group without increasing our empathy for them, our opinions about the group as a whole will remain the same.

This is exactly what happens when we play a game with someone we think we won't like, by virtue of their age or any other prejudicial factor. By increasing our empathy for our fellow player, we increase our empathy for *everyone* who reminds us of that player.

To feel more empathy with others, people have to have positive social interactions in safe environments. Synchronization can't happen if you're preoccupied with negative thoughts or feelings. In fact, research shows that strong prejudice and dislike for someone else's group can actually prevent us from experiencing neurological linkage.[17] But games have an advantage here as well. The NTU researchers theorize that the *equalizing* nature of games makes it easier to connect in spite of existing social tension, anxiety, or mistrust.

When we play a game, we come together on equal terms and equal footing. We agree and trust each other to follow the same rules, to pursue the same goal, and to treat each other fairly. We accept each other as worthy teammates or competitors, regardless of our outside social status.

The equal status and trust that we experience in games, as temporary and as limited as they may be, makes it feel safer to explore social interactions with people we might ordinarily be anxious around or avoid altogether. And it's not just the NTU researchers who have figured this out. Groups around the world are starting to harness the power of play to make allies across cultural borders and boundaries. The Middle East Gaming Challenge, for example, brings tens of thousands of children in the Middle East together to play cooperative video games, online and in person. The organizers' goal is to promote dialogue and confront prejudices that currently exist between Arab and Jewish schoolchildren in Israel. They explain:

Despite being neighbors, these children are all too often exposed to atmospheres of negative stereotypes that, unfortunately, are exacerbated by the two communities' separate education systems. Without a doubt, for many of them the gaming challenge will be a first positive experience shared with someone their own age, in the same corner of the globe, but from an entirely different religious or ethnic background.[18]

When you look at the possible stakes of events like the Middle East Gaming Challenge, it becomes clear why research like the *Wii Bowling* study matters. When we understand how games change relationships, we can see more clearly what it takes to overcome our own biases and prejudices. And we discover just how important it is to synchronize our minds and bodies whenever we want to change someone else's opinion of us from negative to positive.

Surprisingly, and wonderfully, this kind of change does not take exceptional amounts of time or effort. It *does* take a willingness to interact gamefully—by seeking out experiences that put us on equal footing and so make deep synchronization more likely to occur.

The spectacular "mind meld" and biological mirroring effects of video games and other coordinated activities require players to be in the same physical space at the same time. You can't sync over email or text message. But what if you want to strengthen relationships with friends and family you're not able to see in person as often as you'd like? Although you won't get the same mind-and-body connection, you *can* increase your real-life social support systems through online game play. In fact, research suggests that online games are an especially powerful relationship management tool— they make it easier for us to maintain more active social relationships, so we have support from others when we need it most.

Let's see how online play works to help you find real-life allies—and what online games can teach you about how to get social support wherever you go.

Social network games are some of the most widely played *and* widely studied video games in recent years. More than half a billion people have played social network games like *Farmville* (a cooperative farm simulation),

*Candy Crush Saga* (a pattern-matching game in which you share power-ups with your friends), and *Words with Friends* (a variation on the classic board game Scrabble). These games, most commonly played on Facebook or via mobile phones, allow you to play with anyone in your social network—and you don't even have to be online at the same time. In competitive games like *Words with Friends*, players take their next turn whenever they have a spare moment. In cooperative games like *Farmville* or *Candy Crush Saga*, players can contribute toward a collective goal or send their friends helpful power-ups even when their friends are offline.

As these games have gained in popularity, researchers have been curious to find out whether playing a social network game with someone makes people more likely to socialize with them in real life. Study after study has found that it does. When you play a game like *Farmville* or *Words with Friends* with a friend or family member, you not only feel closer to them, you're also more likely to see them in person or to have conversations with them about nongame, real-life events. And if you play cooperative games together, you're more likely to ask each other for, or offer each other, help with a real-life problem.[19]

The more researchers dig into the way social network games work, the more they seem to agree that these relationship-enhancing benefits stem from three key functions: establishing common ground, increasing familiarity, and modeling reciprocity.

*Establishing common ground* simply means sharing a common experience that gives you something to talk about. One of the biggest challenges for many people in maintaining relationships with extended family and friends is a lack of common ground in the present. If we don't have anything in common to talk about, we're less likely to talk at all. But social scientists have found that even something as simple as a Facebook game dramatically improves our sense of having something in the present moment that actively connects us—and therefore something to talk about. Players report that game-related conversations often expand to topics outside the game, such as work and family life. But the game itself remains the foundation of frequent communication, helping us stay actively in touch with people in our social network we would otherwise grow distant from.[20]

*Increasing familiarity* simply means interacting more often. The higher the frequency, the stronger the social bond—as long as the interactions are primarily positive. Social network games seem to be a particularly efficient way to increase familiarity, because they allow two people to interact across time and distance. They remove any obstacles that might stand in the way of face-to-face interactions. And while face-to-face interactions would certainly offer a more powerful social experience (complete with synchronization!), research shows that any increased familiarity improves the odds of offering help or having face-to-face time in the future.

Finally, *modeling reciprocity* means showing other people that we care about them and that they can trust us to offer help. To model reciprocity, we simply have to return a favor or make a simple gesture of kindness. In everyday life, it can be hard to find simple and effective ways to show we care. But in social network games, it's easy. Reciprocity typically takes the form of sending someone a power-up or an extra life—something that will make it easier for our friend to advance in the game. In *Farmville*, for example, you can water your friends' crops or feed their chickens. In *Candy Crush Saga*, you can send your friends extra moves to help them complete a difficult level.

These little boosts of help are almost always free to send someone; there is no cost other than the time it takes to click "send," and the games constantly remind us to do so. Despite the fact that it's so easy to send this kind of help, players report feeling genuinely assisted and looked after by friends and family who regularly give them in-game boosts. Researchers believe that this kind of continual in-game show of support fosters trust and a feeling of responsibility toward each other. And data backs up this hypothesis: people who play online games together cooperatively or as a team report getting more real-life social support from each other. And the support is meaningful—it includes everything from getting advice on a problem and tangible support like monetary assistance, to emotional support like reassurance and listening. [21]

*A SuperBetter Story:*
*The Feuding Families*

"Don't go yet! I have to tell you my story!" These words came tumbling out of the mouth of a beautiful young blond woman who seemed quite intent on speaking with me.

I was at Marquette University in Milwaukee, Wisconsin, and I had just given a guest lecture on game design. Anna, twenty-eight, who was finishing up her bachelor's degree in communications, had waited until all the other students left to try to catch a private word with me.

"This would sound ridiculous to most people, but I know you'll understand," she told me, taking a deep breath. "The Facebook game *Farmville* saved my marriage. Do you have a minute? Can I explain how?" Of course I wanted to hear more.

Anna told me that she and her husband, Aadil, had married several years ago against the wishes of both her parents and his. "Our families would not speak to each other, not before the wedding and not after. It's because of our religion." Anna's parents were from Ukraine. They practiced a very strict Orthodox Christianity. Aadil was from India, his family, Muslim.

"I smoothed things over with my parents so at least they were talking to me, and Aadil did the same with his parents. But the two families have absolutely refused to have any contact with each other. This has been a huge source of pain for us. It's especially hard because we live so far apart from both families." Most of Anna's extended family was still in Ukraine, and Aadil's in India. They stayed in touch with everyone primarily through Facebook.

"We had given up on our families ever getting along," Anna said. "And then one day the strangest thing happened. My mother started harvesting grapes with Aadil's mother!"

Anna was talking about virtual grapes, of course. She had started playing the farming simulation game *Farmville* with her parents a few weeks earlier, "just as something fun to do with them every day, since they're so far away and it's hard to talk across the different time zones." Anna was also playing the game with her husband. "Our schedules are so busy, and I'm always in evening classes when he comes home from work. But we played when we could, and it helped us spend a little more time together."

"So you know how you can improve your farm faster if you get help from your neighbors?" Anna asked me. She was referring to the way Facebook games encourage you to invite your entire social network to play with you, so they can help you in the game. In *Farmville*, real-life friends and family become "neighbors" who can help feed your virtual chickens and water your virtual crops. "Well, I think my mom got really into the game because she was doing whatever it took to level up her farm faster. First she invited Aadil to be her neighbor and help her harvest some crops. That was amazing already. But then one day I was completely shocked, I noticed she had invited Aadil's *mom* to join a co-op mission."

In a co-op, or cooperative, mission in *Farmville*, players have a limited amount of time—usually anywhere from a few hours to an entire day—to accomplish a shared goal together, like planting and harvesting one hundred pounds of grapes. "His mom and my mom were in closer time zones, so I guess it was just easier for them to do missions together than to wait until we were awake in the United States."

By this point in the story, Anna's eyes were welling up. "You have to understand, this was the first social interaction my mom and his mom had willingly had together in three years. It felt like a miracle."

Before they knew it, Anna's parents were regularly inviting Aadil's parents to do cooperative missions together in the game. "They started leaving notes on each other's Facebook pages to plan their missions. And then, I guess since they were already on their pages, they started liking each other's updates and leaving nice little comments. It went from just being about the game to being something more."

The families aren't playing *Farmville* anymore, now that their initial mania for it has died down. But the good news is, they don't need to. "This game has changed everything for us. I don't think we'll ever go back. We're not two families anymore. We're all family to each other now."

Playing games online with extended friends and family helps ensure you have strong social ties and social support when you need it. People you play with are more likely to have your back—and you, theirs. But what if you want to reap the same benefits with people in your life who aren't on your favorite social network, or who might not want to play a game? Although social network games make it easier to establish common ground, model reciprocity, and increase familiarity, you can still use these three techniques to strengthen any relationship—with or without a game.

Here's a quest to help you explore how to translate the power of social network games into the rest of your life.

## QUEST 10: Plus-One Better

**Pick three people:**

1. Someone who would like to hear from you
2. Someone you would like to hear from
3. Someone who might be surprised to hear from you

Do you have your three people in mind? Good. Now—you have a choice. You can complete this quest on a difficulty setting of easy, medium, or hard. "Easy" means you're going to send a message to the first person on your list. "Medium" means you're going to message the first *and* second person on your list. "Hard" means you're going to message all three.

**What to do:** Ask each of the three people, **"On a scale of 1 to 10, how is your day going?"**

It may feel a bit out of the blue to the person who receives it. That's okay. In fact, it's *good.* Your goal is to catch someone off guard with a signal that you care, and that you're thinking about them. Meanwhile, asking for a number from 1 to 10 prompts more reflection than simply asking "How's it going?"—and it often gets you a more honest and interesting reply. (You'll see what I mean as soon as you give it a try!)

Send your message now. Make sure you send it privately—through email, text, or Facebook, for example.

Now you wait—and if they message back a number from 1 to 10, here's what you're going to reply: **"Is there anything I could do to help move it from a 6 to a 7?"** (or . . . "from a 3 to a 4" or "from a 10 to an 11"—you get the idea).

I learned this habit from my friend Michael, a philanthropist and entrepreneur who likes to ask this question (and make this offer) to almost everyone he talks to, day in and day out. He asks me to rate my day every single time I see him. He asks it of servers at restaurants when we eat out. He asked my husband the first time they met, too. After a while, I came to the conclusion that this question is completely awesome. You really can ask it of virtually anyone, close friend or stranger. And it's easy to answer—everyone can think of a number from 1 to 10.

Sometimes they'll answer with just a number. Sometimes they'll offer details to explain their number. It's amazing how much you can learn about what's on someone's mind by how they explain their 1, 5, or 10. And when you offer to do something to bump their number up by just +1, it pretty much *always* makes them smile. *You'll* be surprised by how surprised other people are when you take the time to explicitly offer your support. Consider this reply from my friend Chris, when I sent him the "1 to 10" question the other day: "Better now that you asked. Truly makes a difference. Was a 5, just became a 7."

**Why it works:** This quest is designed to adapt the best features of social games to everyday life. It's quick and easy, and like online games, you don't have to be face to face to do it. It models reciprocity: by offering to make someone's day +1 better, you're communicating that you care and that they can count on you for support. And it increases common ground—if they explain their number to you, you'll know a little bit more about what's going on, which gives you something to talk about. If they don't explain their number, you've still checked in—and every check-in helps increase the familiarity that leads to stronger relationships.

*Tip:* Don't do this quest just once—do it often. Whenever I find myself thinking about someone I haven't talked to in a while, I text them the "1 to 10" question. It's an easy and fun habit to develop and a great way to spark conversation. And if it becomes a playful tradition with some of your friends and family, all the better!

◄►

There are some ways of playing games that do *not* cultivate closer ties and stronger bonds. I want to caution here against one kind of game play in particular: excessive competition against strangers online. This style of game play can actually make it harder for you to cultivate positive relationships in the rest of your life.

Winning a game against a stranger—particularly when playing a video game with strong themes of domination and destruction, like *Call of Duty*—creates distinct physiological and neurological changes. Your testosterone surges, and as a result, you have a diminished neural capacity for empathy.[22] You feel more powerful and aggressive, and you're less likely to be kind or sympathetic to *anyone* you perceive as weak.[23] (Men, it seems, are particularly vulnerable to this effect; women tend to see a smaller spike in testosterone after winning.)[24] Note: This happens only when you play against strangers, not when you play against friends or family.

You might be wondering, what's so bad about feeling hostile toward strangers you'll never meet in real life? It turns out that the feelings of aggression aren't limited to the period of play. Studies show that the effects of a testosterone surge can impact your decisions and behavior for hours afterward.[25] This means that your antisocial feelings toward strangers can spill over and make you more hostile or aggressive toward your real-life friends, family, and coworkers.

It gets worse: while winning against strangers online can temporarily turn you into a bit of a jerk, losing against a distant stranger isn't particularly good for your everyday relationships, either. The most recent game research suggests that much of the aggression that has long been associated with "violent video games" is actually related to feelings of *incompetence* after losing.[26] Players who feel embarrassed and frustrated after losing a game are more likely to display anger and hostility toward others. This can happen when you play a game alone, or with friends and family, but it's much more likely to happen when you play against strangers whom you're unable to synchronize with, mentally or physically.

It's important to be clear: games like *Call of Duty* have *not* been shown to increase hostility or decrease empathy when you play with people you know in real life. In fact, a recent study showed that playing *Call of Duty* competitively against other players in the same physical space actually *decreased* aggression and hostility and *increased* empathy, as much as playing cooperatively did (just as with *Hedgewars*, the game you read about at the beginning of this chapter).[27] For this reason, you don't need to avoid *Call of Duty* or any other game that pits you aggressively against other players.

They have a host of other benefits that I'll talk about more in Chapter 4, such as improved cognitive function and better performance in high-stress situations. Looking at the science, and the potential downside of testosterone-boosting victories, I simply recommend that you spend no more than half of your game play hours trying to beat strangers online. You're much better off, in terms of generating social resilience, trying to beat your friends and family or playing cooperatively with strangers.

Remarkably, and fortunately, negative social impacts seem to occur consistently under only one condition of game play—aggressive, competitive game play *against strangers online.* All other forms of game play tend to strengthen the bond between players and make you, generally, a more likable person to others. Gaming—in person or with friends and family online—is the perfect way to practice your synchronization skills, increase your social intelligence, and develop more empathy for others. These are powerful abilities you can use in any social environment, inside and outside of games.

# MISSION COMPLETE

### *Skills Unlocked: How to Discover New Allies and Strengthen Your Support System*

- To neurologically sync up with someone, play a game together, competitively or cooperatively, in the same physical space. This will activate your mirror neurons, which strengthens your social bonds and increases your social intelligence.
- As often as possible, make time with friends and family for other kinds of synchronizing activity. Anything that naturally leads to physical mirroring, such as walking together, or that requires significant coordination, such as tossing a ball back and forth, will do the trick.
- Start looking for evidence of new allies all around you, by learning to spot the telltale signs of social synchronization. When someone is

subconsciously mirroring your body language or gestures, it means they feel a strong connection to you and are more likely to help you in the future.

- To radically increase the number of potential allies in your life, play games or sync up with people who are different from you—in age, culture, gender, or point of view. You'll not only make new friendships, you'll also increase your empathy for many more people.

- Find new sources of social support by demonstrating reciprocity through social network games or playful communications. Asking for or offering a tiny bit of help, even if it's across time and space, is the most powerful social gesture you can make.

- Try not to spend too much time alone playing competitive games against strangers online. It won't give you any social benefits, and it may negatively impact your empathy and likability to others. If you prefer competitive gaming, make sure to do it on a team, or against your real-life friends and family.

# 3

## You Are the Hero of Your Own Story

### Your Mission

Rewire your brain so it's easier to motivate
yourself, persevere, and succeed.

In video games, we play as heroes. We become conquering space cowboys, warrior princesses, daredevil racecar drivers, or the last survivors of a zombie apocalypse. Even in nondigital games, we strive to be the hero of the day, accomplishing epic feats that amaze. Think about scoring a last-second goal in soccer, or marching a pawn across the chessboard to win a second queen after losing your first.

But do games actually develop our heroic potential? Can games make us more likely to be an inspiration to others, and to achieve extraordinary goals in real life? The evidence suggests yes.

In this chapter, we're going to explore how games of all kinds *increase our character strengths*—like grit, perseverance, compassion, and work ethic. We'll uncover the science behind how games strengthen our real-life willpower and help us change our real-world behavior for the better. We'll look at the neuroscience of game play—how it changes the way our brains respond to challenge and effort, making us less likely to give up when things are difficult for us. And we'll explore why certain games make us more likely to rise to the heroic occasion when someone else is in need.

By understanding exactly how games tap into your natural determination and compassion, you can become better able to tap into these heroic qualities—anywhere, anytime.

Let's start with a game that has a truly audacious goal: to help young people beat cancer.

At first glance, *Re-Mission* looks like a typical fantasy shooter game. You control a superhero robot named Roxxi, who flies through a twisting-and-turning landscape, using powerful weapons to blow up the bad guys. But despite the 3-D graphics and immersive sound effects, *Re-Mission* isn't a typical video game. Look closer, and you'll notice that Roxxi is flying inside the human body, the bad guys are cancer cells, and her weapons include chemotherapy blasters and antibiotic grenades.

*Re-Mission* was created by the nonprofit HopeLab for a special purpose: to improve young patients' adherence to difficult, but life-saving, chemotherapy and antibiotic regimens.

To fight childhood cancers like leukemia, most patients will take oral doses of these medications for two to three years. It's extremely important for patients to try to never miss a dose. Eighty percent of cases where childhood cancer comes back (instead of staying in remission) are associated with missed medication. Fewer missed doses means lower rates of infection, fever, and hospitalization—and most important, better survival outcomes.

Families and patients know this, but young people miss doses anyway, for many different reasons. They can't stand the side effects, such as nausea and fatigue. They get busy with school or sports as they start to feel better, making it harder to follow a strict medication routine. Or after years of treatment, they subconsciously rebel and forget to take the drugs, because they are just "sick of being sick."

*Re-Mission* was designed to prevent these lapses, by helping young patients feel more optimistic and motivated to take their medications. As senior HopeLab researcher and UCLA professor of medicine Steve Cole told me, "Thirty percent of kids miss twenty percent of doses or more. Those kids have twice the risk of having a rebound of the leukemia. This is a completely avoidable risk. We have to somehow get across the message: No matter how bad the disease is, you are fundamentally in control of your health, and no one can save your life if you don't do your part."

Cole and his collaborators hoped that patients would become more committed to their treatment plans if they learned more about chemotherapy in the empowering context of a video game. These lessons were integrated right into the game play. For example, when the virtual patient in the game skips a chemotherapy dose, Roxxi's chemo-blaster weapon starts to malfunction, misfiring every third shot. Skip another chemotherapy dose, and more virtual cancer cells survive each blast. Skip again, and cancer cells become drug-resistant, further increasing the challenge of each level.

So did it work? Yes, overwhelmingly. In a clinical trial, patients who played *Re-Mission* for as little as two hours had greater medication adherence for *three months*.[1]

Electronic pill-cap monitors showed that the game players took 16 percent more antibiotic doses over a three-month period than nonplayers. This means the game effectively eliminated a whopping half of the typically missed doses. And when patients' blood was drawn and tested, *Re-Mission* players had 41 percent higher doses of the cancer-fighting medication in their bodies. They were significantly more successful in keeping up with treatment—and therefore more likely to stay in remission.[2] (The trial was conducted with 375 patients, aged 13 to 29, at 34 medical centers across the United States.)

Interestingly, a full quarter of the study participants reported that they rarely played video games before the trial. Another third had previously played just one or two hours per week. In other words, these were not hardcore gamers who were benefiting from the game. The game worked equally well for novice or infrequent game players as it did for lifelong players—and it is continuing to work for patients worldwide. As a result of this successful clinical trial, *Re-Mission* has been distributed to more than 250,000 cancer patients. And recently HopeLab released six follow-up cancer-fighting games online, including *Stem Cell Defender* and *Nanobot's Revenge*. (They are free to play at www.re-mission2.org.)

HopeLab's games are an incredible, potentially life-saving resource. But even if you aren't battling cancer, the *Re-Mission* research offers a powerful, life-changing insight: *motivation alone is far less important to success and willpower than you think.*

Before the cancer patients played *Re-Mission*, they were already fighting for their lives—presumably a highly motivating state. This was not a group that simply needed more *motivation*. They had it in spades, yet they nevertheless regularly failed to do the things they knew could dramatically improve their chances for a cure.

Somehow the video game *Re-Mission* intervened in a way that converted mere motivation into a much more powerful psychological resource. But what is that resource? And how did the game create it so quickly?

This is exactly what the HopeLab team was wondering after they saw the success from their first clinical trial. Originally, they had hypothesized that *thirty* hours of play would be necessary to make a positive impact on medication adherence. They were amazed when just two hours made such a significant difference. And they had expected players to need continual reinforcement and reminders from the video game every day in order to keep up their behavior change. Yet it turned out that playing the game just once was enough. It was truly a surprising result. What could explain such long-term, real-life behavioral changes after such a short time of virtual play?

The key to solving this puzzle was found in another set of data that the researchers collected during the clinical trial. They weren't just monitoring medication adherence. They also tracked psychological changes during the trial. Players and nonplayers reported the same levels of motivation, stress, cancer symptoms, and physical side effects, but the game players differed remarkably in one area. They reported feeling significantly more powerful, optimistic, and able to positively impact their own health than nonplayers.

Psychologists call this state of mind *self-efficacy*. It's the belief that you, yourself, can effect positive change in your own life.

Self-efficacy is not the same thing as self-esteem, which is a more general positive feeling of self-worth. Self-efficacy means having confidence in the concrete skills and abilities required to solve specific problems or achieve particular goals. It is usually context-specific: you might have high self-efficacy at work but low self-efficacy about public speaking or losing weight.

Self-efficacy is the crucial difference between having lots of motivation but failing to follow through, and successfully converting motivation into consistent and effective action. With high self-efficacy, you are more likely to take actions that help you reach your goals, even if those actions are difficult or painful. You also engage with difficult problems longer, without giving up. But with low self-efficacy, no matter how motivated you are, you're less likely to take positive action—because you lack belief in your ability to make a difference in your own life.

So where did the *Re-Mission* players' new self-efficacy come from? Well, all games are intentionally designed to increase players' feelings of competence, power, and skillful ability over time—in other words, to build up their self-efficacy. Like all video games, *Re-Mission* challenges players to achieve a difficult goal: navigating through a complex, 3-D space and destroying all the virtual cancer cells before time runs out. This goal requires skill, practice, and effort. Players of *Re-Mission*, like players of all games, are typically unsuccessful at first. But quickly, with repeated effort and as they learn how the game works, they start to improve their skills and strategies. Eventually they master a few challenges. And because it's a video game, it gets harder. The challenges get more difficult and complex with each new level. This constantly escalating challenge requires a willingness from players to keep trying, even when they fail. It instills a belief that if they keep practicing and learning, if they put in the hard work, they *will* eventually be able to achieve more difficult goals.

This is the classic path to increased self-efficacy: accept a goal, make an effort, get feedback on that effort, improve a concrete skill, keep trying, and eventually succeed. You don't need a game to set off on this path. But because it is the very nature of games to challenge and improve our abilities, they are an incredibly reliable and efficient way to get there.

And here's the good news: once you have a feeling of self-efficacy about a particular problem, it tends to persist. It's a lasting mindset shift, permanently changing what you believe you are capable of and what goals you believe you can realistically achieve. And this is exactly why *Re-Mission* worked so well. The game created a new source of self-efficacy for young patients, in a situation where it is easy to otherwise feel powerless or overwhelmed. Instead of seeing chemotherapy as a negative experience they were forced to undergo, they came to see it as a powerful weapon they were fully in control of. They understood exactly how it worked, and they weren't afraid to use it!

This shift in mindset alone—from powerless to powerful, from feeling weakened to feeling successful—was enough to supercharge the players' willpower and determination throughout the long course of treatment.

Self-efficacy is increased anytime you learn a new skill or master a new challenge. So let's increase *your* self-efficacy right now—with another quest!

## QUEST 11: The Power Breath

You've probably tried deep, slow breathing to calm yourself down. But there's actually a more useful breathing technique, one that can reduce stress, decrease pain, increase concentration, halt migraines, and prevent panic attacks.

**What to do:** Breathe in while you count slowly to 4. Exhale while you count to 8.

In for 4, out for 8. Repeat for at least one minute. This is a bit more challenging than it sounds! The trick is to always **exhale for *twice as long* as you inhale**.

Give it a try right now. You don't have to do a full minute right away. Try to do it just once: in for 4, out for 8. Got it?

Okay, now try to do it twice in a row.

Good? Now try three in a row. If you can, count a little bit slower, and draw the breath out even more.

Excellent! You've mastered the trick. When you can keep this up for at least one full minute, you will be able to help yourself feel better, almost immediately, in many different stressful or painful situations.

**Why it works:** Breathing at this rhythm increases your *heart rate variability*,[3] the slight differences in the length of time between your heartbeats, from one to the next.

The more variation, the better. In the long term, high heart rate variability protects against stress, anxiety, inflammation, and pain. In the short term, increased heart rate variability has a huge impact on your nervous system. It shifts your body from what scientists call *sympathetic stimulation* (which, when activated by stress, pain, or anxiety, triggers a fight-or-flight mode) to *parasympathetic stimulation* (a calm-and-connect mode).[4]

Just by changing how you breathe for one minute, you can shift your entire nervous system from a stressful state to a highly relaxed state. Muscles relax, heart rate decreases, digestion improves, and state of mind improves. If you're feeling *any* kind of bad, this powerful shift is sure to help.

**But you're not finished with this quest yet!** I want you to think of two different situations where this power breathing technique could help you feel better, immediately. For example, I personally use this technique to stop migraines in their tracks, and to calm my anxiety during turbulence on flights. A collaborator of mine at Nike uses it to relieve muscle cramps after tough workouts.

SuperBetter players have reported using the power breath technique to control their tempers with their kids, to battle the nausea of morning sickness, to fight insomnia, before going into a stressful meeting, and even to put themselves in the mood to make love. How will *you* use it?

**What to do:** Predict **two situations in your life** where power breathing for one minute could help. Make a decision now to use this technique the next time you find yourself in that situation.

**Quest complete:** That's it—congratulations! You've increased your self-efficacy when it comes to battling stress, anxiety, discomfort, or pain. You've learned a new skill, and you've anticipated two specific problems it can help you solve. You've got a superpower—and you know exactly how and when to use it.

Hopefully, you're starting to see how self-efficacy is created—and how it can supercharge your ability to do what's difficult. However, there's still one puzzling thing about the *Re-Mission* clinical trial results. It makes sense that participants in the study would develop more confidence and belief in their video game skills by playing *Re-Mission*. Playing a video game makes you better at that particular game and probably other games as well. But how did confidence in their ability to *beat a video game* translate into confidence to *beat cancer in real life*? It's a hell of a lot harder to win the battle against a real life-threatening disease than it is to destroy virtual bad guys on a computer screen.

To solve this mystery, we need to turn to the neuroscience of video games. Because it turns out that while there are many ways to increase confidence in individual skills, nothing primes the brain for *general* self-efficacy—or the belief that you have the ability to conquer any problem you put your mind to—faster or more reliably than video games.

. . .

*V* *ideo games create a rush in the brain as pleasurable and powerful as*
*intravenous drugs.* It was the first major breakthrough in the neuroscience of gaming, and it was rather shocking. The year was 1998, and a
group of British scientists had just found that playing video games leads to a
massive increase in the amount of dopamine, the "pleasure" neurotransmitter, in the brain.[5] To their astonishment, they found that the increase in dopamine from game play was equal to the boost experienced when scientists
*injected amphetamines intravenously* into the same study participants.

Games impact the brain in nearly an identical fashion to highly addictive
drugs?! On the face of it, this finding might seem alarming—particularly
given that, depending on the study, anywhere from 1 to 8 percent of video
game players consider themselves at least periodically "addicted" to their favorite games.[6] (The most common percentage reported in these studies is
3 percent; in Chapter 4 we'll look at the factors that can lead to excessive
game play and the most effective techniques for treating it.) Indeed, if you're
already familiar with the neurotransmitter dopamine, you've probably
heard about it in the context of addiction. The pleasurable effects of many
drugs, from nicotine to cocaine, are thought to stem from the large amount
of dopamine they release in the mesolimbic pathways, the "reward circuitry"
of the brain.

But the mesolimbic pathways are involved in many brain processes, not
just pleasure and addiction. Dopamine in this region also stimulates memory, motivation, learning, emotion, and desire. In fact, for the vast majority
of people, in the course of ordinary everyday life, increased dopamine in the
reward circuitry is *not* a sign of addiction. More commonly, it's a sign of increased motivation and determination.[7]

Here's how it works. Every time you consider a possible goal, your brain
conducts a split-second, unconscious cost-benefit analysis of whether it's
worth the effort to try to achieve it.[8] How you conduct this analysis depends
less on the facts of the situation than on *how much dopamine is present in*
*your brain.*

When you have high dopamine levels in the reward circuitry, you worry less about the effort required, and you find it easier to imagine and predict success. This translates into higher determination and lower frustration in the face of setbacks. Meanwhile, when dopamine runs low in the reward circuitry—something that happens during a period of clinical depression, for example—you weigh more heavily the effort required, often magnifying it, and you discount the importance of your goals.[9] You also tend to anticipate failure rather than success, which can lead you to avoid challenges altogether.[10]

Obviously, then, when you're tackling a new goal or facing a tough obstacle, it's a huge benefit to have high levels of dopamine. And the benefit extends beyond motivation and determination. High dopamine levels in the reward circuitry are also associated with *faster learning* and *better performance*.[11] That's because when we're goal-oriented, we pay more attention to what we're doing. We also respond more quickly and effectively to feedback, which makes it easier to learn and improve. This is the neurological basis of self-efficacy: high motivation to achieve a goal, combined with the increased determination and faster learning required to master new skills and abilities. This powerful combination makes you more ambitious and justifiably more optimistic about your odds of success.

For many video game researchers (and video game players!), these neuroscience findings make perfect sense. Gamers, after all, spend on average 80 percent of the time failing when they play their favorite games.[12] Without the dopamine rush during game play, surely they would give up much sooner. But the high level of dopamine in the reward circuitry ensures that gamers stay focused, motivated, and determined to succeed. Meanwhile, thanks to the faster learning that occurs with continuous dopamine release, gamers are more likely to improve their skills and eventually achieve their goals.

No wonder frequent gamers work so hard, hour after hour, at their favorite games. *Their brains are being primed for increased self-efficacy with every move they make.* Scientists know that dopamine is released every time we anticipate feedback from a goal-oriented action—whether in daily life or in games. We get a rush of excitement to find out how we did. It just so happens that when we play video games, we take so many goal-oriented actions, so quickly, and get such immediate feedback, that the dopamine rush is as powerful as amphetamine drugs.

It's not always beneficial to be optimistic and determined. In some contexts, a predisposition to try harder for more unlikely or difficult rewards can be counterproductive or even pathological—particularly when greater effort is unlikely to actually help. When it comes to gambling, for example, where luck is more of a factor than hard work, this mindset can lead to terrible consequences. Or in the case of a dopamine rush created by a drug like cocaine or nicotine, extreme motivation to achieve a reward (more of the drug) can lead to a dangerous discounting of the health costs involved with actually getting what we want.

But in many more everyday contexts, especially where hard work is likely to produce better results—such as trying to learn something new, completing a difficult assignment, training for a sport, rehabilitating from an injury, or even just trying to pull ourselves out of depression—a neurological bias toward effortful action can produce powerful and positive results.

But does the dopamine rush translate from video games to real-life challenges and problem solving? Do games rewire our brains to be more motivated and work harder only when we're playing? Or can we translate our increased ambition and self-efficacy to the rest of our lives?

Researchers have found that frequent video gamers *do* indeed put more effort into difficult problem solving outside their favorite games. One recent study showed that gamers exhibited "a dispositional need to complete difficult tasks" and "the desire to exhibit high standards of performance in the face of frustration."[13] When given a series of easy puzzles to solve and difficult puzzles to solve, frequent game players spent significantly more time on the difficult puzzles. Infrequent players, on the other hand, gave up much faster and showed less interest in mastering the challenging task. Overall, the researchers reported, gamers showed much higher *persistence* and *perseverance*. They showed a habitual thirst for challenge and a striving to succeed even under difficult circumstances.

What accounts for this trait development? Previous studies (not on video games) show that individuals who engage successfully in *any* task requiring high effort will continue to extend high effort in future tasks. Working hard and then achieving our goal primes us—neurologically, with more dopa-mine—to work harder. It's the same biochemical process of addiction, but it's a virtuous rather than a vicious cycle.

As a result of these findings, scientists have proposed that higher dopa-mine levels in the brain may actually be the most important driver of a solid work ethic.[14] This is a crucial rethinking of one of the most universally val-ued and admired character strengths. Work ethic is not a *moral virtue* that can be cultivated simply by wanting to be a better person. It's actually a *bio-chemical condition* that can be fostered, purposefully, through activity that increases dopamine levels in the brain. This explains precisely how chal-lenging video games—like *Re-Mission*—could prime us to tackle other ev-eryday challenges with higher effort and more determination.

Adding further evidence to this theory, another recent study suggests that frequent video gamers' brains are indeed changed in a long-term way by the heightened dopamine response. A team of twenty-five scientists from Germany, Belgium, France, the U.K., and Canada reported together that frequent gamers—defined as people who play at least nine hours a week on average—have higher gray matter volume in the "left ventral striatum," part of the reward-processing area of the brain.[15] More gray matter, in general, means that the brain is bigger and more powerful. More gray matter in the left ventral striatum, in particular, means you have more cognitive resources to devote to motivation, determination, optimism, and learning.

It's possible that people who are naturally more motivated by challenge and who are better learners are more attracted to video games—rather than video games increasing these strengths over time. However, most neurosci-entists who study games believe this is *not* the case. They attribute differ-ences between the brains of frequent and infrequent game players to *neuroplasticity*, or the ability of the brain to rewire itself and strengthen different regions based on frequent activity.[16] Daphne Bavelier, Ph.D., and her cognitive neuroscience laboratory at the University of Geneva, Switzer-land, for example, have been studying the effect of action video games on brain plasticity and learning. After more than a decade of research, she be-lieves that games lead to significant *neural reorganization*, resulting in in-creased attention, faster decision making, and more effective learning.[17]

Indeed, Dr. Bavelier has identified video games as potentially the single most effective intervention for increasing neuroplasticity in adults.[18]

Judy Willis, M.D., is another neuroscientist who believes in the power of games to rewire players' brains for the better. A former chief resident at UCLA's neurology clinic, she spent fifteen years seeing patients in her own pediatric neurology practice. Today she works with schools and educators to teach cognitive habits that lead to lifelong success and psychological well-being. Her primary strategy: provide students with daily experiences of self-efficacy, including frequent video game play.

"Neurons that fire together, wire together," she likes to say, quoting one of the basic principles of neuroscience.[19] The more you repeat a thought pattern, the stronger the neural networks that drive it become. And the stronger the neural networks, the more likely you are to repeat that thought pattern in the future. The pattern becomes easier to access, with neurons firing up to one hundred times faster—and because the patterns are repeated so often, the neural networks are less vulnerable to cognitive decline over time.

This means that the self-efficacy we experience when we play games frequently is not just a belief, according to Dr. Willis. It's a way of thinking that is *hardwired into the brain*—a result of repeated activation of specific neurological circuits that train the brain to be motivated by challenge, rewarded by feedback, and more resilient in the face of temporary failure. "This is why nothing builds a success mindset faster or more effectively than video games," Dr. Willis told me. "When you have constant opportunities to try different strategies and get feedback, you get more frequent and more intense bursts of dopamine. Not only do you get minute-to-minute pleasure, but the mindset starts changing in long-term ways. Your brain starts looking at things that weren't achievable before and starts to think they might be achievable with a little effort. It expects to learn and improve and eventually succeed, because that's what it's used to doing.

"When you're constantly experiencing successful goal achievement," she explains, "your brain's cost-benefit analysis changes entirely. You can overrule your brain's default mode that wants you to avoid wasting energy on difficult tasks or challenging goals. Your brain adapts to seek out more challenge, to be less afraid of failure, and to be more resilient in the face of setbacks."

. . .

ifteen years' worth of neuroscience research on games adds up to one big idea: if you want to change your brain for the better—to turn motivation into self-efficacy, to learn faster, and to cultivate more resilience—play more games. Or at the very least, provoke your brain with challenging learning opportunities in the same ways that good games do.

Here is one of Dr. Willis's favorite ways to spike dopamine in the brain. It's not a game, but it's very gameful. She uses this simple technique with patients and clients to help them recover from mental burnout. And it's your next quest!

---

### QUEST 12: Make a Prediction

**What to do:** Make a prediction about something—*anything*—that you can personally verify the outcome of sometime in the next twenty-four hours.

It can be big or small, silly or serious. Just make a prediction—and see if you're right!

**Examples:** Here are some things SuperBetter players have made predictions about.

- The winner of a sporting event
- "The exact amount of money in my bank account at this moment, down to the penny"
- "The number of emails I'll receive in the next hour"
- "What mood I'll be in this exact time tomorrow"
- "Whose snoring will wake me first tonight: husband versus dog. I predict husband!"
- "What song my favorite band will play first at their concert"

- "What score, on a scale from 1 to 10, my best friend will rate the movie we're watching together"
- "How fast I can put the dishes away without breaking anything. Prediction: two minutes, fifteen seconds!"
- "How many hugs I will get from former teachers, coaches, and friends in the next twenty-four hours. I'm visiting my home-town, from thirty years and many miles away, so I think it will be a very high number!"

**Why it works:** Making a prediction is one of the most reliable and efficient ways to prime the reward circuitry of the brain. "Every pre-diction you make triggers an increase in attention and dopamine," says Dr. Willis. That's because every time you make a prediction, two highly rewarding outcomes are possible. You might be right—which will feel good! *Or*, you might be wrong—which will give you informa-tion that will help you make a better prediction next time. Surpris-ingly, this will also feel good—because your brain loves learning. In fact, "the dopamine boost is often greater when you learn some-thing new and useful than when you succeed," Dr. Willis says.

Dozens of scientific studies back up this claim. Gamers get a do-pamine hit even during failure and losses—as long as they have a chance to try again.[20]

So go ahead and make a prediction—any prediction! Whether you're right or wrong, you'll get a dopamine boost. It's a win-win game. Use this trick whenever you're bored, frustrated, or stressed. It's a quick and natural way to provoke curiosity and attention, while strengthening the neural circuitry that promotes determination, ambition, and perseverance. (And if you're with someone who is bored, frustrated, or stressed, ask *them* to make a prediction!)

*Tip:* For an extra dopamine boost, try to get someone else to make a *competing* prediction. The added social stakes will increase your anticipation of a potential reward.

## A SuperBetter Story: The Job Seeker

A few weeks ago I heard from my good friend Calvin. He's thirty-five years old, married, and a computer scientist with a Ph.D. We've known each other since graduate school at UC Berkeley. Over the past decade, Calvin has worked both in the tech industry and in university research labs. Recently, he decided to take a leap of faith and look for a full-time academic position.

"Career adventures are coming fast and frequent at this point," he wrote me in an email. "I've landed interviews at five universities." He sounded upbeat in the letter, but he admitted to being pretty stressed out about one of his interviews at a top research university.

"A friend of mine who interviewed there last year said he was practically crying by the end of the meeting. Apparently, this one professor had started the interview by telling my friend that his dissertation work was complete crap, and that the university had made a huge mistake in inviting him to interview." Not the most encouraging story, considering that Calvin was slated to meet with the same professor!

Job interviews are stressful even in the best circumstances, but when Calvin got to campus for the two-day interview, the tension only increased. "The first few people I met with all warned me about my upcoming interview with this same professor, telling me how notoriously vicious he is with junior researchers. Everyone had a war story about meeting with him. Even the chair of the hiring committee said they had second thoughts about including him on my schedule.

"Needless to say, the night before that day I was pretty nervous. I had to get a grip. I thought 'How can I make this meeting into a game, rather than into something I'm dreading?' So I decided to create a bingo game. I tried to predict the worst possible things he could say to me, whatever would upset me most. I wrote them down, plus the 'free square' in the middle. I folded that bingo card and put it in my pocket when I went in for the interview."

Calvin sent me a photo of the card so I could see his gameful solution for myself. His custom bingo squares included the kinds of moments that would make any interviewee cringe: "Personal attack/critique," "Tests my knowledge/skills," "Points out flaw/error/mistake in my work," "Cites references I'm not familiar with," "Says my work is derivative, obvious," "Dismisses it as not important," "Accuses me of being unprincipled."

And did it help? Unequivocally, yes. "Turns out, he did say lots of those negative things to me, but it didn't bother me at all," Calvin said. "Every time he tried to make me feel small, I got to mentally check off a bingo square. It brought a lot of humor to a really stressful situation."

Calvin won twice. First, he scored a bingo. "The professor got the whole middle horizontal row," he told me. "He really was as bad as everyone said!" But later Calvin scored the real victory: he got a job offer from the university. Ultimately, he decided to take a job somewhere else, but having multiple offers helped him negotiate the best deal.

I'm so impressed by Calvin's clever solution to a nerve-racking situation. He might not have been intentionally hacking into his dopamine pathway, but he was definitely giving himself a dopamine boost every time he filled in a bingo square. And because the mere act of *making* a prediction heightens attention and boosts dopamine, just creating the bingo board put Calvin in a much more determined and optimistic state of mind.

"Worst-case-scenario bingo" may not be a game you look forward to playing—because really, who wants to be in a stressful or unpleasant situation? But if you do need to tap into your determination and grit, this gameful intervention is a brilliant way to prepare your brain for resilience and success. While you're at it, why not create a "best-case-scenario" bingo card for your next big day? Think of all the good things that could happen to you on a trip, or at a big work event, or on a special occasion. After all, you can benefit from determination and optimism on fun days just as much as on tough ones!

Now you know: game play supercharges self-efficacy, work ethic, and determination. So what kinds of real-life goals can you accomplish with these gameful strengths?

One leading-edge research lab at Stanford University has dedicated the past ten years to investigating this question. The Virtual Human Interaction Lab (VHIL), founded and directed by cognitive psychologist Dr. Jeremy Bailenson, specializes in research on how virtual reality experiences can change our real-life attitudes and behaviors for the better. Through dozens of ingenious experiments, they've discovered that just a few minutes in the right virtual environment can increase our willpower and compassion, changing how we think and act for the next twenty-four hours or even the next week.

Here are a few of their most intriguing findings.

Want to exercise more, but can't quite seem to summon up the willpower? There may be a gameful way to trick your brain into moving your body. It's called *vicarious exercise*. All you have to do is watch a video game doppelgänger, or an avatar designed to look just like you, exercising in the virtual world.

It's true. You can build *exercise-related self-efficacy* without doing a single push-up or taking a single step. You just need to spend a few minutes watching your avatar do all the hard work.

In a study conducted by the VHIL, researchers found that participants who watched their virtual doppelgängers running on a treadmill reported feeling significantly higher confidence that they could exercise effectively. More important, after they left the lab, they exercised a *full hour more* than participants who watched their virtual doppelgänger stand around doing nothing. Over the next twenty-four hours, the participants with running avatars walked more city blocks, climbed more stairs, and spent more time in the gym.[21]

However, this technique worked only when the avatars were specially created to look like the participants. Watching a generic male or female avatar exercise had zero effect on participants' real-life movement.

Can seeing a virtual version of yourself succeed trick your brain into believing you've actually done it yourself? This study suggests it can, and that it's an effective shortcut to boost self-efficacy. The Stanford researchers theorize that the virtual doppelgängers create a "mirror neuron effect."[22] (As you'll recall from Chapter 2, our mirror neurons mimic the neural activity of people around us, particularly when we are doing the same activity or feel closely connected to them.) Because participants felt more closely connected to avatars that looked just like them, the mirror neuron effect was stronger. It's quite an astonishing finding—we can create mirror neurons not just with other people but with virtual people as well!

On the heels of this promising study, the same lab decided to try to create an even more effective exercise booster. They kept the virtual doppelgängers and added a new, interactive element. This time participants were asked to lift weights while observing their avatars. Every time they completed a successful lift in real life, their virtual avatar changed shape, appearing more muscular and fit. During mandated breaks in the participants' exercise, however, the avatars changed shape again, becoming heavier and flabbier.

After just a few minutes of this interactive workout, participants were invited to stay for up to thirty minutes and continue their workout.

Compared with a group that lifted weights without a virtual doppelgänger, they completed *ten times* as many exercises. Imagine if you could motivate yourself to do ten times as many push-ups, or climb ten times as many steps, every time you exercised—just by spending a few minutes working out with a virtual version of yourself!

Like many of the other studies we've looked at in this chapter, dopamine bursts seem to be a major factor in creating this positive change. Dr. Bailenson calls it the "instant gratification" of immediate virtual weight loss. "Working out with a virtual doppelgänger means you can see physical rewards of exercise right away," he says, "which is something that doesn't typically happen in the real world. In the real world, it takes days or weeks to notice any positive physical changes." But game avatars that respond to physical activity right away can trigger dopamine boosts that trick the brain into feeling rewarded immediately. This process enables players to build self-efficacy much more quickly than in normal life. And greater self-efficacy, even if it's from a virtual experience, leads to more real-world exercise, right away.

To confirm this surprising phenomenon, the Stanford researchers have conducted five different studies to date. They all show the same thing: vicarious exercise and vicarious weight loss significantly increase self-efficacy, and as a result, real-world exercise.[23]

So what does this mean for you, today? The VHIL virtual doppelgängers aren't available to the public yet—although undoubtedly, vicarious exercise technology will become widespread in the future. In the meantime, this research should be a powerful reminder that self-efficacy, not motivation, is the key to building up your willpower and determination to do things that are difficult. If you need to boost your own self-efficacy without the help of virtual reality, focus on specific skills and abilities that you can increase, even if it's only the tiniest bit each day. Run for one minute longer. Do one more push-up. Walk one more block. The key is to commit to a specific improvement at the start of each workout. Every time you set a slightly more challenging goal and successfully achieve it, you'll activate the neural networks that support increased self-efficacy and determination.

If you want the full avatar experience, however, a simpler version of vicarious exercise may be available to you today. Meredith, forty, an elementary school teacher in Phoenix, Arizona, discovered this trick by accident when she started playing the computer game *The Sims*, a kind of computerized dollhouse in which you create custom avatars and help them achieve their career and family goals. "Not sure what to make of this," she wrote me recently, "but my Sim seems to have inspired me to exercise and talk to my neighbors more." It turns out that Meredith had created a *Sim* version of herself—same hair color, eye color, height, weight, and even fashion sense. And watching her virtual doppelgänger work out and socialize in the computer game triggered the motivation and self-efficacy to do it herself. "The instant results that my Sim gets when she works out or chats with neighbors is so satisfying!" she told me. "Seeing the immediate reward the avatar gets makes it look so easy."

As in Dr. Bailenson's lab, the instant gratification of virtual feedback seems to have triggered real-world self-confidence in Meredith. It also triggered a helpful awareness of priorities. "I think it's the panel that shows the Sims' needs that really inspired me," she said, referring to the way *Sims* games keep score by reminding you that your Sim characters need things like exercise and social activity to be happy and healthy. "I started thinking of what my own panel would be like," Meredith told me. "I realized I needed to spend more time doing the things that make me feel good. Funny how a computer game can teach you something important about yourself!"

We've looked so far in this chapter at heroic qualities like determination, grit, and perseverance. These character strengths help you overcome the kind of tough obstacles and achieve epic goals that can make you an inspiration to others. But there's another kind of heroic quality that increased self-efficacy can provoke: *altruistic* qualities.

In another series of experiments at Dr. Bailenson's Stanford University lab, participants were invited to learn how to "fly like Superman," using a special virtual reality flying simulator.[24] Players would fly through a city landscape, controlling their flight path through their own physical gestures. To give you an idea of what it might feel like to interact with this kind of

simulator, here are the game play instructions given to the study participants:

> Lift your hands over your head to take off. To land, drop your hands to
> your side. Where you point your hands is where you will fly. To move
> faster, move your hands together. To fly slower move your hands apart.

Players were instructed to search the city streets for a crying child. That
child, they were told, is diabetic and needs *you* to deliver insulin to save
his life.

The physicality of the experience was an essential component of this
game's design, for two reasons. First, the researchers wanted to give participants the chance to learn a new and unfamiliar skill. By following the instructions and successfully learning how to control the simulator, players
would experience a burst of self-efficacy. Second, the researchers wanted to
evoke classic mental associations with superhero characters. The ability to
fly through the air using only your own power evokes, for most people, the
idea of a benevolent superhero like Superman. The researchers' hypothesis
was that by having a firsthand experience of effectively developing a superpower usually associated with superheroes, participants would be more
likely to behave heroically toward others in everyday life.

To test this hypothesis, another set of participants were invited to play the
same game, but with a different set of rules. They were told that this game
would take them on a *helicopter ride* through the city. Instead of directly controlling their own flight, they passively experienced a tour of the same streets.
Like the other participants, however, they were instructed to look for a crying
child, so they could land the helicopter and deliver life-saving medicine.

All participants were allowed to keep playing until they successfully
completed their rescue mission. Then—and here comes the clever part of the
experiment's design—the researchers staged a fake accident, which happened after the participants had finished playing the game but before they
left the lab. Would they notice a person in need—a young woman who suffered a spill—and would they come to her rescue?

It turned out that participants who controlled their own flight in the simulator jumped up to help *three times* faster, and helped for *twice* as long, as participants who simply wore the same virtual reality headset and enjoyed a passive helicopter ride through the city landscape. In fact, *every single person* who learned how to fly helped the struggling person, whereas a full 20 percent of the helicopter passengers completely ignored her.

The important take-away from this study is that players who had direct control over their rescue mission were significantly more inspired to help others. Even though all the participants received the same prosocial "help others" messaging, self-efficacy was ultimately a much more powerful boost of altruistic behavior.

This finding was confirmed in another twist of science, when the Stanford researchers invited yet another group of participants to use the flight simulator *without* a rescue mission. This group of players learned how to "fly" but were not asked to find a crying child or deliver life-saving medication. This nonrescue group, despite not receiving any "help others" messaging, also was quicker to jump to the rescue and spent more time helping than were the helicopter passengers with a rescue mission. The direct experience of a superpower was enough to change their real-life behavior, even without the subconscious priming of a fictional rescue mission.

The superhero *story*, it turns out, doesn't matter as much as the superempowering experience of having full control over a successful outcome. If you want to tap into *your* own heroic nature, give yourself the chance to master new skills and experience success—whether it's in a game or a sport, in the kitchen or the garage. Whenever you feel strong and capable, you're more likely to use those strengths and capabilities to help others.

Superpower simulators aren't the only gameful way to unleash your heroic altruism. Here's a quest inspired by one of my favorite scientific papers from the past decade, written by researchers at MIT's Sloan School of Management and New York University's Stern School of Business, and conducted with Princeton University psychologists. The paper, titled "From Student to Superhero," documents a simple psychological trick you can use anytime, anywhere, to increase your own real-life heroic behavior.

## QUEST 13: The Superhero Mirror

Your quest instructions come straight from a psychology lab at Princeton University:

"For this task we would like you to describe the characteristics of a superhero. Think of a superhero, and list the behaviors, values, lifestyle, and appearance associated with these characters."[25]

Go ahead and do this now.

**What to do:** Take at least two full minutes to list everything you can think of that describes a generic superhero: what motivates them, how they treat others, what they do in the face of danger—you get the idea.

You don't need to be a comic book genius to complete this quest, just do your best! And remember, don't describe any superhero in particular. Instead, **try to list characteristics that describe many, if not most, superheroes.**

For the biggest impact, don't just think of your answer. **Write it down,** or record it into your phone. At the very least, talk out loud to yourself—it will help you focus and fully lock in the benefits of this quest.

**Why it works:** Just thinking about what it takes to be a superhero makes you more likely to act like one in the future. You're more likely to volunteer to help others and donate your time to a worthy cause.

Here's the data on this quest: the MIT and NYU researchers found that study participants who completed the same quest *you* just completed were far more altruistic afterward. When asked to sign up to tutor local at-risk youth, twice as many participants who thought about superheroes volunteered as participants who did *not* think about superheroes (51 percent compared with 24 percent). Among those who volunteered, the superhero group volunteered twice as many hours (an hour a week versus half an hour a week, on average). Most surprisingly, a full three months later, the superhero participants were *four times* as likely to actually show up for a volunteering session.

How could just a couple minutes' worth of reflection trigger significant behavior change over a three-month period? Well, psychologists know from numerous studies that when we're asked to think about the positive traits of a particular social group (such as the selfless, fearless behavior of superheroes), we invariably compare ourselves to the admirable group—and we usually start by looking for similarities. We subconsciously measure ourselves against their values and virtues—and because almost everyone wants to live up to highly admired social standards, we naturally look for ways to fit the bill. It's like holding up a mirror that reflects back only the best parts.

It's a bit of a "positive bias"—we all want to think that we're amazing, wonderful people, even if we're not. But it's still a neat and useful psychological trick. Take advantage of your own bias by spending a few minutes thinking about the values and virtues of a group of people you admire—whether they're professional athletes, firefighters, emergency room nurses, teachers, activists, CEOs, or artists. Every time you do just that, you become twice as likely to jump at the chance to be like these heroes when the opportunity arises.

**One important caveat:** This quest seems to work only when you think about an entire group of heroes, not one in particular. If you single out one particularly amazing person, you are more likely to

compare yourself *unfavorably* with his or her virtues or achievements. That's because, psychologists have found, we tend to look
for similarities between ourselves and admirable groups, but we
tend to notice *differences* between ourselves and admirable *individuals*. Thinking about these differences can actually decrease your
motivation and self-efficacy! So be sure to focus on general qualities of groups you admire and not on individual heroes.

*Tip:* To really benefit from this quest, you should look for an opportunity *right now* to be more like your heroes (or superheroes,
whoever inspires you most!). If you make a mental commitment to
do something concrete while the positive social standard is still at
the top of your mind, you're more likely to follow through in the future. Researchers describe this as "committing yourself to future
behavior while a temporary goal is more salient," or top-of-mind. If
you're thinking about heroes or superheroes right now, you're more
motivated to adopt an altruistic goal. Adopting that goal *right now*
makes it much easier for you to make the time and energy to
achieve it, whether it's tomorrow, next week, or even months from
now. So make a tiny commitment right now to do some good in the
world, and you'll fully reap all the benefits of this quest.

The science of games reveals that we have more power to motivate and
improve ourselves than we realize—to make positive change, to adopt new
habits, to be better people, to do what is otherwise hard. Games show us
how to strive for epic goals that inspire us—and in doing so, they help us
build the strengths that inspire others.

# MISSION COMPLETE

### *Skills Unlocked: How to Build Heroic*
### *Character Strengths*

- If you want to make a change for the better or achieve a tough goal, don't worry about motivation. Instead, focus on increasing your self-efficacy: confidence in your ability to solve your own problems and achieve your goals.

- The fastest and most reliable way to increase your self-efficacy is to learn how to play a new game. Any kind of game will do, because all games require you to learn new skills and tackle tough goals.

- The level of dopamine in your brain influences your ability to build self-efficacy. The more you have, the more determined you feel, and the less likely you are to give up. You'll learn faster, too—because high dopamine levels improve your attention and help you process feedback more effectively. Keep in mind that video games have been shown to boost dopamine levels as much as intravenous amphetamines.

- Whenever you want to boost your dopamine levels, play a game—or make a prediction. Predictions prime your brain to pay closer attention and to anticipate a reward. (Playing "worst-case scenario bingo" is an excellent way to combine these two techniques!)

- You can also build self-efficacy vicariously by watching an avatar that looks like you accomplish feats in a virtual world.

- Whenever possible, customize video game avatars to look like you. Every time your avatar does something awesome, you'll get a vicarious boost to your willpower and determination.

- Remember, self-efficacy doesn't just help you. It can inspire you to help others. The more powerful you feel, the more likely you are to rise to the heroic occasion. So the next time *you* feel superpowerful, take a moment to ask yourself how you can use your powers for good.

# 4

## You Can Make the Leap from Games to Gameful

### Your Mission

Smash the boundaries that keep your gameful strengths separate from your real life.

So far we've looked at findings from more than one hundred scientific studies that reveal the natural gameful abilities we all possess: to control our attention, thoughts, and feelings; to connect and bond with virtually anyone; and to supercharge our willpower and determination.

But not everyone who plays games will succeed in translating these strengths from games to daily life. In fact, many gamers seem to suffer—academically, socially, or in their physical and mental health—as a result of excessive play, leading many to worry about "video game addiction." How is it possible that some frequent game players benefit from play while others struggle?

It's a paradox I've spent years researching, and I'm not the only one. Consider the following headlines. These are all actual results from peer-reviewed research on the impact of playing video games.

"Study Shows Videogames Linked to Depression and Lower Life
Satisfaction"[1]

"Study Shows Frequent Gamers Experience Greater Levels of Happiness
and Life Satisfaction"[2]

"Gaming Linked to Lower Grades, More Drug Use in Teenagers and College Students"[3]

"Video Game Play Linked to Higher Grades, Less Drug Use in High
School and College Students"[4]

"Videogames Linked to Poor Relationships with Friends, Family"[5]

"Videogames Improve Family Relationships, Particularly Between Fathers and Daughters"[6]

It's maddening, isn't it? I've read literally hundreds of scientific papers on
this topic, and many of them convincingly argue that playing games will
make you more depressed, anxious, and socially isolated. But many more
just as convincingly argue that playing games frequently will make you happier, healthier, and more ambitious, with stronger social support to boot.

It's not that either group of researchers is wrong. They're both right.

When you examine all the factors behind the diverging results, as I have,
again and again you'll come across one reason why only *some* gamers learn
how to effectively apply these strengths in real-world contexts, such as work,
school, health, or family. So what makes the difference?

It's not, surprisingly, a matter of which games you play, or how much
time you spend playing them. Instead, it depends entirely on *why* you play
games.

*Do you play to escape your real life, or do you play to make your real life
better?*

(If you're not sure which *you* do, keep reading—this chapter will help you
figure it out.)

If you typically play games to escape your real life—that is, to ignore your
problems, to block unpleasant emotions, or to avoid confronting stressful
situations—you will have a very difficult time translating your game skills to

real life. An escapist approach to play really does increase depression, worsen social isolation, and make you *less* likely to achieve real-life goals.[7] That's because the more stressful your life gets, the more you play games— and the less time and effort you put into action that could help solve your real-life problems. Your problems therefore get worse, so you spend more time gaming to escape them. It's a vicious cycle.

If you know someone who is addicted to games, they are almost certainly playing with an escapist mindset. In fact, researchers have found that "the use of games to escape daily life" is the number-one factor that predicts excessive or pathological game play. [8]

However, if you *play with purpose*—with a positive goal, such as spending quality time with friends and family, learning something new, or energizing yourself after a long day—you are much more likely to bring gameful ways of thinking and acting into everyday contexts. You're not playing to avoid problems—you're playing to bring benefit. You clearly see the connection between gaming and its impact on your daily life, so you're better able to activate your gameful strengths in real-world contexts.

Researchers have found that this kind of purposeful play builds self-confidence and real-world problem-solving skills.[9] More important, it has the opposite impact of escapism: it helps you be happier, better connected, and more successful in real life.[10]

The difference between struggling and flourishing turns out to be quite simple. You don't have to play different games, or even spend less time playing games, to benefit. *You simply have to stop thinking of games as a distraction from real life and start thinking of them as a source of genuine strength, skills, and power.* It sounds almost too easy to be true, but the research is persuasive. Let's take a look.


Although virtually all gamers experience a deep level of immersion when they play, it turns out there are actually two different kinds of immersion: *self-suppressive* immersion and *self-expansive* immersion.[11]

When you self-suppress, you're trying to *prevent* bad thoughts, feelings, or experiences. You're avoiding rather than seeking.

Almost everyone self-suppresses from time to time, even though it's not the healthiest psychological coping mechanism. Some people self-suppress by reading a juicy novel, or completing a hard workout, or binge-watching a television show. Any escapist activity can be self-suppressive, helping us mentally block out a stressful reality we're trying to avoid.

More dangerously, many people self-suppress with addictive substances, such as alcohol, drugs, or food. This kind of habit can spiral quickly out of control: addiction only adds to the problems and stress you're trying to suppress, so you spend even more time trying to escape them.

Even people who self-suppress rarely, or who try to escape through a relatively benign activity like reading or running, may experience a downside to this coping technique. While self-suppression works in the short term, leading to a *temporary* improvement in mood and well-being, it hurts us in the long term. Every time we succeed in feeling better by escaping reality, we become less likely to face our stress or challenges in the future. We reinforce the idea that the fastest way to feel better is to avoid rather than to engage. Over time self-suppression actually diminishes our sense of self-efficacy and control over our lives. We no longer see ourselves as people who can effectively solve our own problems.[12]

When you self-expand, on the other hand, you're trying to *promote* positive thoughts, feelings, and experiences. You're actively creating something good in your life. You focus on what you want more of, not on what you want less of. Self-expansive activity looks exactly like self-suppressive activity: reading a book for an hour, going for a five-mile run, playing a video game all afternoon. You can't tell whether someone is self-suppressing or self-expanding just by looking at what they're doing, or how much time they spend doing it. You can find out only by asking about their motivation and mindset.

If someone has a *negative* motivation—"I don't want to deal with anyone right now" or "I just don't want to think about it"—they're self-suppressing. If they have a *positive* motivation, like learning something new, improving a skill, achieving a goal, reenergizing, or strengthening a relationship, they're self-expanding.

Self-expansive activity is a healthy and positive coping mechanism, even though it also involves ignoring "real life" for a while. That's because when you self-expand, you build confidence and self-efficacy. You start to look at your favorite leisure activities—whether they're sports, games, hobbies, or other pastimes—as powerful tools you can use to get stronger and improve your life. This self-efficacy spills over into daily life. When you feel successful at creating positive thoughts, feelings, and experiences for yourself in your leisure time, you are more likely to put in the effort and creativity to seek positive outcomes in challenging everyday situations.

In some cases, however, the line between self-expansion and self-suppression seems unclear, particularly when it comes to highly immersive video games. In Chapter 1, for example, we looked at the use of virtual reality games like *Snow World* to block pain, or video games like *Tetris* to prevent flashbacks. Are these uses self-suppression? The goal, after all, is to avoid physical pain or mental anguish, which sounds like negative motivation. But ultimately, it boils down to how players think about what they're doing. If they feel *powerful* and *proactive*, then their game play is self-expansive. If they think, *I have the ability to control how I feel right now*, or *I have the power to influence whether I suffer traumatic flashbacks*, they have a *positive* motivation. They are building self-efficacy. But if they are simply seeking refuge—*I can't deal, this game is my only escape*—they are indeed self-suppressing. By playing with this self-suppressive mindset, they diminish their own capacity to solve problems and improve their lives.

In edge cases like this, players must understand that they are using games to tap into their own strengths, not to avoid their problems. The behavior may be the same, but the mindset is different—and the mindset is what determines whether gameful strengths will be used effectively not only in play but in all of daily life.

So what exactly do you have to do to move from a self-suppressive mindset to a self-expansive mindset? It's quite easy—you simply need to identify the benefits you seek from games, then consciously embrace play habits that give you what you seek. This purposeful approach to play is all it takes for your gameful strengths to flourish.

If your favorite games are sports or puzzles, or board or card games, you probably have some benefits in mind already. Playing sports not only improves physical health but also builds character and contributes to emotional well-being. Puzzles are widely considered to be a good way to stay cognitively sharp as we age. Board and card games are often praised for promoting family together time, or as a way to enjoy face-to-face interaction with friends. Basically, if your favorite kind of game is anything *but* a digital game, you likely can already identify some benefits, because nondigital games are for the most part accepted by society as a healthy and positive activity.

However, even if you derive great pleasure from playing your favorite digital games, you may not have a very good idea of how exactly they are building up your real-life strengths (beyond what you've learned in the first three chapters of this book, that is). That's because for the past three decades, discussion about video games has mostly focused on their potential harms rather than their potential benefits.

Fortunately, in 2014, the scientific journal *American Psychologist* published an extensive analysis of "The Benefits of Playing Video Games."[13] This paper summarizes the findings from seventy other scientific studies, including many of the studies you have already read about in this book.

So far, in our discussion of the benefits of playing video games, we've focused on the ones that directly contribute to your ability to be stronger and more successful in the face of stress and challenge. But there are many others. Knowing these additional benefits can help you play with greater purpose. So here they are for your consideration. Which of these benefits ring true to your own experience? (If you're not a frequent game player, you can share this list with any passionate gamers in your life and see which ring true for them.)

## COGNITIVE BENEFITS

Games can make you smarter, particularly fast-paced action and racing video games like *Call of Duty, Forza,* and *Grand Theft Auto*. Individuals who frequently play action video games enjoy the following cognitive benefits:

- Improved visual attention and spatial intelligence skills, which predict higher achievement in science, technology, engineering, and mathematics
- Faster and more accurate decision making in high-stress, time-sensitive contexts
- Improved ability to track multiple streams of information simultaneously—up to three times as much information as an infrequent game player
- More efficient neural processing generally—the brain uses fewer resources during difficult tasks[14]

Strategic games, such as *StarCraft, Mass Effect,* and *Final Fantasy,* also improve concrete problem-solving skills that predict academic success and higher achievement in daily life. These benefits include:

- More effective information gathering
- Faster and more accurate evaluation of options
- Stronger ability to formulate and follow strategic plans
- Greater flexibility in generating alternative strategies or goals[15]

Finally, all genres of video games have been linked to greater creativity. Kids who spend more time playing games—including games with violent content—score higher on tests of creativity that involve storytelling, drawing, and problem solving.[16]

It's worth noting that significant scientific evidence for the cognitive benefits of traditional, entertainment-focused video games is considerably greater than that for so-called brain-training games that are marketed specifically as improving cognitive function. In fact, in 2014, seventy neuroscientists cosigned a public statement calling attention to the fact that in the peer-reviewed scientific literature, brain-training games—the best-known example being Lumosity games—have *not* been found to produce long-term cognitive benefits.[17] More important perhaps, studies that have directly compared the benefits of mainstream video games like the sci-fi puzzler *Portal* and the fantasy role-playing game *World of Warcraft* to brain-training games have found that the traditional video games improve cognitive performance significantly more than the brain trainers.[18] The researchers I've talked to about these results suggest a simple explanation: traditional video games are more complex and harder to master, and they require that the player learn a wider and more challenging range of skills and abilities. Therefore, if you are particularly interested in cognitive benefits, I encourage you to play ordinary video games that are challenging and new to you, and not to spend your limited game play hours on simple "brain trainers."

# EMOTIONAL BENEFITS

Playing video games helps change your mood and improve your emotional state, particularly puzzle games such as *Angry Birds* and *Bejeweled* and platform games such as *Super Mario*. Playing your favorite games gives you the power to

- Improve mood immediately
- Ward off anxiety
- Experience more frequent positive emotions, such as delight, curiosity, surprise, pride, wonder, and contentment[19]

Video games also help you learn to manage difficult emotions. This is especially true of very challenging, scary, or emotionally intense games, such as *BioShock, Resident Evil,* and *Silent Hill.* Frequent players of these games become

- Better able to deal with frustration and anxiety in high-pressure situations
- More skillful at controlling extreme emotions like fear and anger[20]

Gamers even develop some unusual emotional "superpowers." Perhaps the most surprising power has to do with dreaming. People who frequently play first-person games (which graphically show you the game world from the point of view of the hero, like *Minecraft*, *Halo*, and *Portal*) develop two rather amazing skills:

- They can halt nightmares in their tracks, controlling themselves in their dreams the way they control a character in a video game.
- They experience more frequent "lucid dreaming," or dreams in which they realize they're dreaming and purposefully enjoy the dream—for example, the opportunity to fly.[21]

# SOCIAL BENEFITS

Multiplayer and massively multiplayer video games can teach important social skills, beyond the ally-building skills we examined in Chapter 2. People who frequently play team-based games, such as *Call of Duty*, *League of Legends*, and *Team Fortress*, show

- Stronger cooperative mindsets in daily life
- Improved communication and collaboration skills [22]

Meanwhile, people who frequently play games that require them to organize groups and lead others in like-minded efforts, such as *Guild Wars* and *World of Warcraft*, are rated by others as

- Better leaders
- More effective motivators

They are also more likely to engage in civic behavior, such as volunteering and raising money for charity.[23]

. . .

These are just a few of the benefits that you can purposefully reap by playing games. The key to adopting a self-expansive mindset is to be perfectly clear on why you play. What are you seeking, and how does it benefit you in daily life?

This question has many good answers—answers that are potentially as unique and varied as the 1.23 billion people on this planet who play video games for at least one hour per day. What's *your* answer?

Here's a quest to help you find out. It's designed specifically for people who frequently play games (of any kind, including sports, board games, and card games). However, if you're not a frequent game player, you can replace "games" with any kind of "hard fun"—that is, any favorite hobby or pastime that regularly challenges you to learn and improve. If you don't have any hard fun hobbies yet, you can skip this quest for now.

*If you have a gamer in your life who you worry may be playing excessively, use this quest to start a conversation with them about how to play with purpose. It's the first and most important step to getting a negative gaming habit under control.*

## QUEST 14: Play with Purpose

Playing with greater purpose is easy. Just follow this **simple three-step method**.

1. **Choose a game.** Name a game that you often play.
2. **Find the benefit.** What's *one* benefit you think you get from playing this game? It might be a skill or talent you build, or a positive change in how you feel, think, or interact with others. (For ideas, review the benefits listed in this chapter!)
3. **Connect it to a purpose.** What real-life goal, or what situation

in daily life, could this benefit help you deal with more effectively?

It may feel awkward at first to answer these questions, especially if you're used to thinking of games as just "fun" or a waste of time. But give it a shot!

**Examples:** For inspiration, here are some SuperBetter players' responses to this quest:

## Nancy, 64, Colleyville, Texas

*The game: Criminal Case* on Facebook.

*The benefit:* "I like the feeling of making progress and solving the crimes. I feel mentally quite sharp!"

*The purpose:* "I can have more confidence in my memory, which puts me in a better mood and helps me feel less shy in social settings."

## Jacob, 23, Pittsburgh

*The game:* "I usually play *FIFA* [a soccer video game] after work."

*The benefit:* "I have more energy after I play. It's like a jolt to my system."

*The purpose:* "After about thirty or forty minutes of playing, I can 'switch gears' and be better company for my girlfriend. She gets the best of me instead of the worst of me."

*Merilee, 38, Indianapolis*

*The game:* "I play *Just Dance* on the Wii with my kids."
*The benefit:* "I'm getting exercise on days that I don't have any free time for myself."
*The purpose:* "I'm staying fit even when I'm busy, plus I'm helping my whole family be physically active, which is important to me."

*Joshua, 13, Edmonton, Alberta, Canada*

*The game:* "My favorite game is *Minecraft*."
*The benefit:* "I get to be creative. I can make whatever I can imagine!"
*The purpose:* "When I have to be creative for school projects, I never draw a blank. I'm good at thinking up new things to make because I practice all the time in *Minecraft*."

Now it's your turn. Choose a game, find the benefit, and connect it to a purpose.

**Quest complete:** Were you able to complete the three steps? If so, well done. You're starting to realize the powerful strengths and skills you're building when you play—and knowing your strengths is the first and most important step toward using them in daily life.

The more you play with purpose, the more resilience you'll have against all kinds of self-suppression in the future. Like all cognitive habits, self-suppression can become hardwired into your brain. Each time you self-suppress, you strengthen the neural networks that urge you to escape again in the future.

Learning to keep this cognitive habit in check is important, because self-suppression is closely related to another psychological behavior that can wreak even more havoc on your life: *experiential avoidance*. Also sometimes referred to as *experiential escape*, it's an unwillingness to accept or directly deal with distressing thoughts or emotions, coupled with attempts to escape or avoid anything that might trigger distressing thoughts and emotions in the future.[24]

Here are some examples of experiential avoidance: A young woman experiences anxiety on a turbulent flight; for years afterward, she avoids taking long-distance trips and goes to extreme lengths to avoid flying. A son feels guilty whenever he visits his aging mother in her assisted living apartment, so he stops visiting her. In both of these cases, instead of learning to manage their anxiety or discomfort, the person simply tries to avoid its trigger. The more they try to escape potential distress, the more positive experiences and relationships they are likely to miss out on in the future.

This kind of escapist mindset can lead to profound depression, social isolation, and even self-harm. At the very least, being unwilling to do things that might potentially trigger a negative thought or feeling severely restricts and limits your goals, ambitions, and life experiences.

Experiential avoidance is something you'll learn more about in Chapter 7, when we talk about "bad guys" and how confronting them regularly can make you stronger and braver. For now, it's enough to know that playing with purpose will help you develop the psychological habits necessary to avoid escapism of any kind and to live with greater purpose, even in the face of risk, adversity, or challenge.

There's one more important thing to understand about self-suppression or escapist game play: it often reaches a tipping point. Eventually, beyond a certain limit, avoiding the reported negative consequences of excessive video game play, such as more depression and anxiety, lower grades, and social isolation, becomes very difficult.

What is the tipping point? I've spent five years investigating this issue, looking at everything from military studies of how much time troops spend playing video games, to player surveys of when their play starts to feel detrimental to their health and happiness. Here's what I've found, again and again: at around twenty-one hours a week of digital game play, things start to go south. *Twenty-one hours a week is the tipping point.*[25]

People who play video games three or fewer hours per day tend to reap the benefits of play. They report having a good balance between their game pursuits and their real-world goals. However, for both children and adults, playing *more* than three hours a day takes too much time away from non-game work, study, physical activity, and relationships. These areas of life start to suffer, and the vicious cycle of self-suppressive play kicks in.

However, here's the good news: once you get your gaming hours under twenty-one hours per week, the benefits start kicking back in. This is a crucial finding. If you are seeking a practical intervention for yourself or for someone you care about, you don't have to eliminate games or even reduce them severely. You just need to get the total hours per week below twenty-one. For gamers who worry about playing too much, this change in habit is far less intimidating than giving up games completely.

Playing fewer hours per week won't automatically switch someone to a self-expansive mindset. However, it will get them safely under the self-suppressive tipping point—which will ultimately make it much easier to stop escaping and to develop a healthier relationship to immersive play.

◄►

Despite what we now know about the harms of escapism, a whopping 41 percent of frequent game players still say they "play video games to escape daily life."[26] No wonder so many gamers have not yet made the leap from games to gameful! They're convinced that games are just a distraction. This belief is not only incorrect—it's actively harmful. Another study of game addiction found that "playing without a sense of purpose to the activity" was the best predictor of problematic or excessive game play.[27]

Well-meaning parents, spouses, and educators make the situation even worse by admonishing gamers to "put down the game and do something real," or to "stop wasting so much time." This kind of nudging, while well intentioned, conditions gamers to believe that play has no purpose, no meaningful connection to success in daily life. This kind of artificial psychological barrier makes it almost impossible to develop a self-expansive mindset.

If you have an avid game player in your life, the best thing you can do for him or her is to start a conversation about the benefits of play and the psychological strengths of gamers. Instead of asking him or her to put the game away, here are some powerful questions to ask:

- What are you most proud of achieving in this game so far? How did you accomplish that? What strengths or skills did it take?
- What makes this game hard? What are your strategies for winning? How did you come up with those strategies?
- How long have you been trying to complete this level or mission? What keeps you going? Where do you find the motivation to not give up?
- What do you think this game makes you good at? Is there another part of your everyday life where you could apply the same skill or talent to solve a problem?
- I read today that gamers are better at [X] than nongamers. Did you know that? Do you think that's true for you?

And then the most powerful question to ask any gamer (because connecting is always better than escaping):

- Can I play with you?

I've made it my mission to explain the difference between playing to escape and playing with purpose to as many gamers as possible—through my TED talks, my first book, in interviews, on Twitter, and anywhere else I can reach them. Through this work, I've had the opportunity to meet many gamers—and parents and spouses of gamers—who, simply by changing their mindset, have been able to make the leap from just playing games to being gameful in everyday life.

Paul's story, relayed to me by his father, is typical. At fifteen, Paul seemed addicted to online video games. He attended classes at his Chicago-area high school, but he ignored his schoolwork, preferring to play *League of Legends* every night until three in the morning. His physical health deteriorated from lack of sleep. His GPA dropped to a D+ average. His parents tried to intervene, taking away his computer, but it backfired: Paul didn't come home at night and found other places to play. His father told me that the situation seemed hopeless.

Then one day Paul's father showed him a video of one of my talks. They started a conversation about the psychological strengths that gamers develop—strengths that Paul surely had. His dad asked him how he might use these strengths for good in the real world. From this conversation alone, Paul began to make big changes. He didn't stop gaming, but he became curious about what he could achieve with his gameful strengths—particularly his determination, his online research skills, and his team leadership.

Paul started using these strengths to set and achieve real-life academic goals. He took a gameful approach to college applications, approaching each step in the process like a quest. He planned and celebrated every "achievement" he unlocked, from finding five colleges he could picture himself happy at, to collecting three letters of recommendation, to finishing a first draft of a personal essay. He assembled a team of people to help him in his college quests, including his high school counselor, his parents, and graduated classmates. Today, Paul is thriving as an engineering major at Dartmouth—still playing games every night, but not until three in the morning. As his dad proudly told me, "It's all because he finally understood, and because we as his parents finally understood, that his love of games isn't a weakness. It's a source of strength."

Paul's story is a dramatic one. Most people don't need to make such a 180-degree turnaround in their relationship to games. However, almost everyone can benefit from understanding the huge difference it makes in our lives when we stop playing to waste time or forget our troubles and start playing with purpose.

Amelia McDonell-Parry, thirty-six, a writer in New York City, is a great example of how even small efforts to connect game strengths with daily life can lead to big positive changes. Amelia spent the summer of 2013 playing the wildly popular pattern-matching game *Candy Crush Saga* for hours on end. She played so often, in fact, that she regularly experienced visual flashbacks. "I close my eyes," she said, "and I see the *Candy Crush* playing field. *Candy Crush* combos infiltrate my dreams."

Amelia wanted to make those hours count for something more than a high score, so she decided to think about what the game had taught her about her strengths and weaknesses. The most important lesson she learned, she decided, was this: "Don't be afraid to ask others for help." She describes her "aha!" moment:

> Friends who also play *Candy Crush* can give you additional lives and help get you access to the next set of levels, if you can put aside your pride and ask for it. At first this made me uncomfortable. I generally don't like asking others for assistance and prefer to figure things out on my own. Having an issue with an article I'm writing? I troubleshoot it myself. Need to put together a piece of IKEA furniture? I don't care that the directions say it's a two-person job! I'm doing it by my lonesome! Having a really rough day? No, I don't want to talk about it, I just want to cry in a corner by myself, thanks. But sometimes in life, you need a shoulder to cry on, a tidbit of advice, an extra set of hands, or a spare *Candy Crush* life from that Facebook friend you haven't seen or spoken to in ten years. Don't be afraid to ask for any of these things when you need them.[28]

Amelia's breakthrough realization was that she could do in her daily life exactly what she learned to do so effectively in her favorite game. Asking for help and cultivating allies was a skill the game taught her, and it didn't remain limited to the game. This is a quintessential example of making the leap from games to gameful.

The most convincing evidence I've seen that almost anyone can bring gameful strengths to daily life—even individuals who rarely have time to play games!—is the SuperBetter community. There hundreds of thousands of people have learned how to bring their gameful strengths to real-world challenges. They've harnessed their natural gameful abilities—to control their attention, to turn anyone into an ally, and to supercharge their willpower and determination—to bring more motivation, creativity, positive emotion, and social support to their most important real-life goals.

You've completed Part 1 of the book, which means *you* are now ready to make this same leap. You understand the science of games. Now it's time to actively use that science to change your life. It's time to play SuperBetter.

## MISSION COMPLETE

### *Skills Unlocked: How to Make the Leap from Games to Gameful*

- Being gameful means bringing the strengths and skills you develop during game play to real-life goals and challenges.

- Not every gamer is successful in transferring their gameful strengths to daily life. The biggest obstacle? An escapist mindset, or playing games to avoid or forget about real life.

- The solution is to *play with purpose*: identify the benefits you get from games, and seek them out every time you play.

- Make a list of benefits you seek when you play. They might include specific positive emotions you like to feel, cognitive skills you want to develop, or ways you want to strengthen your relationships.

- Identify the skills and abilities that you develop by playing your favorite games, and look for opportunities to use those strengths in everyday life.

- If you have an avid game player in your life, talk to them about their gameful strengths. Share with them some positive research on games. Encourage them to see their love of games as a source of strength, not a weakness.

- To maximize benefits and minimize potential harm, keep video game play—or any escapist activity—to twenty-one hours a week or less. Leave plenty of time to enjoy and take full, real-world advantage of your improved mood, energy levels, relationships, cognitive skills, and self-confidence.

# PART 2

How to Be

Gameful

W e all already have the power within ourselves to think and live gamefully—and to become stronger, happier, and braver as a result. It's just a matter of putting that power into concrete actions, within a gameful structure.

SuperBetter gives you that structure, in seven simple rules to play by whenever you want to tackle a challenge or make a positive change in your life. Those seven rules will make it easier for you to draw on your natural gameful strengths—the four strengths discussed in Part 1:

- Your ability to control your attention and therefore your thoughts and feelings
- Your power to turn anyone into a potential ally and to strengthen your existing relationships
- Your natural capacity to motivate yourself and supercharge your heroic qualities, like willpower, compassion, and determination
- Your ability to play with purpose: to confidently face challenges head-on instead of trying to escape them

The seven SuperBetter rules you'll learn in Part 2 have been validated through scientific study and data analysis. The stories presented come from the more than 400,000 players who have tested the SuperBetter method to improve their own lives. The recommendations are drawn from an analysis of more than 10,000 unique challenges tackled by players—from "finding a new job" to "having a healthy pregnancy" to simply "getting back on my own two feet."

More formally, the University of Pennsylvania conducted a randomized, controlled trial of the SuperBetter system. (The study was led by Ann Marie Roepke, Ph.D. candidate, the researcher who coined the term *post-ecstatic growth*.) The study determined that playing SuperBetter for thirty days significantly reduces symptoms of depression and anxiety and increases optimism, social support, and self-efficacy. The study also found that people who followed the SuperBetter rules for one month were significantly happier and more satisfied with their lives.[1]

Additionally, the Ohio State University Wexner Medical Center conducted a clinical trial of the SuperBetter system to help rehabilitate young patients with concussions.[2] This study, three years in the making, was funded by the National Institutes of Health and was designed to find out the best ways to use the SuperBetter method in a medical setting. Quantitative results from the trial and interviews with patients and doctors strongly support the finding that a gameful approach improves optimism, decreases anxiety and suffering, and strengthens family relationships during rehabilitation and recovery. The study was led by OSU College of Medicine faculty member Lise Worthen-Chaudhari, who has twenty years' experience in rehabilitation research and who says, "I haven't seen anything else that does what SuperBetter does so well, in terms of increasing social support, motivating patients to do things to take care of themselves, and giving caregivers concrete and positive ways to help."

You can learn more about both the Penn study and the OSU trial in "About the Science" at the end of this book.

So how will *you* get superbetter? Just take it one gameful rule at a time. Each chapter in Part 2 includes:

- One rule for how to be gameful
- Stories about successful SuperBetter players and how they followed this rule

- One major scientific principle that supports this rule, with a quick dive into the research
- Practical tips for following the rule in daily life

In Part 2 you will meet many SuperBetter players who in interviews share their stories of growth and triumph. (And I have stories to share, having used the SuperBetter rules not only to heal from a mild traumatic brain injury but also to train for my first marathon and to successfully complete IVF treatment—which resulted earlier this year in the birth of twin daughters!)

SuperBetter players, as you'll see, come from all walks of life and play for all kinds of reasons. They are people like:

Josh,* twenty-five, a computer programmer who suffered with depression for years but never had the courage to tell any of his friends or family about his struggle. In his own words: "SuperBetter helped me finally tell two people what I've been going through, my brother and a close friend. That may not sound like a lot, but for me it's huge. I've never spoken to anyone about my depression. It has been this huge secret, a huge weight. Just being able to finally talk about this alone has helped so much. I would not have had the courage to do this outside the context of this game."

Beckie Tran, thirty-six, who suffered from insomnia for twenty years and cured herself by playing SuperBetter for two months. In her words, she went from being "a chronically sleep-deprived half-person" to being "someone who sleeps like a baby every night—something I thought I would never, ever, *ever* achieve."

Joyce Curwin, sixty-seven, recently retired, who wanted to "find a new spark in life"—and especially "a way to be sexy to my husband again." Playing SuperBetter for thirty days was the perfect springboard for her new life, helping her jump-start a writing practice and leading her husband to remark that she was, indeed, "looking sexier than I have in decades! What could be better than that?"

---

* Some players are happy to have their names and identifying details included in their stories; their full names are listed here. Others have asked to be identified by their first names only, or to have a few identifying details changed.

Kamalah, thirty, a bank officer who had a very difficult time working through her grief over her father's unexpected passing. She followed the seven SuperBetter rules for a month to find a better balance between her sadness and her desire to live joyfully. "I was completely stuck before I tried SuperBetter. It was like I had no control over what I was thinking or feeling. I'm not sure why it worked exactly. I think SuperBetter made it possible for me to start finding the positive again, even though it didn't take the sadness away. It helped me honor my father by living more fully again."

Eric, thirty-eight, a lifelong gamer who started following the SuperBetter rules "to lose weight and get in shape." After losing twenty-five pounds in six weeks of play, he said, "I guess I was surprised to realize that I could do small things every day to make a big difference. I was avoiding even trying because I didn't really think I could do it. By treating it like a game, it wasn't such a big deal, and I didn't have to worry about failing. That's the kicker. I finally stopped worrying about failing, and that's what made me successful."

Sonja Rauwolf, forty-two, a stay-at-home mom who introduced her friend with a new diagnosis of multiple sclerosis to SuperBetter. "I wanted to show her that I was willing to be there for her. I wanted to do something concrete. I feel it has greatly improved our relationship already. By playing together, I now have an easy way to show my support. Even if it only takes me a minute a day to check in on the game, to let her know we're in it together."

Phillip Jeffrey, thirty-one, a photographer and cancer patient who is living with a rare, advanced blood cancer. He plays SuperBetter as "Phillip the Creative Cancer Fighter." Although this fatal disease has no known cure, Phillip decided to use the SuperBetter rules to help get the most out of each day and to combat the draining side effects of chemotherapy. He says, "Playing SuperBetter has been one of the most positive experiences of my life. It gives me a sense of purpose and control over how I feel. Even on bad days, I am committed to completing at least one quest. I get out of bed every single day because of this game. It has added so much meaning to my life, playing this game, and reminding myself that even with cancer, I can be creative, I can be accomplished." Three years later he has experienced several periods of remission and is still completing quests.

Marilyn, fifty-four, a middle-school teacher who "doesn't have any major problems—I just want to get SuperBetter." She isn't currently facing any big obstacles in her life, but she does want to feel happier, healthier, and more confident. She is like many of the 400,000 people who have helped us study the SuperBetter method: she wants to live more fully, build resilience, have more happy years ahead, and become stronger in the face of any potential challenges in the future.

Part 1 explored the science of why games make you so good at tackling tough challenges. Part 2 will teach you how to apply these gameful skills to everyday life.

Whether you're getting superbetter from a trauma, an illness, or an injury, or you just want to become the best possible version of yourself, this part of the book will teach you everything you need to know to use your gameful strengths to unlock the powerful benefits of post-ecstatic and post-traumatic growth.

Are you ready to lead a life truer to your dreams and free of regret? If so—let's play!

# 5

## Challenge Yourself

### How to Be Gameful Rule 1

Challenge yourself. There are thousands of ways to get happier, healthier, stronger, and braver. Decide what real-life obstacle you want to tackle, or what positive change you want to make first.

Here's an interesting fact about games: we almost never feel hopeless when we play them.

It's true. Psychologists have studied the top emotions during game play, and genuine anxiety and pessimism are extremely rare. Even when we're losing or struggling, we're vastly more likely to feel determined and optimistic than panicked or powerless.[1] This is true even of professional athletes and poker players whose careers and livelihoods are on the line when they play.[2] That's because—as you'll learn in this chapter—the psychology of games naturally makes it easier for us to manage anxiety more effectively, to focus on opportunity rather than threats, and to fear failure less.

Why? Because when we play a game, we focus on goals and growth. We seek out challenges voluntarily, and we savor the difficulty. We play not to avoid losing but to find out what we are capable of. And we believe that victories even against great odds are possible.

What if you could bring this gameful mindset to your *real-life* obstacles? Is it possible, or even wise, to feel the same optimism, courage, and curiosity in everyday life, where the stakes are higher and failure has significantly more consequences?

Yes, it absolutely is possible *and* wise to bring a gameful mindset to real-life obstacles. It's called adopting a *challenge versus threat* mindset—and as you'll see in this chapter, the research shows it works.

◄►

A *challenge* is anything that provokes our desire to test our strengths and abilities and that gives us the opportunity to improve them. Crucially, a challenge must be accepted. No one can force you to tackle it. You have to choose to rise to the occasion.

Here are some of the challenges SuperBetter players have tackled successfully by adopting a gameful mindset:*

- Battling stress at the job from hell
- Getting debt-free
- Donating my kidney
- Working on my stammer
- Being pregnant while on bed rest
- Liking myself and believing others like me, too
- Doing the Gospel work
- Recovering from a bad breakup
- Twenty-one-day sugar detox
- Coping with migraines and fatigue
- Adult ADHD
- Becoming awesome at being self-employed
- Preparing for divorce
- Less lazybones

---

* Success in SuperBetter is defined as achieving at least one epic win, a special kind of goal that you'll learn more about in Chapter 11.

- Not falling into funks or flying off the handle
- Raising a happy, successful child with autism
- Completing my first triathlon
- Being a better man
- PTSD from a car accident
- Recovering from a stroke
- Coming out to my family
- Quitting smoking
- Rape aftermath
- The fight against cancer
- Recovering from the death of my life partner of twenty years
- Embracing life with enthusiasm
- Transforming into a survivor

Some of these challenges are entirely self-chosen, a positive life change that the player wants to make. Many of them, however, are challenges no one would ever choose for themselves—an injury, an illness, a trauma, a loss. You might think that *these* kinds of challenges would be resistant to a gameful approach. They're too serious, too painful, too life-or-death to "play around" with. Fortunately, this is not the case. In fact, a gameful approach to problems works even better for the *uninvited challenges* that life throws at you than for the positive changes you decide to make.

That's why I recommend tackling something that is truly an urgent goal for you—whether it's living free of anxiety, finding a new job, changing your diet, flourishing despite chronic pain, or jump-starting your love life. Tackle an important problem in your life, even if it seems overwhelming right now or out of your control.

In fact, tackle it *especially* if it overwhelms you or feels out of your control. Gameful thinking and acting work extremely well in situations where we can easily become hopeless and give up. Indeed, according to data from more than 400,000 SuperBetter players, the *more* overwhelming the problem or daunting the challenge seems to you, the more effective the gameful method seems to be. That's because everything about it helps you develop more control and exercise more power in situations where you feel powerless or have self-doubt. So don't hold back. Pick a tough challenge for yourself that you feel will truly change your life.

If you're seeking **post-traumatic growth**, your challenge could be:

- To manage an injury or illness more effectively
- To get through a difficult ordeal as best you can
- To solve a problem for yourself or your family
- To recover from a trauma
- To overcome any kind of obstacle

Here are the ten most common post-traumatic growth challenges that SuperBetter players have chosen to tackle (ranked in order, with number one being the most common):

1. Beating depression
2. Overcoming anxiety
3. Coping with chronic illness or chronic pain
4. Finding a new job or overcoming unemployment
5. Surviving a divorce or family separation
6. Healing from a physical injury, including traumatic brain injury
7. Bouncing back from a school or career setback
8. Recovering from PTSD
9. Thriving with a learning disability or neurological disorder (*often tackled by a parent and child together*)
10. Grieving the loss of a loved one

If you're seeking **post-ecstatic growth**, on the other hand, your challenge might be:

- To adopt a new habit
- To develop a talent
- To learn or improve a skill

- To strengthen a relationship
- To make a physical or athletic breakthrough
- To complete a meaningful project
- To pursue a lifelong dream
- To make any other positive change in your life

Because everyone has different dreams and talents, post-ecstatic goals tend to be more varied. Some of the more popular ones we've seen among SuperBetter players include eating healthier, finishing a degree, writing a book, sleeping better, "doing something that scares me," starting a business, getting better at managing stress, losing weight, running a 5K or a marathon, learning to meditate, starting a family, saving for and planning a dream trip, helping a friend with a personal challenge, making a difference for a good cause, being a better parent, and being a better husband or wife.

You may be facing serious adversity or trauma in your life right now, but that doesn't mean you can't pursue post-ecstatic growth. Many SuperBetter players have successfully reduced anxiety, depression, and pain by pursuing a meaningful personal goal or dream. You may feel more motivated and optimistic right now about tackling a positive goal than about focusing directly on an illness or trauma. That's totally okay! There's no right or wrong challenge to tackle first.

Have you got an obstacle in mind? Good. But before you dive in, there's a skill you need to master. It's called *cognitive reappraisal*, and it means changing how you think and feel about a stressful problem in your life.

How does it work? There's actually a very simple trick—a scientifically validated method—that I can teach you right now. It helps you turn *anxiety* into *excitement*, and it's the easiest form of cognitive reappraisal to learn.

It turns out that anxiety and excitement are, physiologically, the exact same emotion. Whether you are anxious about something or excited about it, your body responds in a nearly identical "high arousal" state. You have excess energy, you may feel butterflies in your stomach, your heart rate may increase, and so on.

This means that when you're feeling anxious about a problem, it's much easier to try to get *excited* about solving it than to try to *calm down*. In order to calm down, you would have to slow your heart rate and reduce your adrenaline. That's not easy, especially when you're facing a stressful situation. But to get excited, you don't have to change how your body feels at all. *You just have to change how your mind interprets what you're physically feeling.* You can reappraise the adrenaline rush and the increased heart rate as signs that you're actually enthusiastic and eager or even exhilarated.

It's easy to do. Based on mind-body science, Harvard Business School researcher and psychologist Alison Wood Brooks has devised an incredibly simple trick to turn anxiety into excitement.[3] Are you ready to learn it? All you have to do is this:

Think about something that usually makes you nervous—not something truly traumatic, but an everyday situation where you personally would like to experience more confidence and less negative stress. Perhaps it's public speaking, or taking a test, or asking for a raise at work, or flying, or going to a party alone. Even better, if you have something specific on your horizon that's making you nervous—a tough conversation you need to have, a doctor's appointment, getting feedback on your work, a first date—concentrate on that. Whatever it is that gets your nerves going, keep imagining it, and wait until you feel the telltale butterflies in your stomach.

As soon as you feel your nerves, say *I'm excited* or *Get excited* to yourself. Out loud. Say it a few times. *I'm excited. Get excited!* That's it—that's the whole trick. According to Dr. Brooks's research, this is literally all it takes to make people less anxious, more optimistic, and more successful in solving problems or undertaking stressful tasks. When we're not thinking anxious thoughts, we're free to use that mental effort and physical energy to be creative, focus on the problem, and otherwise get stuff done. This explains why, in Dr. Brooks's lab, participants not only felt more optimistic but also performed better at high-stress tasks (like singing in front of judges) when using this technique.

The key to making the *Get excited!* technique work is to be open to the possibility that you are, in fact, at least a little bit excited about whatever you think you're anxious about. Could something good come about as a result?

Is there any reason to be hopeful about what might happen? If so, you truly might be excited, not anxious.

This is not just a mind game you're playing with yourself. The line between feeling anxiety and experiencing excitement is exceedingly thin. Your body reacts the same way to both, and your brain can't always tell the difference. This means that most of the time, *you have a real choice between feeling anxiety and feeling excitement.* Game players and athletes exercise this choice all the time. It's why a football player can feel excitement instead of terror when someone is chasing him down the field, trying to violently tackle him.

Don't hesitate to use this power to your advantage, especially when it's as easy as saying two little words. It will not only make you feel stronger and happier in the moment, it will also improve your ability to tackle tough obstacles and achieve your goals.

The *Get excited!* technique works best for situations where the stakes aren't too high and you simply want to get a better grip on your nerves. But you can also use your powers of cognitive reappraisal for much more serious problems.

When faced with a truly significant adversity, you can use cognitive reappraisal to view it as a challenge you're capable of meeting, rather than as a threat that will overwhelm or harm you. This is called replacing a *threat mindset* with a *challenge mindset*.[4] And it's the number-one rule of living gamefully.

In a threat mindset, you focus on the potential for risk, danger, harm, or loss. You feel pressured to prevent a negative outcome rather than to achieve a positive outcome. A threat mindset often occurs when you have low self-efficacy—that is, if you feel it's outside your control or ability to change the situation or to avoid negative impacts.

In a challenge mindset, you focus on the opportunity for growth and positive outcomes. Even though you acknowledge that you may face risk, harm, or loss, you feel *realistically optimistic* that you can develop useful skills or strategies to achieve the best possible outcome. You prepare yourself to rise to the difficult occasion by gathering resources and drawing on your personal strengths. People with high self-efficacy find it easier to adopt a challenge mindset. So do people who spend a lot of time playing games.[5] In fact, "challenge-seeking" is one of the most common personality traits of frequent game players.[6]

Every time we play a game, we approach it with a challenge mindset— and *you're* going to learn how to bring this mindset to real-life goals and obstacles. But first let's talk about why a challenge mindset matters.

Psychologists have been researching challenge versus threat mindsets for more than thirty years, studying how they impact people's ability to handle stress and adversity. Here are the main differences they've found:

When you operate under a threat mindset, you're more likely to develop anxiety and depression in addition to whatever struggle you face. As a result, your ability to perform under pressure suffers. Meanwhile, instead of developing helpful coping skills or finding new resources, you're more likely to engage in escapist and self-defeating actions, like social isolation, drug and alcohol abuse, or simply ignoring your problem until it gets even worse.[7]

With a challenge mindset, however, you experience less anxiety and depression, and you adapt to change more effectively. You don't try to escape your problem. Instead, you take advantage of important resources like social support and your own competence. You increase your skills and become better able to solve your problem. In short, you're much more likely to achieve the best outcome possible in your current situation.[8]

The differences between a challenge mindset and a threat mindset aren't just mental. They also determine how your *body* reacts to the stress.

In a threat mindset, your arteries constrict, and your heart has to work much harder to pump blood throughout your body. In the short term, this increases your chances of suffering a heart attack. Over time, if you spend months or years operating under a threat mindset, your heart may weaken from having to work so much harder.

With a challenge mindset, by contrast, your arteries expand, and you experience much more efficient cardiac output. You have improved blood flow, with much less effort. In other words, a challenge mindset keeps your heart healthy and relaxed.

In a threat mindset, your fight-or-flight instinct kicks in, which activates your sympathetic nervous system. If your sympathetic nervous system is engaged continuously for hours, days, weeks, or longer, your immune system can become compromised, and you may experience more illness.

With a challenge mindset, however, your nervous system finds a better balance between the sympathetic (fight-or-flight) and the parasympathetic (calm-and-connect) responses. This balance helps you avoid nervous exhaustion and burnout.

Finally, a threat mindset leads to an increase in the stress hormone cortisol and the metabolism hormone insulin. Increased cortisol and insulin are associated with weight gain, difficulty building muscle, and diabetes.

In short, a threat mindset is not just a psychological barrier—it's also damaging to your physical health. Adopting a challenge mindset, on the other hand, increases both your mental *and* your physical resilience.

N ow that you know how important a challenge mindset is, it's time to figure out how close you are to achieving one. The best way to do that? A quest!

## QUEST 15: Challenge vs. Threat

Think about your biggest personal challenge, goal, or source of stress at the moment. We're going to call this your *obstacle*. By answering twenty questions about your obstacle, you can figure out whether you're likely to tackle it with a threat or a challenge mindset.

**What to do:** Put a check mark (or highlight) any statement that you agree with. If you disagree with a statement, skip it.

1. I'm eager to tackle this obstacle.
2. Thinking about this obstacle stresses me out.
3. I'm worried that this obstacle might reveal my weakness.
4. I can become a stronger person because of this obstacle.
5. There is someone I can turn to for help with this obstacle if I need it.
6. Tackling this obstacle seems like an exhausting prospect.
7. This obstacle is probably going to have an overall negative impact on my life, no matter what I do.
8. I get fired up when I think about tackling this obstacle.
9. This obstacle threatens my or my family's health and happiness.
10. I'm worried that I lack the resources needed to overcome this obstacle.
11. This obstacle gives me a chance to find out what I'm really made of.
12. I feel like this obstacle represents basically a hopeless situation.
13. I get excited when I think about the possible outcomes of tackling this obstacle.
14. I don't mind struggling with this obstacle, or sometimes failing, because the outcome is important to me.
15. I think I have or can acquire the abilities needed to successfully tackle this obstacle.
16. If I succeed, my choosing to tackle this obstacle will have a positive impact on my or my family's health and happiness.
17. This obstacle probably requires more strength than I have to deal with it effectively.
18. If I fail to overcome this obstacle, it will have significant negative consequences for me and my life.

19. It's beyond anyone else's power to help me with this obstacle.

20. I'll probably learn something by tackling this obstacle as best I can.

**Scoring:** How many of the following statements did you *agree* with? 1, 4, 5, 8, 11, 13, 14, 15, 16, 20. This is your challenge score. How many of the following statements did you *agree* with? 2, 3, 6, 7, 9, 10, 12, 17, 18, 19. This is your threat score.

To reap the benefits of a challenge mindset, you should strive to have a challenge score that is higher than your threat score. The bigger the difference between the two numbers, the better.

If you're already 100 percent in a challenge mindset, with a threat score of zero, fantastic. More likely, you're somewhere on the spectrum between threat and challenge.

Your goal, by the time you finish this chapter, is to move yourself at least one or two points closer to a full challenge mindset and away from the threat mindset.

Here's something important to keep in mind: different people will appraise the same exact situation as a threat or a challenge, depending on how they evaluate the opportunities for harm versus growth. *The actual stressful circumstance you face does not determine whether you view it as a challenge or a threat.* It's how you choose to engage with the stress that makes the difference.

Indeed, researchers have so far found *no limits* to the kinds of stressful situations in which a person can successfully develop a challenge mindset. According to more than three decades' worth of studies, whether you are dealing with economic hardships or a medical crisis or even living in a war conflict zone, achieving a challenge mindset—no matter how objectively threatening the circumstances—is possible.

Here are just a few of the types of stress for which scientists have documented profoundly significant benefits from cultivating a challenge mindset:

- College athletes who had a challenge mindset at the beginning of a season performed better and won more games the entire season.[9]
- Students who adopted a challenge mindset immediately before taking a test scored significantly higher on the test.[10]
- HIV and cancer patients have much lower rates of depression and anxiety if they see their diagnosis as a challenge, not only as a threat.[11]
- Couples with fertility struggles who adopt a challenge mindset report fewer fights, less distress, and closer marriages.[12]
- Men and women who develop a challenge mindset toward managing negative emotion are better able to control their anger.[13]
- During the transition from primary to secondary school, children who have a challenge mindset experience more social and academic success and fewer behavior problems.[14]
- Bereaved spouses who identify specific challenges to tackle during their grieving process have better physical health, and less anxiety and depression.[15]
- Civilians and soldiers who have a belief in their ability to successfully meet the challenge of war zone stress are less likely to develop post-traumatic stress symptoms.[16]

There's one important point I want to make clear: a challenge mindset doesn't require you to think positively all the time, or to ignore your pain or losses. It's more about investigating your own strengths and abilities and trying to increase them.

Similarly, having a challenge mindset does *not* mean living in denial of potential negative outcomes. It simply means paying *more* attention, and devoting more effort, to the possibility of positive outcomes or personal growth. It means not accepting the negative as inevitable—or if a negative outcome is inevitable, not allowing it to completely define your experience.

With a challenge mindset, you're committed to looking for something more than the negative, something that will bring meaning and purpose to your struggle.

So how can you move from a threat to a challenge mindset? Here are three techniques to try:

1. **Write down the ten expressions of a challenge mindset** (statements 1, 4, 5, 8, 11, 13, 14, 15, 16, 20 in Quest 15) and **put the list in a place where you will see it every day.** Looking at this list will give you a daily reminder of what a challenge mindset feels like. This can be extremely helpful, especially if it doesn't come naturally in your current situation. You can also try reading the statements out loud like a mantra once a day. That won't make them automatically true, but it *will* give you a chance to reflect on the possibility that they might become true. Indeed, the more you speak them, the more likely you are to make choices or changes that foster a challenge mindset.

2. **Ask yourself,** *What's the best that could happen?* When we operate under a threat mindset, we tend to spend a lot of time pondering *What's the worst that could happen?* (And we usually come up with lots and lots of answers.) To balance out this cognitive habit, ask yourself the opposite, and see how many answers you can come up with. It will help you stay open to the potential for some kind of positive outcome or post-traumatic growth.

3. **Say that you're getting superbetter** *at* **something, not** *from* **something.** Just the way you talk about your SuperBetter journey can influence whether you adopt a threat or a challenge mindset. Getting superbetter *from* something implies a threat, but getting superbetter *at* something implies the opportunity for growth.

    If you're pursuing post-ecstatic growth, this phrasing should come naturally. *I'm getting superbetter at writing a novel. I'm getting superbetter at world travel. I'm getting superbetter at triathlons. I'm getting superbetter at running for city council.*\* But for post-traumatic growth, it may require a bit of rethinking. For example, instead of getting superbetter *from* anxiety, you might be getting superbetter *at* being brave, or finding peace, or preventing panic attacks, or whatever represents to you the positive change or growth you want to experience. Instead of getting superbetter *from* insomnia, you might get superbetter *at* sleeping. Instead of getting superbetter *from* a concussion, you might get superbetter *at* healing your brain.

Eventually, as you continue to get superbetter—and as you learn the other six rules of living gamefully—you'll naturally strengthen your challenge mindset. That's because the other rules are designed to help you increase your personal resources or help you focus on the potential for growth and positive outcomes. Collecting power-ups will give you more physical and emotional resources. Battling bad guys will allow you to develop new mental resources. Completing—and designing your own—quests will help you acquire new skills and abilities specific to your challenge. Recruiting allies will increase your social resources. Seeking epic wins will help you focus on opportunities for growth and positive impact. And adopting a secret identity and keeping score will highlight your progress and growing strength. So even if you feel unprepared at this moment to bring a challenge mindset to your most pressing problems, don't worry. Keep going. Achieving a challenge mindset is the inevitable outcome of engaging with obstacles more gamefully.

In the meantime, here's another cognitive reappraisal technique—and a quest—to help you start bringing out the challenge, and squashing the threat, right now. It's called *Find the unnecessary obstacle.* It's significantly more difficult to master than Dr. Alison Wood Brooks's *Get excited!* technique—but you're up for a challenge, right?

To master this next technique, you need to learn my favorite definition of a game. It comes from the late philosopher Bernard Suits, who famously

---

\* Believe it or not, this was a real SuperBetter player's challenge. I met the councilman at a local business luncheon, where he told me that he had used the game to help him handle the stress of the election cycle!

wrote: "Playing a game is a voluntary attempt to overcome *unnecessary obstacles.*"[17]

Think of the game of golf—a classic case of unnecessary obstacles. In ordinary life, if your goal were to put a small ball in a small hole, you would simply walk up to the hole and carefully drop the ball in. But because golf is a game, you agree to stand very far away from the hole—the first unnecessary obstacle. And to make it even more difficult, you agree to use a long stick (your golf club) to try to aim the ball toward the hole—the second unnecessary obstacle. There is no logical or necessary reason to approach the goal of getting a small ball into a small hole in this way. We do it simply for the pleasure of engaging wholeheartedly with a difficult challenge. We do it for the enjoyment of testing our abilities and improving them.

*Every* game works the same way. Every game offers us the opportunity to accept a challenging goal that, by design, will stretch our capabilities and help us develop new skills. This is why there is such a strong correlation between a gameful mindset and a challenge mindset. *When we play a game, we volunteer to be challenged.* No one forces us to try to solve a game's puzzles, or defeat another team, or reach a certain score. Because we are fully in control of whether we accept a game's challenge, we don't experience anxiety or depression when we play—despite the very real possibility of loss or defeat. Our primary experience is of agency, not of threat.

But in daily life, we don't always get to choose our own obstacles. The challenge you are facing now may be an obstacle you would *never* have volunteered to tackle if you had a choice. This makes it harder to be gameful. It's not easy to focus on the possibility of a positive outcome when you feel blindsided by the threat.

Cognitive reappraisal, however, can help you regain a sense of agency and choice. It can empower you to find the unnecessary obstacle within the uninvited challenge you face.

The key is to *identify an obstacle that you feel capable of tackling within the larger challenge,* an obstacle that other people might not choose to tackle.

To see how this works, let's try a quest.

## QUEST 16: Find the Unnecessary Obstacle

Think about the biggest uninvited difficulty you currently face, or any personal setback or disappointment you've experienced in your life.

**What to do:** Use your imagination to answer this question: What would be the *worst* possible, least helpful reaction that you—or anyone else in your shoes—could have to it?

You don't have to be completely realistic here. Let your mind go to extremes for just a moment. Here are some examples from SuperBetter players:

- "Lost my job / Turn to a life of crime."
- "Have Lyme disease with chronic flare-ups / Give up and never get out of bed again."
- "My book manuscript was rejected by every publisher I sent it to / Never write a word again."
- "Having trouble getting pregnant / Drown my sorrows every night in ice cream and pick fights with my husband until we can't bear to have sex with each other."
- "Had a bike accident and concussion / Confine myself to a small, padded room for the rest of my life to avoid further injury."
- "Got laid off / Go on a social media rampage badmouthing my former employer and all my workmates (making other companies much less likely to hire me in the future)."
- "Recently lost my mother / Drop out of school, let myself be consumed by grief, stop eating, and waste away, until my mother starts haunting me from the other side about how much it hurts her that I've given up on my dreams."

As you can see, some people approach this quest with a sense of humor. Others find it helpful to just be honest and plainspoken about the worst reaction they might have. Two common reactions to this quest are simply "Someone else in my shoes might just give up and do nothing," or even, "The worst thing I've considered doing is killing myself." If that's what popped into your mind, it's good to acknowledge it and work with it.

Now: What is the opposite of that worst reaction?

**Examples:**

- "Turn to a life of crime / Turn to a life of service."
- "Give up and never get out of bed again / Get out of bed every single day, even if it's just for a minute."
- "Never write again / Write something every day."
- "Drown my sorrows every night in ice cream and pick fights with my husband / Eat healthy to prepare my body for a baby and say something kind to my husband at the end of each night."
- "Confine myself to a small, padded room / Find three new outdoor spaces to spend time in while I recuperate."
- "Go on a social media rampage / Every day find one company or person whose work I admire and say something positive about it on social media. Who knows, if they see it, it might help me build my network."
- "Drop out of school, waste away, and be haunted by my mother / Every day try to make my mother proud."
- "Give up and do nothing / Do something. Anything. Do one damn thing that shows I haven't given up."
- "Kill myself / Keep living."

Whatever the opposite of your "worst possible, least helpful re-action" is, consider adopting it as your unnecessary obstacle. Challenge yourself to do something that requires more strength and determination than what someone else might do in your shoes.

**Why it works:** Completing this quest has two benefits. First, when you imagine the worst possible reaction you could have to adversity, you highlight your agency in the situation. You do have options. And as long as you're *not* doing that worst possible, least helpful thing, you can challenge yourself to do something better. It may not feel like total agency and choice, but it involves *some* agency and choice—and that's enough to activate a challenge mindset.

Meanwhile, imagining the *opposite* of the worst possible reaction gives you a specific positive and purposeful goal. This goal is now something you can aspire to achieve. You may not have chosen your current adversity, but you *are* choosing to challenge yourself to engage in a way that improves your chances for growth and success.

The more concrete you can make your unnecessary obstacle, the easier it will be to embrace it as a challenge. One SuperBetter player found that having a very specific goal made all the difference between a challenge and a threat mindset.

## A SuperBetter Story: The Broken Artist

Rowan, forty, is a freelance artist in Missouri who recently developed extremely painful tendinitis in her right arm—"my drawing arm," she explained in an online discussion forum for SuperBetter players. The injury caused her quite a bit of anxiety. "I need to get better so I can keep working. This is my dream job. Also, my art business is my sole income."

Rowan expected her arm to heal quickly, but it didn't. "This injury has entered the realm of chronic pain," she wrote. "It's quite disheartening if I allow it to be, and I have." Knowing that she needed to change her mindset, she decided to look for the unnecessary obstacle.

What was the *worst possible* reaction she could have to her injury? "Ignore the pain and try to work through it." What was the *least helpful* thing she could do? "Continue grinding down the tendon until the arm is permanently damaged." So what was the opposite of all that?

"I'm learning to do things with my left hand to give poor ol' righty a break," she announced one day. This became her new, unnecessary obstacle: *Learn how to do ten new things with her nondominant hand.*

Rowan started practicing each day and looking up videos online showing how to do things one-handed. "I'm amazed at how many things I can do with my left hand that I never tried before, like open a jar with one hand." Granted, opening a jar wasn't her ultimate goal—returning to work was. But pretty soon the benefits of a challenge mindset—including a sense of optimism and the ability to spot opportunities for growth—kicked in. "I'm rethinking everything," she wrote. "I am focusing now on the fact that I have one perfectly healthy arm and that I can make that arm stronger."

Rowan had found the perfect unnecessary obstacle for her. It was small enough to feel manageable but challenging enough to provoke her curiosity and stretch her abilities. More important, it was genuinely helpful in her current situation. By challenging herself to learn this new skill, she was actively helping her dominant arm heal faster. And if for some reason her right arm *never* healed, strengthening her left arm would create new windows of opportunity for her in the future.

As the weeks progressed, her mood improved, and she stopped

feeling helpless or hopeless about her situation. She realized she might have to live with tendinitis in her right arm. But by focusing her efforts right now on a smaller, voluntary obstacle, she is actively improving her chances of continuing her successful career as an artist.

Hopefully, you're starting to feel skillful at cognitive reappraisal. But sometimes, no matter how hard you try to reappraise a problem, it still seems more like a threat than a challenge. This is natural. Some problems really do have higher stakes or trigger unavoidable grief or anger. It can feel unnatural and absurd to try to view a major illness, the loss of a loved one, the incarceration of a family member, or severe economic distress as an opportunity for growth. These kinds of adversity and loss strongly resist reappraisal, especially when you're just beginning to cope with them. Even though any form of adversity contains potential for post-traumatic growth, looking for that "silver lining" too soon can feel wrong, disloyal, or inappropriate—and rightly so.

If you find yourself in this position right now, you still have more power than you realize. If you're facing a threat or a loss that you simply cannot, in any way that feels genuine and sincere, view as a challenge, there is a gameful technique you can employ. It's called "adopting a strategy goal," and it can help you get many of the benefits of a challenge mindset, *even if it feels more natural and appropriate to operate (at least for now) under a threat or loss mindset*. Here's how it works.

Anyone in the face of an obstacle or struggle can adopt three types of goals: a difficult goal, a do-your-best goal, and a strategy goal.[18] To explore the differences among these three types of goals, let's use two examples of potential obstacles: running a marathon and trying to get out of credit card debt.

Adopting a *difficult goal* means trying to achieve something very specific and very challenging. It's the kind of goal you could reasonably expect to fail at, even if you try your best. A marathon runner's difficult goal might be "I want to run this marathon in under four hours, which would be faster than I've ever run one before." A credit card debtor's difficult goal would be "I want to be 100 percent debt-free a year from today." In ordinary or low-stakes life circumstances, such as running a marathon for fun, difficult goals can be highly motivating and effective. But in a high-stakes situation, like getting out of debt, difficult goals are more likely to add to your negative stress, making it harder for you to thrive.

Adopting a *do-your-best goal* means putting forth your best effort, without concern for the results. You generally hope to do well, but you have no specific expectations for what you might achieve. The marathon runner's do-your-best goal would be "Try to finish this race without walking, but if you have to walk, that's okay, too. Just do your best!" The credit card debtor's do-your-best goal might be "I'll pay more attention to what I'm spending and try to avoid buying things I can't afford." Do-your-best goals can alleviate performance anxiety, which can be beneficial in some circumstances. But generally speaking, unless your biggest problem is a crippling fear of failing to meet your own standards, a do-your-best goal is not particularly motivating or helpful.

Adopting a *strategy goal*, on the other hand, means being determined to discover and master strategies that will help you be successful. Instead of focusing on a specific outcome (as with a difficult goal) or a general effort level (as with a do-your-best goal), you put your attention on learning and improving concrete skills and strategies that will help you do better in the future. The marathon runner's strategy goal might be "I'm going to try out a new strategy in this race. I'll run the first half slower than my practice pace, so I have lots of energy left in the tank for the second half of the race." The credit card debtor's strategy goal could be "Every week for the next six months, I'm going to adopt one new strategy for saving money that I can put toward paying down my debt. This week the strategy is to pack my lunch instead of eating out at work. Six months from now I'll be doing twenty-five things to help me get debt-free." When you adopt a strategy goal, you can be successful regardless of whether you win the race or even finish it; and regardless of whether you're 100 percent debt-free in a year or just well on your way. You're successful as long as you're learning and improving.

Researchers have figured out that *for someone operating under a threat mindset, a strategy goal is absolutely the best kind to adopt.*[19] When the stakes are high or the loss severe, a strategy mindset will increase your resilience and improve your coping abilities.

Why does this work? By focusing on developing and practicing effective strategies, you're going to build up new strengths and abilities. These strengths and abilities will be a real resource for you. They will help you be braver, happier, healthier, or more successful within the reality of the threat or loss you're facing. Your strategies may not change that reality, but they will help you find and maximize your power to do and feel the absolute best you can, given the obstacle you face.

Adopting a strategy goal is also like adopting a mini-challenge mindset. You're challenging yourself to learn and improve, even if the overall situation still feels overwhelming or is objectively out of your control. A mini-challenge mindset will help trigger some of the physiological and psychological benefits of a challenge mindset, like less depression and anxiety, and lower cortisol and insulin levels. (And as a bonus, as you learn and master each new strategy, you'll experience the neurological benefits of goal achievement, such as the increased determination and optimism described in Chapter 3.)

So here's the upshot: if you've tried all the quests in this chapter and you don't think a challenge mindset is realistic for you at this moment, don't worry. You can still adopt a strategy goal. In fact, I have a specific strategy goal in mind for you:

Keep learning and practicing as many strategies as you can to increase your four types of resilience—in other words, your physical, mental, social, and emotional strengths.

Here's a SuperBetter story about a man who experienced success with this very strategy goal.

## A SuperBetter Story:
## The Man in Search of Purpose

Dennis, sixty-six, lives in rural Kansas. For the past forty years, he has worked in higher education, overseeing grant programs for low-income students and serving as their academic adviser. He is also a SuperBetter player. He recently wrote me to describe a major loss he's facing, and the strategy he's adopted to cope with it gamefully.

"I'm getting close to retiring and, frankly, it is (was) scaring the bejesus out of me. I've worked hard to help underprepared students find success in college. For a good number of years, I've been heavily focused on this task. But now my wife and I are talking about retirement in *real* terms—with dates associated with it. Don't get me wrong, I would love to live near my grandchildren and be a significant part of their lives—that's the upside. But I'm having difficulty coping with the change. It feels like a loss of purpose.

"For the past six months I've found myself exhibiting signs of depression at home. I had worked myself into a frozen state unable to deal with the practicality or emotionality of this change. Then I found SuperBetter. I decided my strategy was to work on the 'physical' and the 'mental' at the same time.

"So I got up once every hour and did at least one small thing on a project I had been ignoring. I noticed this started to make for pretty good evenings. The projects I have undertaken vary from simply watering plants, organizing my laptop/reading section, and doing stretches, to larger projects like vacuuming the house, pulling weeds in the yard, or like the last three nights, deep-cleaning the carpets on the first floor. (Second floor begins this weekend.) One of my larger ongoing projects now is journaling my thoughts and formulating plans.

"The point of this for me is that I have been able to shift away from an inward, downward spiral and refocus my attention outward. I was finally just now able to put together a plan for retirement and talked with my wife about it. I am beginning to consider how I change from assisting students to assisting other people in volunteer roles. I am becoming more excited to think about this transition.

"There are two other strengths to build as I go. For my emotional strength, I put a photo of a smiling baby on my work desktop. I simply cannot help but smile when I look at it. This is the same photo I've used with students over the past decades, usually to help them with test anxiety. I've always told them that when they see someone else smile, they smile inside for a short time. Now I realize I can use the same trick in my own life.

"Oh, and I really don't need to worry about the social—I am madly in love with my wife and we travel frequently to see our grandkids. But it's good for me to pay attention to how much strength I already have in this part of my life."

Dennis, like many folks who are getting superbetter, keeps me apprised of his progress by email. He always refers to his gameful activity not as playing but as "my four resiliences work." This is a perfect example of cognitive reappraisal in action! For a man retiring from a truly meaningful job, it's good work and not necessarily play that will truly energize and engage him. And it does seem to be making a big positive difference. As he wrote me just today: "What can I say? The four types of resilience are changing me and my life. I'm pleased to see progress and know that I will have further insights over time."

Dennis's attitude is the perfect example of adopting a strategy goal. He is focused on making progress and getting stronger one day at a time.

*You* can adopt a strategy goal right now. You learned about the four types of resilience in the Introduction, and you've been completing quests all along the way that bolster them. You can decide right now to continue to learn and practice new ways to build more physical, mental, social, and emotional re-silience as you cope with whatever adversity is currently causing you pain or difficulty. At SuperBetter, we call this challenge simply "getting superbetter."

◄►

Most of the advice in this chapter has been geared toward helping you adopt a challenge mindset in the face of obstacles that others might view as a threat. But what if you're not facing any truly significant obstacle in your life currently?

If you're seeking transformative growth, you need to put yourself in a position to be seriously challenged. It's just as important for *you* to choose a challenge as it is for someone who is facing a personal setback, illness, in-jury, or loss. After all, wrestling with a significant challenge is how you ex-perience the "gains without pains" (or at least fewer pains) that Ann Marie Roepke calls post-ecstatic growth.

But how do you choose the right activity to maximize your chances of experiencing post-ecstatic growth? While becoming a parent for the first time and running a marathon are two classic examples, most people at any given moment in their lives are not necessarily in a position to do either. So I asked Dr. Roepke what other kinds of challenges a SuperBetter player should choose if they're seeking post-ecstatic growth.

In reply, she designed the following quest, based on her research, clinical practice, and personal experience. Give it a try!

## QUEST 17: Go for Gains Without Pains

Looking for inspiration? Here are the top three questions that can help lead to post-ecstatic growth.

**What to do:** Ask yourself one, two, or all three of these questions to figure out the perfect challenge for your SuperBetter journey.

1. **What would I do if anxiety and fear weren't holding me back?**
"Positive experiences don't always feel 'positive' through and through," Dr. Roepke says. "Often the things that people cite as their best experiences actually involve struggle and pain, not just love and inspiration. Think of the two classic post-ecstatic growth examples: having a baby and training for a marathon! There may actually be a blurry line between so-called positive and negative experiences, between post-ecstatic growth and post-traumatic growth. It could be that our lives are richest when we have a blend of struggle and pain on one hand, and comfort and inspiration on the other—just like athletes are at their best when they have a blend of exhausting work on one hand, and nourishment and rest on the other. The juxtaposition of dark times and bright times—a sort of psychological chiaroscuro—may help us grow the most."

2. **What have been the most energizing and inspiring moments in my life so far?** "Most of us have a few flashbulb memories of important experiences, and we can use these for insight and inspiration," Dr. Roepke advises. "Maybe these memories happened a long time ago, and they might seem irrelevant to us now, at a first glance. But we can look past the superficial features of that experience, isolate the important ones, and design a new experience that scratches the same itch."

3. **What do I want to be remembered for after I've lived a long, full life?** "Think of what you would want people to say about you in your obituary, or in a toast at your ninetieth birthday party. What will you have stood for? What will you be loved for? What will you have done that's bigger than you? If you can answer this question, you'll have a better idea of the kinds of

activities that will be personally meaningful enough to you to facilitate real growth."

Questions like these can help you zero in on the kinds of positive challenges that eventually lead to growth. But as Dr. Roepke reminds us, "There's a difference between facilitating an experience and forcing one. In some ways, trying to make yourself have a growth experience is like trying to make yourself fall in love. There's an uncontrollable, unpredictable element to some things in life, so we'd be wise to relax into whatever form our experiences take." In other words, don't worry about finding the perfect post-ecstatic growth challenge. Just pick any tough and meaningful obstacle to wrestle with, and you'll build the skills to grow from challenges now *and* in the future.

Now that you've mastered Rule 1 for living gamefully—*Challenge yourself and purposefully engage with potentially life-transforming obstacles*—it's time to choose your first SuperBetter challenge.

## QUEST 18: Choose Your Challenge

The SuperBetter method works best when you focus on just *one* challenge at a time. If you could be stronger, happier, healthier, or braver *in one specific way*, what would it be?

I'm getting superbetter at:

_____.

*Tip:* The phrasing is important! You're going to get SuperBetter *at* something, not SuperBetter *from* something.

### *Skills Unlocked: How to Choose Your Challenge*

- There are two ways to respond to a stressful situation: with a threat mindset or a challenge mindset. A threat mindset can increase anxiety and depression, and it takes a toll on your physical health. A challenge mindset, however, will improve your ability to successfully achieve your goals *and* reduce the suffering that can accompany stressful or traumatic experiences.

- It's natural to react to adversity with a threat mindset, but you aren't stuck with one. You can use the cognitive reappraisal skills you learned in this chapter (like *Get excited!* and *Find the unnecessary obstacle*) to rethink your emotional reaction to any stressful or traumatic situation.

- If you're struggling to adopt a challenge mindset, try repeating the challenge mindset statements from Quest 15 like a mantra. Ask yourself, *What's the best that could happen?* Say you're getting superbetter *at* something, and not *from* something.

- Having a challenge mindset doesn't mean that you're happy to be facing your current obstacle, or that you don't wish things were different. It just means that you recognize your own resilience—and that you want to actively explore ways to make things better.

# 6

## Power-ups

### How to Be Gameful Rule 2

Collect and activate power-ups—good things that
reliably make you feel happier, healthier, or stronger.

Power-ups are essential to most video games. They're the bonus items that give you more strength, more power, or extra life. Think of the power pellets in *Pac-Man* that allow you to gobble ghosts, or the care packages in *Call of Duty* that restore your soldier's health, or the super seeds in *Angry Birds* that supersize the birds in your slingshot, making them capable of knocking down bigger, stronger walls.

What if we could collect and activate power-ups in real life? Good news: we can. And it's easier than you think.

Here are a few of my favorite real-world power-ups:

Watch videos of baby animals on YouTube. Look out a window for thirty seconds. Hold my husband's hand for six seconds. Eat ten walnuts, because they're good for my brain. Try to make my dog smile. Send a text message to my mom. Listen to a song from one of my favorite Bollywood movies. Do ten push-ups even if I'm exhausted—in fact, especially if I'm exhausted, because I like how strong it makes me feel. I think to myself: *Screw you, exhaustion! Look at what I can do!* I call them screw-you push-ups, and they feel awesome. (Confession: I just did a set, to fight writer's block!)

What do all these power-ups have in common? I can do them easily, at no cost, and they never fail to make me feel at least a little bit better, no matter what else I'm thinking or feeling or battling that day.

This is one of the most powerful weapons in the arsenal of someone who is living gamefully. It's the ability to feel better, anytime, anyplace, *no matter what*.

Just as you would use a power-up in a video game to get through a particularly difficult level, or to accomplish a seemingly impossible task, you can use real-world power-ups to give you a boost during difficult times.

Different power-ups work for different people. This chapter is about experimenting with and collecting the power-ups that work for *you*.

A *power-up* is any positive action you can take, easily, that creates a quick moment of pleasure, strength, courage, or connection for you. *Collecting* a power-up simply means identifying it as something you want to try. *Activating* a power-up means actually doing it in your daily life.

The concept is simple enough: do little things that will give you a burst of energy, a positive emotion, social support, or motivation. But power-ups are about more than just feeling better in the moment. They also *change your biology* in extraordinarily important and long-term ways, helping you become far less vulnerable to stress and much more likely to experience post-traumatic or post-ecstatic growth. In the pages ahead, you'll learn all about the biology of positive change. But first let's give *you* a chance to power up.

## All-Time Favorite Power-ups

Over the past three years, SuperBetter players have collected and activated more than a million power-ups. Which are their favorites? Here are the all-time most activated and shared power-ups, by resilience type. If you think you could use a quick boost of physical, emotional, social, or mental resilience, by all means, try one or more of these power-ups right now!

### PHYSICAL RESILIENCE

**Drink a glass of water!** There's almost nothing it doesn't help, from improving mood to building muscle to controlling appetite to increasing energy to boosting the immune system.

### EMOTIONAL RESILIENCE

**Sing your lungs out!** Just pick a favorite song you know most of the lyrics to, and sing it at the top of your lungs. "At the top of your lungs" is the crucial part—it turns singing into an aerobic activity, which can trigger a release of endorphins, the happy hormones. So don't hold back—you've got to really belt it out to get these benefits!

### SOCIAL RESILIENCE

**Love spree!** Check the clock or start a timer. You've got *three minutes* to like, favorite, or leave a positive comment on as many social media posts from friends and family as you can. If you're not on social media, use your three minutes to send quick "you're awesome" or "thinking of you" emails and text messages to as many people as you can. You've only got three minutes, so don't think—just spread the *love*!

## MENTAL RESILIENCE

**Future boost!** Name two specific things you're looking forward to in the next week, big or small. This dopamine-boosting power-up is inspired by the ancient wisdom "Always have two things to look forward to." If you can't think of two things in the next seven days that you're genuinely looking forward to, now is the time to schedule them.

Once you've chosen your challenge, collecting and activating power-ups is the most important part of daily gameful living. That's because in order to rebound from stress and tackle major life obstacles successfully, you need what scientists call *high vagal tone*. And power-ups are the best way to get it.

Vagal tone refers to the health of your vagus nerve, which stretches all the way from your brain to your intestines. The vagus nerve touches your heart, lungs, voicebox, ears, and stomach, helping to regulate virtually every important function in your mind and body, from your emotions to your heart rate to your breathing rate to your muscle movement to your digestion.[1]

Because the vagus nerve is so essential to so many biological and psychological functions, its health is an excellent measure of your mind-and-body resilience. Nearly twenty-five years of research, in fact, has consistently shown that the tone, or strength, of the vagus nerve is the single best measure of how effectively a person's heart, lungs, and brain respond to stress.[2]

If you want to get a more concrete feel of what vagal tone is, try this trick: place your fingers on the pulse point on the side of your neck. Feel your pulse for a few seconds to get a sense of its speed. Now start to breathe in and out as slowly as you can.

You should notice that your pulse subtly quickens on the inhalation and slows on the exhalation. It might be easier to notice if you mentally count each beat of the heart. Take a minute now to feel this.

This subtle difference between your pulse when you inhale and exhale is what scientists call *respiratory sinus arrhythmia*, or RSA for short.[3] *Arrhythmia* literally means "without a steady beat"; most people associate the term with potentially dangerous heart conditions in which the heartbeat changes erratically. However, a variable heart rate—within certain bounds— is absolutely healthy, normal, and necessary. If your heart rate *didn't* increase during inhalation and decrease during exhalation, you would be at a higher risk for heart attack, stroke, aging-related cognitive decline, and stress-induced illness.[4] In fact, the more pronounced the difference between your inhalation and exhalation heart rates, the better.

The bigger the difference, the stronger your RSA—and therefore the stronger your vagal tone. The stronger the vagal tone, the better able you are to control your emotions and thoughts, the more physical pain you can withstand, and the less likely you are to suffer a variety of ailments, from diabetes and irritable bowel syndrome to social anxiety, loneliness, depression, and post-traumatic stress disorder.[5]

Dr. Stephen Porges, a neuroscientist at the University of North Carolina at Chapel Hill, was the first researcher to identify vagal tone as a physiological marker of stress vulnerability, and he has continued to research it for decades. He argues that increasing vagal tone is the best all-around mental and physical health intervention possible. That's because, he explains, what determines your mental and physical health is not the presence or absence of a stressful life event or even how you *react* to such an event; it's your *neurophysiologic state*, or mind-body strength, before a stressful life event occurs. Depending on how much strength you've built up, you will either be more resilient and therefore better able to experience growth, or more vulnerable and therefore likely to experience negative impacts.

B y now you're probably wondering how strong your vagal tone is and whether there's a way for you to measure and compare it with others'.

If you were a participant in a formal scientific study, researchers would measure your vagal tone using sophisticated laboratory equipment: echocardiogram (ECG) electrodes would track your heart rate, while "pneumatic bellows" strapped around your chest would measure the rise and fall of your breath. This would produce a very precise RSA number that could be deemed high, low, or average.

Assuming you don't have this equipment lying around at home, you're not going to get an accurate RSA number just by taking your own pulse. But don't give up yet: there's another way to put a number to your vagal tone, one that doesn't require any special equipment at all. In fact, it doesn't even measure your breath or heart rate. Instead, it measures your rate of emotions—specifically, *how many positive emotions you feel in the course of a day compared with how many negative emotions you feel*. Although this measure, known as emotional ratio, may seem highly subjective, scientific studies have shown it to predict vagal tone quite effectively. The higher the ratio between positive and negative emotions you feel daily, the stronger your vagal tone.[6]

The relationship between emotional ratio and vagal tone was first discovered by leading psychologist and mind-body scientist Dr. Barbara Fredrickson, director of the Positive Emotions and Psychophysiology Lab at the University of North Carolina. Dr. Fredrickson was investigating the underlying body mechanisms that account for the association between positive emotion and physical health. For decades, researchers have known that experiencing more positive emotions in everyday life is correlated to better physical health. Longitudinal studies of hundreds of thousands of people have documented that experiencing feelings like curiosity, hope, laughter, and wonder seems to make people more resilient to illness and injury. In fact, people who experience positive emotions on a more frequent basis are not only happier; they also live ten years longer. And along the way, they get fewer colds, experience fewer headaches, show less inflammation in the body, feel less pain, and have lower rates of cardiovascular disease. Emotions linked to stronger social connections—such as gratitude and love— seem to be especially powerful drivers of better health and longevity.[7]

Happier people are healthier not just because they don't have health problems to worry about, but also because, as research shows, positive emotions provide protection. People who experience more positive emotions re-cover faster from whatever illnesses and injuries they do suffer—and are better able to avoid chronic conditions like high blood pressure and high blood sugar that wear down health over time.[8]

What accounts for this mind-body connection? Dr. Fredrickson's psy-chophysiology lab was the first to figure it out: the vagus nerve, which con-nects the mind to so many important organs in the body, is the most likely candidate for what mediates the relationship between emotions and physi-cal health. For many years, researchers have observed that people with a stronger vagal nerve seem to have more control over their emotions and to experience more positive emotions daily. This fact, combined with decades of research on the relationship between vagal tone and physical resilience, convinced Dr. Fredrickson that the vagus nerve was the missing link be-tween positive emotions and better health.

This hunch quickly paid off: in a series of studies, she and her colleagues demonstrated that interventions designed to increase positive emotions (like the power-ups described in this chapter) directly improved the health of the vagus nerve, which in turn improved the RSA numbers that represent the body's resilience to stress. Not only that, but the stronger the vagus nerve became, the better able participants were to feel and provoke positive emo-tions on a daily basis.[9] This created what Dr. Fredrickson refers to as an "upward spiral dynamic" between positive emotions and physical resilience. Improving your vagal tone makes it easier for you to have positive emotional reactions to everyday life events, and with every positive emotion you feel, your vagus nerve gets stronger. This is why measuring the positive emotions you feel daily turns out to be such a valid and effective alternative measure of vagal tone.[10]

Now that you know how it works, let's measure *your* vagal tone with a quest inspired by the technique used in Dr. Fredrickson's lab.

## QUEST 19: What's Your Number?

To calculate your positive emotion ratio, let's do a quick count of all the emotions you've felt since you woke up today. (If you just woke up, think about yesterday instead!)

**What to do:** Take a look at the following list of emotional experiences. If you've felt this emotion today, put a check mark by it.

If you felt it *really* strongly, or for a very long time, and not just for a fleeting moment, feel free to put two, three, four, or even five check marks by it. For example, if you finished a big project this morning and felt extremely proud about it, you might decide that just one check mark by "pride" isn't enough to represent how you feel—maybe it's worth two or three. Or if you spent most of the morning *really* angry about a serious injustice you personally experienced, it might be worth five check marks by anger. If the feeling was mild or fleeting, one check mark is fine.

## POSITIVE EMOTIONS

Amusement, laughter

Pride, accomplishment

Love for someone else

Interest, curiosity

Hope, optimism

Inspiration, motivation

Peacefulness, serenity

Awe, wonder

Gratitude, thankfulness

Excitement, energy

Connection, being part of something bigger than myself

Joy, bliss

Pleasure, contentment, satisfaction

Surprise (positive)

Looking forward to something

Savoring a pleasant memory

## NEGATIVE EMOTIONS

Anger

Boredom

Depression

Disgust

Embarrassment

Fear

Guilt

Frustration

Hatred for someone else

Hopelessness

Sadness

Shame

Dissatisfaction

Loneliness

Dread or anxiety about
something in the future

Rehashing a negative experience

**Scoring:** Count up all the check marks by a positive emotion (PE). This is your PE total. Then count up all the check marks by a negative emotion (NE). This is your NE total. Now divide your PE by your NE. This is your positive emotion ratio. For example, if you have six check marks by positive emotions and four check marks by negative emotions, your ratio would be 6/4, or 1.5.

*Tip:* If you find you have a hard time remembering how you felt over the past twenty-four hours, Dr. Fredrickson recommends that you keep a log of your activity for the *next* twenty-four hours. Write down everywhere you go, what you do, and who you talk to. At the end of the day, go back through the list and use it to help you recall any emotions you might have felt. This option requires more work but it has the benefit of being more accurate.[11]

Now that you know your positive emotion ratio, what does it mean?

Generally speaking, you want more positive emotions than negative emotions—and the *higher your ratio, the stronger your vagal tone*. If your ratio is 1:1 or lower (meaning you have as many or more negative emotions as positive ones), you're more vulnerable to stress and less likely to experience post-traumatic or post-ecstatic growth. If your ratio is higher than 1:1, you're probably already experiencing significant resilience, but raising your ratio to 2:1, 3:1, or more will make you stronger.

To give you an idea of how your positive emotion ratio can relate to positive life outcomes and resilience to stress, consider these findings from scientific studies:

- Marriages thrive when couples rate their personal interactions as having a positive emotion ratio of 5:1. Couples who rate their interactions closer to a 1:1 ratio, however, more often than not will separate or divorce.[12]
- People who are suffering from clinical depression tend to report positive emotion ratios of 1:1. After successful treatment, their ratios typically rise to between 2:1 and 4:1.[13]
- Employees who calculate their own positive emotion ratios between 3:1 and 4:1 are evaluated by their employers as being more creative and effective at work.[14]
- Cancer patients who report a positive emotion ratio of higher than 1:1 coped with stress better in a variety of ways, experiencing less depression, denial, guilt, and suicidal ideation. (But no significant benefits were observed for increasing the ratio beyond 3:1.)[15]
- Civilians exposed to missile attacks who had a baseline positive emotion ratio of 2:1 or higher were less vulnerable to anxiety, depression, and post-traumatic stress disorder.[16]
- Seniors who increased their positive emotion ratio over a two-year period subsequently experienced less negative stress and felt more in control over aging-related problems. Seniors who had a high positive emotion ratio also suffered fewer declines in attention and memory.[17]

Understand that positive emotion ratios are not precise mathematical formulas. You can't calculate your resilience to stress with the exactness of the circumference of a circle or the boiling point of a liquid. At the same time, myriad studies show that having more positive emotions, on average, than negative emotions is highly beneficial. And if you can have double, triple, or even quadruple, you may benefit increasingly. But there is no optimal or ideal number you're trying to reach. There's no magic tipping point at which your life will go from very difficult to full of joy, good health, and success.

Instead, think of your positive emotion ratio as a baseline you can maintain or build on, if necessary. If you want to increase your resilience to stress and improve your chances of experiencing post-traumatic or post-ecstatic growth, simply increase your ratio. Whether you're increasing your number from 1 to 2, or 2.5 to 3, or even just 3 to 3.1, you'll strengthen your vagal tone—and as a result, you'll experience a wide range of mind and body benefits.

So why are power-ups such an important tool for increasing your positive emotion ratio and strengthening vagal tone? Interestingly, Dr. Fredrickson's lab has found that trying to directly decrease the number of negative emotions you feel provides virtually *no* benefit. People with high vagal tone experience just as many negative emotions daily as people with low vagal tone—in fact, some research suggests they may feel even more. The difference between high and low vagal tone is in the number of positive emotions you can pile up to balance out and offset the negative emotions. This is good news, because it's much easier to find little ways to feel happy and connected than it is to block or prevent negative emotions entirely.

The research also shows that when it comes to positive emotion, frequency is more important than intensity.[18] Little positive things matter and pile up. You don't have to make major improvements in your life or experience huge bursts of powerful, all-consuming positive emotion to increase your resilience. Instead, the most effective strategy is to collect as many microbursts of positive emotion as you can throughout the day.

. . .

When I was recovering from my concussion, power-ups gave me control, even on the darkest days, to do something, *anything*, to help me get stronger. When I look back at that difficult time, I credit using power-ups as the most important and effective step I took to break free of the cycle of anxiety and depression.

Here are other SuperBetter players talking about their favorite ways to quickly boost resilience—and what power-ups have meant to them.

---

### *How to Power Up: Player Favorites*

•————•

The power-ups below have all been rated highly effective by the Super-Better community.

## PHYSICAL POWER-UPS

**Sunshine on your shoulders:** Go outside and let the sun touch your skin for at least five minutes.

"This power-up was recommended to me by a nurse at the hospital where I'm getting treatment for a traumatic brain injury. She said to think of it as harvesting vitamin D from the sun. I have to admit, even on days when it feels like I can't do anything right, this is something I can do."[*] —Devon, twenty-four, whose challenge is to recover from a traumatic brain injury

**Dance break:** Stop whatever you're doing and dance to a favorite song.
"I use this with my six- and eight-year-old girls, especially when they're fighting with each other or giving me a hard time. Whoever is in the worst

---

[*]Clinical trials have shown that increasing vitamin D levels improves brain healing. Activated vitamin D is a neurosteroid; it can stimulate new neuron growth and protect existing neurons.

mood gets to pick the song we all dance to. It's good for our physical health, and it really pulls everyone out of the drama." —Therese, thirty-three, whose challenge is to be a calmer, happier mom

**Make new bacteria friends:** Eat yogurt or pop a probiotic pill to strengthen the ecosystem in your gut. This one's not just about digesting better. The friendly bacteria in yogurt and probiotic supplements communicate directly to your brain through your vagus nerve, sending signals to your brain to secrete anxiety-reducing and mood-boosting neurotransmitters.[19] The higher your vagal tone, the better this power-up works!

"I thought this was a really weird idea at first, but I also know from personal experience that stress and anxiety seem to make my stomach problems worse. So I love the idea that now my intestines can tell my brain to chill out, instead of my brain always telling my intestines to freak out!" —Jackie, forty-five, whose challenge is to end IBS once and for all

## MENTAL POWER-UPS

**Brand-new day:** If you're having a terrible, horrible, no-good, very bad day, get back into bed, pull the covers up, and close your eyes for one minute—then roll out of bed as if you've just woken up for the first time.

"This helps me when I've been procrastinating a lot and I'm starting to beat myself up over it. I feel bad that I've wasted the whole day, so I get back in bed and jump out and ask myself, 'Liz, what do you really want to do today?! Okay, let's go do it!'" —Liz, twenty-three, whose challenge is to figure out what she wants to do with her life

**Stop, challenge, choose:** This is a willpower booster. Stop before eating, and challenge your choice—is there any one thing you could do to make this meal or snack a tiny bit healthier? Now choose to make one small positive difference based on your health or weight-loss goals.

"This is a lot easier than dieting. I make one decision, whenever I eat, to do one small thing better. I put one squirt less of ketchup to cut back on sugar, or I make myself eat one bite of something green before I eat anything else. Instead of focusing on what I shouldn't do, I look at what I can do. It's fun to challenge myself. Plus I feel good about every single meal instead of feeling guilty because I know I did at least one thing right." —Phuong, thirty-one, whose challenge is to get to a healthy weight

**Digital Detox:** Power down and walk away from anything with a screen—your phone, a tablet, a computer, the TV. Don't turn it back on or pick it up for ten whole minutes. See who or what captures your attention in the physical world. (No, you can't cheat and use your phone to check the time! Find a clock!)

"I'm a self-diagnosed workaholic. I'm trying to get superbetter at giving my wife and our son more of my attention at home. I'm doing the digital detox when I walk through the door." —Marco, forty-one, whose challenge is to find a work-life balance

## EMOTIONAL POWER-UPS

**Hug yourself:** Give yourself a hug or a pat on the arm or back, while telling your body what a great job it's doing—just the way it is.

"I feel like I'm always fighting with my body, always mad at it, always disappointed by it. I activate this power-up when I need to take a minute to treat my body the way I would treat a dear friend's, with compassion and kindness and warmth." —Mia, twenty-one, whose challenge is to stay in college with myalgic encephalomyelitis

**Find your voice:** Read one of your favorite poems or quotations out loud.

"I read Maya Angelou's poem 'Still I Rise' out loud. By the time I get to the final three lines, 'I rise, I rise, I rise,' I feel like nothing can stop me." —Terry, forty-eight, whose challenge is to reduce her stress so she can serve her community better

**A mighty act of self-care:** Attend to one simple and easy task that helps you take care of yourself. Brush your teeth or hair, put away one piece of laundry, stretch for one minute, or get dressed in something you love.

"There are some days where this power-up feels like it's literally the only thing I've accomplished. But you know what? That's okay. I'm working on my depression and it feels good to acknowledge when I take care of myself." —Mike, twenty-eight, whose challenge is to manage his depression

## SOCIAL POWER-UPS

**Cheer 'em on:** Pick one person and send them words of encouragement or support about something they're doing or going through today.

"This one's my fave. By the time I pick someone, think of something, and tell them, *I* feel great." —Jack, forty, whose challenge is to be healthier for his family

**Matching socks:** Any time you activate compassion and express care for another human by noticing a commonality between the two of you—you power up! It could be as simple as noticing you're both wearing the same color socks!

"I do this when I find myself feeling aggravated or annoyed or judgmental of someone else. I can always find at least one thing we have in common, like the fact that we're both women so we probably face similar pressures to be thin and beautiful, or we're both with our pups at the vet, so we both want the best for our animal. It doesn't mean we're going to become best friends or anything, but it softens my heart whenever I do it." —Louisa, thirty-eight, whose challenge is to just get superbetter

**Listen to a friends-and-family playlist:** Send an email, or write a social media post, asking all your friends and family to pick one song for you to add to a music playlist. Pick a theme or occasion for the playlist, like a holiday, or "survive my commute," or working out, or just "calm my nerves." Whenever you listen to the playlist, you'll know that it's made up of music handpicked just for you. Make a new playlist whenever you need another musical hug. (*Tip:* You can use a streaming audio service like Spotify or a video-sharing site like YouTube to make your playlist.)

"I asked my friends and family to make me a Good Times playlist to listen to during chemo. I asked them to pick a song that reminded them of one of the best times in their life, and to tell me the story behind it. It gives me something special to think about during treatment, which can last as long as four hours. I felt like I knew them all better whenever I listened to it."
—Lisa, fifty-two, whose challenge is to survive breast cancer

As you're hopefully starting to see, it's easy to brainstorm and collect power-ups. But there is one catch: it's easier to provoke positive emotions when you already have a strong vagus nerve. Consequently, it's *harder* to strengthen your vagal tone when you're not currently experiencing many positive emotions. This is particularly true of power-ups that focus on building emotional and mental resilience.[20]

It's a bit of a catch-22: the happy get happier, and everyone else has a much harder time of it. If your ratio is 1:1 or lower, power-ups that work well for someone with a relatively high positive emotion ratio might not work for you—yet.

But don't worry if you find yourself in this situation. While you may be more resistant to mental and emotional power-ups right now, studies show that physical power-ups (such as exercising, getting good sleep, and consuming omega-3 fatty acids) and social power-ups (such as spending more time with friends and family and participating in a faith community) are still effective for people with low vagal tone.[21] When your ratio goes up, you'll be more responsive and open to positive events and experiences—so a wider range of power-ups will start to work better. In the meantime, if your ratio is currently near or below 1:1, collect and activate as many physical and social power-ups as you can.

. . .

So, the more power-ups, the better? Not quite. There can be too much of a good thing, even when it comes to getting stronger. If your ratio reaches an extreme like 30:1 or higher, researchers caution, it may be an indication of mania—the mental disorder characterized by extreme euphoria and risk-taking activity. (If you already know you're prone to periods of mania, you might consider a rapidly climbing ratio to be an important warning signal.)[22]

More generally, a high ratio could also indicate an absence of negative emotion—which, you might be surprised to know, psychologists also consider a problem. Without any negative emotions at all, you lack sufficient motivation to recognize and deal with problems in your life. Indeed, according to Dr. Fredrickson, a very high PE could be a sign of psychological denial.[23]

If you're feeling virtually no negative emotion in your day, you may be having an unusually good day—or you may just be trying to hide from the bad parts. As you'll see in Chapter 7, it's important to be open to negative experiences and feelings. So if your PE ratio hits the double digits, take a closer look and make sure you're not simply ignoring the difficult stuff.

In the end, is there a positive emotion ratio that is *just too high*? There are no hard and fast numbers that scientists can point to—no tipping point at which power-ups become dangerous or counterproductive. Just be aware that your goal is *not* to keep increasing your positive emotion ratio higher and higher forever. Instead, find a happy range that works for you—it might be 2:1, or it might be 10:1. When you find *your* happy range, you may never want to go any higher—and that's perfectly fine.

Every power-up you collect is a resource you can use to change how you feel, when you need it most. So let's start building those resources—and increasing your control—right now, with a quest.

## QUEST 20: Collect Your First Five Power-ups

The world around you is *full* of power-ups. All you have to do is spot them. So let's start looking.

**What to do:** Collect your first five power-ups. Remember, anything that makes you feel happier, stronger, healthier, or better connected counts as a power-up.

You can collect any of the power-ups already shared in this chapter. Or, if you'd like to personalize your list, here are some brainstorming questions to help you out:

- What song makes you feel powerful?
- What food makes you feel energized?
- Who or what helps you feel calm and relaxed?
- Is there a mantra that makes you feel more motivated?
- What physical activity energizes you?
- What reliably inspires you when you read it or watch it?
- What memory brings you great satisfaction when you recall it for thirty seconds?
- Is there something small you like to do to help others?
- What photo, video, or image always makes you smile?
- Is there a daily habit that makes you feel better when you remember to do it?
- Is there a place or space that you can get to easily that brings you joy or comfort?
- Who is the best person to call, text, write, or visit to get a quick pick-me-up?

**My power-up list:**

1.

2.

3.

4.

5.

**Quest complete:** Congratulations! You've collected your first five power-ups. Eventually you may build up a supercollection of one hundred or more! The bigger your power-up collection, the more control you have every single day to feel better—no matter what stress, pain, or adversity you're facing.

**Bonus quest:** I challenge you to activate one of your five power-ups right now before you continue reading!

Now that you've got your first power-ups, here's how to make the most of them.

**Try to activate at least three power-ups every day.** If it helps, think of it as one in the morning, one in the afternoon, and one in the evening. (If you want to activate more than three a day, by all means, go for it! Power up every single hour, if you need the boost.)

**Keep collecting.** The more power-ups you know how to activate, the stronger you'll get. Collecting power-ups is a mental habit, a way of seeing the world around you. To start developing that mental habit, *challenge yourself to find one new power-up every day for the next week*, and you'll have a total of one dozen at your disposal.

**Trade.** Most SuperBetter players say their favorite power-ups are ones suggested to them by a friend or family member. The easiest way to collect them is to ask this simple question: "What's something you can easily do in five minutes or less that makes you feel happier, healthier, or stronger?" Ask it of as many people as you can.

Use social media to trade and collect even more power-ups. Post one of the brainstorming questions from Quest 20 on Facebook, Twitter, or your favorite discussion forum. Or if you're a visual person, ask friends to show you their favorite power-ups by sharing photos on a platform like Instagram or Pinterest. (Finding out what makes other people in your life feel better is also a great way to boost your social resilience.)

**Always experiment!** Part of the fun of collecting power-ups is discovering new tricks and finding surprising sources of strength. Don't be shy to try a new power-up. You never know what might work for you. If it doesn't make you feel better, no problem—you never have to try it again! Power-ups are a chance to be creative and learn new things. The more open you are to new power-ups, the better.

**Retire power-ups if they're not working for you.** A power-up may not work forever. Pay attention and make sure you're getting the biggest boost possible. If the boost is less than it used to be, you may need to refresh your power song, your mantra, your energy food, or your "always make me smile" photo with a new one.

**Boost all four types of resilience.** Make a point to collect and activate power-ups that help you build up mental, physical, emotional, *and* social resilience. Most people have a blind spot in their daily lives—a type of resilience they're less likely to develop. Figure out what yours is, and make a conscious effort to collect and activate power-ups for that type.

Finally, keep in mind that powering up isn't something you do just to improve yourself. You can share the power with others.

If you have children in your life, powering up is a highly effective way to help them practice emotional regulation and to develop positive habits. The ability to self-provoke positive emotion is an important life skill that, if learned early, builds lasting resilience in children. Studies have shown, for example, that high vagal tone improves attention in school, protects children from parental conflict, and reduces the amount of the inflammation-related stress hormone cortisol they produce during stressful challenges.[24]

Fortunately, most children grasp the concept of real-world power-ups easily, thanks to their ample experience with video games. Here's a story about one SuperBetter player who discovered her young daughter's natural ability to build her own resilience gamefully.

## A SuperBetter Story: The Empowered Daughter

Reva, thirty-six, a self-defense instructor who lives in Phoenix, started playing SuperBetter last year to deal with a mysterious and difficult to diagnose autoimmune illness. She recently wrote me to share her delight that her entire family wanted to get in on the game—particularly her seven-year-old daughter.

"SuperBetter has been so beneficial in getting me through the beginning stages of this chronic illness diagnosis that I haven't been able to stop talking about it for the past several months. My daughter, Aditi, who is very curious, has had so many questions about SuperBetter! I've mostly just told her that it's a game that I play to accomplish my goal of feeling better. I've also explained that unlike the other games we play on our iPhone and iPad, it has specific uses that may be more suited for grown-ups. But she was not going to give up easily!

"Yesterday we took a drive to visit my mom. Her house is a bit of a drive from mine, so I told Aditi that she could bring her iPad. On the way home, her iPad battery died, and while I was recharging it, she asked to play a game on my phone. I could see through my rearview mirror that she was very engaged in her game, but I didn't think to ask what she was playing. I figured it was the usual *Pac-Man*, *Makeup Girls*, or *Fruit Ninja*. It wasn't until we arrived home that she told me she had played SuperBetter. In fact, not only had she played, she had created her own power-ups!

"This week we had a situation where an older boy, who is a friend, cornered her alone and told her that he liked her and had a crush on her. It made her uncomfortable, and she didn't know how to react. We discussed boundaries and how others need to respect them, and to inform a parent or adult if you feel uncomfortable.

"So I was amazed when she showed me the 'Boundaries' power-up she had created, turning the unpleasant incident into an empowering lesson she had learned. ("Boundaries! Say a boy likes you. Does it make you feel weird? Have boundaries! And tell your parents.") She also created a 'Dance' power-up, about one of her favorite activities to stay healthy ("Dance! You should always dance. It is good for your body, and plus you get to dance to your favorite song.") She even included her own pictures from my camera roll!

"I am so impressed by her ability to take the few details I mentioned about the game, primarily in conversation with my husband, and make them useful and relevant to her life, without any direct input from me."

Reva's experience reflects a wider phenomenon: young children today are strikingly fluent in the language and concepts of game play, thanks to the ubiquity of digital games. Aditi's natural ability to turn her own stressful experience into a way to be stronger shows just how easily kids can adopt a gameful mindset to build resilience. You may find that power-ups are a wonderful way to talk to your kids about how to handle stressful situations, and how to be happy and healthy.

There are infinitely many power-ups you can choose for yourself. But I want you to try one more power-up in particular, one that has been scientifically tested and demonstrated to be supereffective. It's called *social reflection*, and it works even for people with extremely low vagal tone. This is important, because as you recall, people with low vagal tone can actually be resistant to many power-ups. Besides physical exercise, social reflection is the *only* power-up proven in studies to boost the vagal tone and positive emotion ratio of people who are suffering from extreme stress, burnout, trauma, or depression—that is, people with a positive emotion ratio of less than 1:1.[25]

Let's learn this power-up right now, with a quest inspired by the research of Dr. Bethany Kok, a scientist at the Max Planck Institute of Human Cognitive and Brain Sciences.

## QUEST 21: Try the Social Reflection Power-up

Social reflection is the *king* of power-ups. It's the one that can boost your resilience no matter how troubled, hopeless, or uninspired you feel.

**What to do:** Shortly before you go to sleep, think about the three social interactions in which you spent the most time today. They could be at home, at work, at school, at church, or in any public or social setting. They might be in person, on the phone, on video chat, or even just an extended conversation by email or text message. They could be interactions with individuals or with a larger group— such as participating in a sports practice, a discussion group, a work team, a fitness class, or a club meeting, or even just sitting in a café, theater, or hall full of other people.

If you spent most of your time alone today, you might think of more fleeting interactions, such as with a cashier at the store or a stranger you made small talk with. Depending on how you spent your day, they might even be three different interactions with the same person. (This often happens to me when I'm working from home, and the only person I speak to or see all day is my husband!)

Okay, have you got your three social interactions in mind? Now think of them *all together* and ask yourself how much you agree with the following statements:

1. During these three social interactions, I felt close to the other person or people.
2. During these social interactions, I felt "in tune" with the other person or people.

Rate your agreement on a scale of 0 to 10, with 0 representing "I completely disagree with this statement" and 10 representing "I agree completely." You should have two numbers after completing this power-up, a number between 0 and 10 for each of the two statements.

**Why it works:** Dr. Kok and her colleagues theorize that reflecting on your social interactions helps in several ways. It gives you an opportunity to savor any positive interactions you had, which increases positive emotions. It helps you identify potential allies for the future, increasing your social resources. And if your social interactions were fewer or less satisfying than you'd like, it gives you the chance to notice that, so you can plan to be more social tomorrow.

**How to use it:** The power of this simple technique comes from repetition. You'll need to activate this power-up **each night for at least three days** before the benefits start to kick in. According to Dr. Kok's research, the biggest impact will occur if you keep up the habit for a month or longer. That's a lot to ask—but for now **make a commitment to try it for three days in a row**.

To make sure you don't forget, *right now* set an end-of-night cal-

endar appointment on your phone or email, or put a Post-it note reminder on your toothbrush or your bedside so you'll be sure to see
it each night. After all, there's no point in collecting a power-up if
you forget to activate it!

### Skills Unlocked: How to Power Up Anytime, Anywhere

- Power-ups are simple positive actions you can take to feel better, stronger, healthier, or more connected anytime, anyplace.
- Power-ups strengthen your vagal tone, which is a physiological measure of how well your heart, lungs, and brain react to stress. The stronger your vagal tone, the more resilient you are—and the more likely you are to experience post-traumatic or post-ecstatic growth.
- You can measure your vagal tone by comparing the number and intensity of the positive and negative emotions you feel in a day. This is your positive emotion ratio. Tracking this ratio over time will help you see the impact of your power-ups on your vagal tone.
- If you're having a very difficult time, and experiencing very few positive emotions on a daily basis, focus on social and physical power-ups until it's easier to activate mental and emotional ones.

# 7

## Bad Guys

### How to Be Gameful Rule 3

Find and battle the bad guys—anything that blocks
your progress or causes you anxiety, pain, or distress.

W e all know how bad guys work in video games—they're the obstacles that force us to be creative and clever, like the relentless
chocolate fountains that block our moves in *Candy Crush
Saga*. They require us to try harder and jump higher, like the ubiquitous
turtles we have to avoid in *Super Mario Bros*. The really tough bad guys
might prompt us to call in a friend for advice or a little backup. (Which first-
time *Minecraft* player hasn't needed some help figuring out how to avoid
those pesky creepers?) Many nondigital games have bad guys, too, even if
we don't call them that: the sand traps in golf, for example, or defenders in
basketball, or the letter J in Scrabble.

Bad guys in everyday life work just the same way—they make things
tougher on us. But in making it harder for us to achieve our goals, bad guys
also help us develop skills and strategies that ultimately make us smarter,
stronger, and faster—so we can achieve bigger goals in the future.

That's why we battle bad guys: to get better. As the poet T. S. Eliot famously wrote, "If you aren't in over your head, how do you know how tall you are?"

This is not just a feel-good sentiment—it is a validated, scientific finding. In order to become happier or healthier, we need what researchers call *psychological flexibility:* the courage to face things that are hard for us. We must be open to failure and negative experiences—not just in games but in everyday life. We must know when to retreat and regroup, until we feel ready to try again.

Living gamefully helps you develop this flexibility. SuperBetter players have battled more than half a million real-life bad guys. And according to our data, SuperBetter players feel better—stronger, happier, more confident, and more optimistic—after reporting a battle, *whether they win or lose.*

Here are just a few of the real-life bad guys battled by SuperBetter players:

"Mrs. Volcano. She erupts inside of me and makes me yell horrible things at my little children and husband who I adore to bits."

"The Elevator Sirens. They call to me seductively whenever I'm trying to be more active and take the stairs. They say, 'You deserve a nice relaxing ride, come to me, come to me.'"

"Lord Impossibility. If I plan anything good, he comes and tells me it's impossible. 'You're not good enough, you have no luck, it's too difficult, you don't have enough money, you never completed any of your plans, you're quitting everything as soon as it calls for diligence. Look around you, can you see any people who can do it? Well, you can, but they are healthier, richer, smarter, younger, older than you, etc.'"

"My Four Devil Foods: pizza, soda, marshmallows, and hot chocolate. It feels really liberating to not worry so much about *all* the food in the world that I shouldn't eat, and just work on battling the four big ones. I already took a Sharpie to the marshmallow bag and drew a scary face on it. Next time I really want a piece of fluffy sugar junk, I will be faced with a *terrible monster that I must destroy...* by not eating it."

"The Regret Parade, in which all the things that I have done in my life that I regret scroll past at random, in my head."

"The Late Night Computersaur and the Late Night TV-saur. These guys are tough. Not only do they strike at night, when I'm most vulnerable to the onslaught of distraction, but they can also battle for several hours at a time. You know they are close when you smell the distinct odor of Netflix and XBox."

"The Sad Nap. That's when I go to bed in the middle of the day because I'm bored or depressed, not because I'm actually tired. They tend to last a long time, and they screw with my sleep later on, which starts a Sad Nap cycle that's hard to get out of."

"The Pain That Doesn't Go Away. I have rheumatoid arthritis that is very difficult to treat. For me, defeating this bad guy doesn't involve making the pain go away, because it hardly ever does. Instead, it means making the day manageable and not using the pain as an excuse to be unhappy."

"Snuff the Tragic Dragon. This is basically just self-pity. But guess what? It's not a big, powerful monster. It's ridiculous, and I can laugh at it."

As you can see, there are all kinds of bad guys: mental, emotional, physical, and social. They can be counterproductive thoughts or bad habits (mental); unpleasant emotions that zap your energy, focus, or motivation (emotional); actions that make you feel unwell, or symptoms that cause you pain or limit your activity (physical); or negative ways of interacting with others that make it harder for you to find and keep allies (social).

In short, a real-life bad guy is anything that tries to stop you from doing what you want or need to do to get superbetter. *Spotting* a bad guy means identifying it as a potential source of trouble or distress. *Battling* a bad guy means experimenting with different strategies for dealing with it effectively. *Succeeding in battle* means not letting it stop you from having a good day or making progress toward your goals.

You'll notice that in all the examples above, the bad guys have names that are worthy of a truly legendary foe. It isn't necessary to get this creative, but it *can* help you spot and battle the bad guys more effectively. As one player explains, "My bad guys all have their own distinct names and identities. Otherwise I feel like I'm swatting the air. Also, the names help separate them from me. It's no longer all the dark stuff I'm carrying around and can't drop."

My roster of bad guys changes constantly. Yours should, too. By regularly confronting your bad guys, you'll eventually get strong enough, smart enough, or skillful enough to vanquish them forever. Something that's a bad guy for you today likely won't be a bad guy for you six months from now.

For example, when I was playing to get superbetter from my concussion, my real-life bad guys included bright lights, crowded spaces, and reading or writing for more than a few minutes at a time. These bad guys triggered my symptoms, so I had to avoid them. But little by little, I built up my tolerance to them, and eventually, my brain healed. Now I no longer have to avoid them. That's one way to vanquish a bad guy: get strong enough that it doesn't bother you anymore.

When I was training for my first marathon, my bad guys included painful blood blisters and throbbing shin splints. The only way to beat these bad guys was to get smarter about training. Instead of giving up or skipping runs, I learned better ways to run and cross-train. (I also learned about wool socks.) That's another way to vanquish bad guys: to be clever and outsmart them.

When I was trying to get pregnant with my husband, it wasn't easy for us. We went through fertility treatment, and I had to do all kinds of things that scared me: inject myself with hormones, get blood drawn every day for weeks, and even have surgery. But these things weren't my bad guys—they were actually positive steps toward my goal. The real bad guys were the thoughts that made me anxious or pessimistic while I took those crucial steps. The biggest bad guy I battled during fertility treatment I nicknamed "Madame Esmeralda"—the psychic in my mind who kept looking into her crystal ball and predicting that everything would go horribly wrong. She never once predicted that everything would go right! So I had to tell Madame Esmeralda to shut up and stop trying to predict the future—it was better for my mind and my body to stay focused on the present. This is yet another way to vanquish a bad guy: learn a new skill to overpower it. My anxiety lowered considerably when I learned to turn off catastrophic thinking (or always expecting the worst)—and I know this had a positive effect on how successfully my body responded to the treatment. (In the end, Madame Esmeralda's predictions all proved wrong—and my husband and I are the proud parents of twin girls!)

In this chapter, you'll learn how to spot your own bad guys and develop the courage to do daily battle against them. You'll practice simple techniques for becoming stronger, smarter, and skillful enough to conquer your bad guys permanently.

To begin, let's introduce you to four of the bad guys that tend to trap and torment SuperBetter players the most.

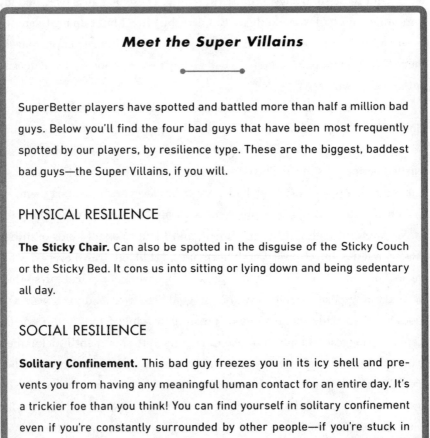

### *Meet the Super Villains*

SuperBetter players have spotted and battled more than half a million bad guys. Below you'll find the four bad guys that have been most frequently spotted by our players, by resilience type. These are the biggest, baddest bad guys—the Super Villains, if you will.

### PHYSICAL RESILIENCE

**The Sticky Chair.** Can also be spotted in the disguise of the Sticky Couch or the Sticky Bed. It cons us into sitting or lying down and being sedentary all day.

### SOCIAL RESILIENCE

**Solitary Confinement.** This bad guy freezes you in its icy shell and prevents you from having any meaningful human contact for an entire day. It's a trickier foe than you think! You can find yourself in solitary confinement even if you're constantly surrounded by other people—if you're stuck in your head, distracting yourself with digital devices, or keeping all your thoughts and feelings to yourself.

## MENTAL RESILIENCE

**The Too-Headed Monster.** You know you're in the clutches of this bad guy when you find yourself making an "I'm too" statement. "I'm too tired to . . . ," "I'm too depressed to . . . ," "I'm too scared to . . . ," "I'm too stupid to . . . ," "I'm too slow to . . . ," "I'm too fat to . . . ," "It hurts too much to. . . ." This kind of statement is usually an excuse to talk yourself out of doing something you really want or need to do to get superbetter.

## EMOTIONAL RESILIENCE

**The Guilty Twin.** This bad guy twists positive feelings of gratitude into negative feelings of guilt. It happens more easily and often than you might expect. According to researchers at UC Berkeley's Greater Good Science Center, guilt is actually gratitude's evil twin emotion.[1] If we feel unworthy of someone else's kindness or forgiveness, we can actually make ourselves feel guilty about something good.

So what should you do if any of these bad guys are lurking in *your* life? We tapped the insights of psychologists, doctors, and researchers at Stanford University, UC Berkeley, Ohio State University, and the University of Pennsylvania to come up with the most effective battle strategies possible.[2] If you recognize any of SuperBetter's biggest Super Villains, try out our recommended battle strategy right now!

**The Sticky Chair strategy:** Battle this bad guy by getting up for a count of five. (For an extra boost, when you get to five, say out loud or think to yourself, "I'm free!") When you're finished counting to five, you can sit or lie back down if you really want to. But once you've escaped the Sticky Chair's clutches, you may find that you want to stay unstuck at least a little while longer!

**The Solitary Confinement strategy:** To battle this bad guy, blast through the isolation with a warm ray of human contact: send someone a "thinking of you" message, start a conversation, give a stranger a smile, pick up the phone and tell someone what you're feeling, give someone a high-five or a hug. Or leave your digital devices at home and just go somewhere you can be around other people without distraction.

**The Too-Headed Monster strategy:** Whatever your excuse—as an experiment, just for today, get rid of the "too" and *do it anyway*! Instead of saying, "I'm too tired to cook dinner," say "I'm tired, *and* I'm going to cook a healthy dinner anyway." Instead of saying "I'm too depressed to get out of bed," say, "I'm depressed, *and* I'm going to get up and dressed anyway." Instead of saying, "I'm too slow to run a 5K," say, "I'm slow, *and* I'm going to go running today anyway." When you do battle using this strategy, you'll figure out that *you don't have to change how you feel or what you think about yourself* to do something good that makes you stronger, better, happier, or healthier. So don't let your "too-headed monster" stop you. Acknowledge it, and do whatever you want anyway.

**The Guilty Twin strategy:** If you find yourself feeling guilty, ask yourself: are you actually twisting profound gratitude about the good someone else has brought to you, or the forgiveness they've shown you? If so, then remind yourself that you *are* worthy! And to ease your guilt, thank that person. Thank them for their time, their effort, their support, their thoughtfulness—or just thank them for valuing and loving you enough to forgive your mistake. Express your gratitude—in writing or in person—to turn the "guilty twin" back into its better half.

Although bad guys like these four Super Villains can seem like nothing but trouble, you benefit enormously from confronting them. Every time you battle a bad guy, you increase your awareness of what's really standing in your way, and you broaden your repertoire of potential strategies. These are precisely the two key components of psychological flexibility: increased awareness of the difficult stuff and a willingness to experiment with different responses to it.[3]

As you will recall, psychological flexibility is the courage to face things that are hard for us. Developing this courage is a two-part process.

First, you must increase your awareness, or *mindfulness*, of anything that might block your progress or cause you pain, difficulty, or distress. Being mindful means paying close attention to negative thoughts, feelings, and experiences. You don't try to deny, avoid, or suppress them. Paying attention to the negative helps you deal with it more effectively. After all, you can't solve a problem or change a behavior if you pretend it doesn't exist.

Over time, mindfulness also helps you accept that negative sensations and experiences are a natural part of everyday life. This includes the inevitable temporary setbacks and failures you'll face as you try to overcome tough challenges and achieve meaningful goals. Eventually, you'll start to notice that bad guys, no matter how powerful or persistent, do not necessarily prevent you from having a good day or leading a meaningful and satisfying life. This realization is a pivotal step toward post-traumatic or post-ecstatic growth. Studies show that transformative personal growth is much more common among individuals who are both mindful and accepting of the negative as a part of their daily life.[4]

Then, once you're fully aware of your bad guys, you can work toward developing multiple strategies for dealing with them. Psychologists call this having a *flexible response*. Instead of relying on a single dominant strategy, you develop many ways to respond effectively. You vary your response based on which bad guy you're facing, what resources you have available at the moment, and whatever else might be compromising your motivation, physical ability, or attention.

Having multiple strategies makes you much more resilient to setbacks. When a bad guy takes you by surprise, or when multiple bad guys gang up on you at the same time, you'll be much more agile and flexible in your response. And if one strategy doesn't work, you're less likely to give up entirely. You'll simply pay attention, change your strategy, and keep trying to make progress. The more strategies you have, the more likely you are to keep taking action toward your goals, no matter how much difficulty, unpleasantness, or uncertainty you face.

*Spot the bad guys* and *Battle the bad guys* are gameful descriptions of these two essential mental strengths. When you spot a bad guy, you're being mindful of the negative. When you battle a bad guy, you're developing a flexible response.

So why do these two mental strengths matter? Studies have shown that people with greater psychological flexibility experience fewer psychological problems, more positive emotions, greater career success, closer relationships, and an overall higher quality of life.[5] People with psychological flexibility have also been shown to cope better and recover faster from all kinds of injuries, illnesses, griefs, economic difficulties, career setbacks, and personal losses.[6]

On the other hand, a psychological *inflexibility*—or a tendency to ignore, deny, or avoid things that are hard for us—is linked to worse coping and longer recovery times, and higher rates of self-harm and addiction.[7] Psychological inflexibility also increases the chances of developing post-traumatic stress disorder after a traumatic experience.[8]

To understand how one simple mental strength can make such a huge difference in outcomes, it helps to take a closer look at one of the most interesting areas of research related to psychological flexibility: the development of chronic back pain and disability after an acute back injury.

Researchers have known for years that some people who experience acute back pain recover successfully and lead full lives, while others experience ongoing pain that eventually leads to disability. Surprisingly, it's *not* the type or severity of back injury, or the degree of pain initially experienced, that best predicts who will recover and who will continue to suffer. Instead, it's the psychological flexibility of the patients at the time of their injury.[9]

The more psychologically flexible a patient is, the faster they return to work, the more they exercise, and the fewer pain symptoms they report over time. But the less flexible they are, the less likely they are to ever return to full employment, and the more likely it is that back pain will continue for months or even years to interfere with their ability to lead full lives.

Two decades' worth of pain and psychology studies help explain this phenomenon. It turns out that a fear of pain, discomfort, or failure can cause people who are ill or injured to enter a downward spiral of withdrawal from ordinary activity. In an effort to avoid triggering pain or experiencing failure, they severely limit the actions they take—avoiding physical activity, travel, or work, for example. This can be a helpful and natural reaction at first. But if these self-imposed limits are not challenged and tested often, they become artificial barriers to full living. Individuals become less likely to challenge themselves and therefore less likely to discover that they have, in fact, gotten stronger or can still do things that are important to them even while in pain.

To compound the potential downward spiral, restricting daily activity gives individuals more time and attention to pay to their physical symptoms. This can lead them, quite understandably, to become even more convinced that their injury or illness is so severe as to require *further* restricting activity.[10] This has been shown to be true not only for back pain but also for migraines, chronic fatigue syndrome, fibromyalgia, irritable bowel syndrome, chronic anxiety, and many other potentially debilitating chronic conditions.[11] In all these cases, avoiding pain and failure leads to more suffering and disability, not less.

The only way to avoid this kind of downward spiral, clinical psychologists have shown, is to stay fully engaged with your goals and your life, even when you're facing extremely negative thoughts, feelings, or experiences.

In other words, you have to acknowledge and battle your bad guys. You can't ever let them persuade you to give up or to stop looking for ways to lead a good life.

The biggest Super Villian I ever faced was the suicidal thoughts I had during my concussion recovery. They were persuasive and persistent, and I had never dealt with anything quite like them before. It took me almost a week to recognize that these suicidal thoughts weren't just fleeting feelings—that something was happening in my brain, that some flip had been switched, and these thoughts were getting stronger and not going away.

I remember telling my husband, "I don't want you to freak out, but I keep hearing this voice in my head that I should kill myself." I was able to recognize the seriousness of this enough to want to talk about it. "I don't actually want to kill myself," I promised him. "But I keep having these thoughts. I'm trapped in this dark place, and I don't know how to get out."

By the time I became Jane the Concussion Slayer, I realized I needed to actually do something about the problem. So I asked my husband to do an Internet search for scientific articles about concussions and suicidal thoughts. Was this common? I wanted to know. If so, how long would it last? What should I do about it?

Within minutes, we found an article that described suicidal ideation as extremely common in traumatic brain injuries—up to one in three people with a concussion will go on to have suicidal thoughts. It's a complication of the altered brain chemistry that occurs while the brain is trying to heal itself. It typically passes, the researchers wrote, in a few weeks or months.

I can't remember another time in my life, before or after, when I have felt more relief than I did in that moment. I instantly saw my suicidal thoughts for what they were: not a rational reaction to my circumstances, not an option I should seriously consider, but rather merely a side effect of my brain trying to heal.

I remember saying to my husband, "It's not me, it's just a symptom!" I realized I didn't have to believe the voice in my head telling me to kill myself, because it didn't represent my true thoughts or feelings. It wouldn't be easy, but I would have to tough it out for a few more weeks or months and let my brain heal itself. I didn't have to fix the suicidal thoughts. I just had to acknowledge them and wait for them to pass.

The truth was that I wanted to live *and* my brain was going to tell me I wanted to die. I held this contradiction in balance until my brain healed and the thoughts went away. I didn't know it at the time, but what saved me was the strength of psychological flexibility.

N ow that you know what psychological flexibility is and why it's so important, let's talk about how to measure and increase it.

Researchers have developed several scientific questionnaires to measure psychological flexibility; the Acceptance and Action Questionnaire is the most popular.[12] It tests your willingness to have negative thoughts, feelings, and experiences while remaining committed to your most important goals.

How flexible are you right now? Let's find out! For your next quest, I've selected some of the most important items on the Acceptance and Action Questionnaire. (If you'd like to take the entire forty-nine-question inventory, check out the reference in this endnote for a link to an online version.[13]) Let's see which items you agree with—and which mental muscles still need to be stretched!

## QUEST 22: Touch Your Mental Toes!

Measuring your psychological flexibility isn't quite as easy as bending over and touching your toes. But it can be done!

**What to do:** Take a moment now to see how many of the following statements from the Acceptance and Action Questionnaire you wholeheartedly agree with. If you're not sure about a statement, skip it.

- It's okay to feel depressed or anxious sometimes.
- I take action on a problem, even when I fear I may fail or get it wrong.
- I don't avoid situations that make me feel nervous.
- It's okay if I remember something unpleasant.
- I can move toward important goals, even if I don't feel good about myself.
- I don't have to get rid of every scary or upsetting image that comes to my mind.
- I would rather achieve my goals than avoid unpleasant thoughts and feelings.

How many of these statements did you wholeheartedly agree with? If you agreed with *at least one*, good news—you already have some psychological flexibility, and you can work to increase it. Every time you spot and battle a bad guy, without judging yourself negatively, you're stretching it just a little further.

If you didn't agree with any of them, don't worry. By identifying and engaging with your bad guys on a daily basis, you'll be doing what it takes to increase your acceptance of negative experiences while taking action toward your goals.

And if you already agreed with every statement on this list, congratulations—you are tackling your SuperBetter challenge with extreme psychological flexibility! Battling bad guys will help you stay flexible and take full advantage of the strength you already have.

*Tip:* Copy this list and put it in a place where you can read it every day to remind yourself of the mental strengths you're trying to build. (If you really want to stretch yourself, read the list out loud once a day like a mantra.) Pay special attention to the statements you *don't* already agree with wholeheartedly. These are the areas where you can improve the most. Be sure to test yourself again after a couple of weeks of battling bad guys—you'll almost certainly see your flexibility growing.

Now that you have a better sense of how much psychological flexibility you're starting with, let's put it to use—and start taking the gameful actions that will help you increase these crucial mental strengths.

As you know, the first step toward psychological flexibility is greater awareness, or mindfulness. When you're mindful, you have the ability to observe and describe specific things that are causing you distress or difficulty.

Every time you spot and name a bad guy, you're building this skill. So let's start increasing your mindfulness right now—with a bad-guy-spotting quest!

## QUEST 23: *Spot Three Bad Guys*

If you want to get superbetter, you can't hide from the bad guys. You have to spot them and look them squarely in the eye, so you can figure out how to battle them more effectively.

Remember, a bad guy is any habit, symptom, thought, feeling, or behavior that makes it harder for you to get superbetter.

**What to do:** Create your bad guy list. Did you recognize any of the bad guys already shared in this chapter? If so, add them to your lineup now.

If you'd like to **hunt down a few new bad guys,** here are some brainstorming questions to help you out:

- What habit do you want to break?
- What distracts you from getting things done?
- What causes you physical pain or discomfort?
- What makes you nervous or uncomfortable?
- What zaps your energy?
- What thought or feeling runs through your mind that makes you question your goals or abilities?
- What has a doctor or therapist recommended you do less of, or avoid?
- What makes you feel stressed out, if you let it get to you?
- What symptoms make your day harder for you?
- What moods make you want to just stay home and do nothing?
- What triggers are you trying to steer clear of?
- What behavior would you like to stop?

**My bad guy lineup:**

1.

2.

3.


**Quest complete:** Well done! You've identified three of your biggest bad guys. Just by naming them, you've taken a huge step toward neutralizing their power.

*Tip:* Many SuperBetter players find that giving their bad guys a silly or creative name helps them tackle them with a more positive mindset. But you don't have to give your bad guys clever names—just identifying them is a huge accomplishment.

You've got some bad guys in your sights. Now let's talk about how to battle them effectively, with flexible response.

In order to ensure that you always have a purposeful and positive action to take in response to a bad guy, you'll need to prepare and experiment with multiple strategies. But where should you start?

I've spent three years working with and studying SuperBetter players, trying to figure out the most effective strategies for vanquishing bad guys. I've learned that there are five potential ways to successfully battle any bad guy. You can Avoid, Resist, Adapt, Challenge, or Convert.

Let's look at each strategy one at a time, with the help of some examples from experienced SuperBetter players. Keep in mind that the most successful SuperBetter players experiment with *all* five strategies before deciding which ones work best for particular bad guys.

## 1. Avoid

This is the most straightforward strategy. If it's a bad habit, you try not to do it. If it's a symptom of pain or illness, you try not to feel it. If it's an unpleasant or counterproductive thought, you try not to think it. Here's an example of how it works:

*Bad guy:* The first bite.

*Avoid it strategy:* Don't take the first bite!

"I'm trying to lose weight. I tell myself I'll have just one bite of something I'm not supposed to eat. Before I know it, I've eaten a ton. But if I don't start, I don't have to stop!" —Michelle, forty-five.

Although avoidance is the easiest strategy to understand and adopt, it's also—perhaps surprisingly—the *least* useful. That's because it's impossible to always avoid negative thoughts, feelings, or experiences. And no one has perfect willpower. If it's in your control to avoid something, and there are no personal costs to avoiding it, by all means try this strategy. But you will absolutely want and need to develop additional strategies so you can make progress and have a good day even when you slip up, or when you're simply unable to avoid the inevitable pains and difficulties of a full and meaningful life.

## 2. Resist

Resisting is a way to actively wrestle with the bad guy and try to stop it in its tracks. If you have an unhelpful thought, you try to change it. If you're in pain, you try to alleviate it. If you're isolating yourself from others, you try to connect. If you're procrastinating, you leap into action. Here's an example:

*Bad guy:* Thinking constantly about little things that go wrong, instead of moving on.

*Resist it strategy:* Spend thirty seconds doing something productive, to interrupt the thought cycle.

"When something goes wrong, I just can't let it go. I've been trying this strategy, and it's working for me. I tell myself I only have to spend thirty seconds being productive. Usually that's enough to get me out of the stew. But even if I go right back to sitting around feeling sorry for myself, at least I've done one thing." —Jason, twenty-five.

The resist strategy is much more powerful than simply trying to avoid a bad guy. When you resist a bad guy, you use your unique skills and strengths to prevent the bad guy from having too much of a negative impact. This strategy works even when you can't control your circumstances.

It's important to resist bad guys without judging yourself negatively. It's not your fault that a bad guy appeared; bad guys appear to everyone, every day. Instead, congratulate yourself for having the mindfulness to spot the bad guy at work and the courage to confront it directly.

## 3. Adapt

Adapting means making a significant change, or finding a long-term solution to the bad guy. You might not be able to avoid or resist the bad guy when it gets you, but you may be able to come up with a clever or creative work-around that massively limits its ability to affect you.

*Bad guy:* Forgetting to take my medication.

*Adapt to it strategy*: Set three daily reminder alerts on my phone, for seven, eight, and nine p.m.

"I have a new prescription for my depression. I keep 'forgetting' to take it, which I think is just me avoiding making a commitment to seeing whether this drug will actually help me or not. This strategy gives me three chances to take my pill. If I decide not to, at least I've consciously made the decision not to take it and not just halfheartedly 'forgotten' about it. This strategy was suggested to me by one of my allies. With three alarms, there is basically no way that I will just 'forget' to take my pill anymore, so I have definitely vanquished this bad guy." —Cliff, thirty-three.

Other people are a great resource for coming up with adapt strategies— ask around. It's as simple as saying, "If you had this problem, what would you do to solve it?"

## 4. Challenge

Challenging a bad guy means asking yourself: Is this actually bad for me? Is it possible that I don't have to make this feeling or thought or habit go away before I can lead a happy, healthy, meaningful life?

*Bad guy:* No self-confidence.

*Challenge it strategy:* Ask yourself: "So what if I lack self-confidence? Does it really matter?"

"My biggest fear in life right now is that I won't be able to complete my college education and get a good job. I have full-on panic attacks about it. I'm full of self-doubt, and I lack the confidence to believe that I can actually do it. But my allies are helping me think about it differently. Maybe I worry so much because I really care. It's not necessarily a bad thing. It shows how motivated I am. Also, I do want to be more confident in life. But having doubts or fears doesn't have to stop me. I can still show up to class. I can keep applying for internships. I think that taking steps toward my goal is more important right now than fixing how I feel." —Julian, twenty.

This is a strategy you should adopt early and often. Be open to the possibility that your bad guys have less power or influence over you than you thought. Something that made you feel nervous or unwell in the past may be perfectly fine today. Or if something always makes you feel stressed, anxious, exhausted, or physically uncomfortable, can you simply acknowledge those feelings and accept them? Do you really need to feel calm, or rested, or pain-free to pursue your goals? This is the single most powerful kind of psychological flexibility you can achieve. It's the freedom to keep important commitments and pursue your daily dreams, regardless of whether you can lessen pain, discomfort, and distress or eliminate them from your life.

## 5. Convert

Converting means finding a way to turn your bad guy into a power-up. For example, if you're feeling pain, it could help you experience more compassion for others who are in pain. If you're feeling angry, you could use it as a source of energy and channel it into something productive. Can you imagine any situation in which having your bad guy around would *help* you instead of hurting you?

*Bad guy:* Addiction to drama.

*Convert it strategy:* Be inspired by other people's drama to do better myself.

"I keep getting into friendships and relationships with people who bring all kinds of drama into my life. This distracts me from putting my time and energy into my own plans. Eventually, I want to bring more positive people into my life. But some people are in my life for good no matter what. They're family. I can't change them, but I can get inspired by them to do better and be better. They are inspiration to develop my own drama-free qualities, like patience and forgiveness." —Therese, thirty-six.

Converting a bad guy into a power-up isn't always easy, but it's worth the extra effort. It's the most profound stretch you can make in your psychological flexibility.

## A SuperBetter Story: The Dream Warrior

Mia, twenty-nine, is proud to call herself a survivor.

At twenty-six, she escaped a violent and abusive marriage. But years of physical abuse and sexual assault had left her in a constant state of high alert, always full of adrenaline and certain she was in danger. She found herself socially isolated and, understandably, had a hard time trusting new people. Her therapist diagnosed her with post-traumatic stress disorder.

Mia was determined to reclaim her life. With the support of her therapist, and in addition to regular counseling, she started playing SuperBetter to work through her symptoms of PTSD. During this time, she learned as much as she could about the disorder, not only to help herself but also to help others. She started a blog to encourage other victims of domestic violence to seek safety.

She was making great progress, but one bad guy still haunted her. In life, she was a survivor—no doubt about it. But in her dreams, she was still a victim. As she explained on her blog: "I have nightmares almost every night about being attacked. Last night I dreamed that a stranger attacked me in my home and was trying to kill me. The nightmares are so intense, they feel real. I often wake up screaming."

Mia declared nightmares her number-one bad guy. And she started asking allies for help. Over the next few weeks, she started experimenting with different strategies.

One of the first suggestions she received from an ally was to learn lucid dreaming. "The idea is that you train yourself to recognize when you are dreaming. So when you are asleep and suddenly you realize, 'Hey wait this is a dream,' then you have the power to change what you are dreaming about."

Mia took this idea to her therapist, who gave her concrete tips for learning to control her nightmares. She learned a simple exercise called Alternative Endings. Here's how it works: During the daytime, you think of a scenario that frequently occurs in your nightmares—for example, being chased by a dangerous man. While you're wide awake, you vividly imagine alternative endings to this scenario. You might imagine your pursuer getting smaller and smaller, or slower and slower, until he is no threat to you at all.

Over the next six weeks, Mia got better and better at stopping the nightmares in progress. "I've always been a vivid dreamer, I just never really realized how much I could influence the dreams. I still have dreams with disturbing things, but they don't jar me like the nightmares. Taking control of my dreams consciously has really helped."

But Mia also realized that while lucid dreaming was a good way to *adapt* to the problem, it wasn't a total cure. The nightmares sometimes were harder to control, and she still occasionally woke up sweating, crying, and shaking. She needed to be flexible in how she battled them—so she decided to try out a challenge strategy.

To challenge her nightmares, she asked herself, "What if they aren't all bad?" She played with a new way of thinking: "Maybe nightmares are just reminders so we don't get too comfortable and not alert about the bad things that could happen to us. Nightmares are just my brain's way of understanding and dealing with trauma and healing. They're not trying to torment me. They're trying to help me." Although this cognitive reappraisal didn't stop the nightmares, it helped Mia stop beating herself up for having them. More important, it gave her a way to look for possible benefits from nightmares—a previously unthinkable idea. If her nightmares were just a reminder, could she use them to change her waking behavior in a positive way?

One day she updated her allies: "I've been going along fine for the past couple months, and then last night I had a terrible nightmare, one of the ones where I wake up bawling my eyes out and screaming. I was dying in my nightmare, blood all over the place. I was in a whole hell of a lot of pain, and no one was around to help me. I felt so much remorse for being alone dying with no one to help me."

Using her new strategy, Mia decided to treat this terrible dream like a helpful reminder. What important message could it have for her? "I've been feeling really isolated from my friends lately," she realized, "and I think that's what this is about." She put aside the haunting imagery of the dream and embraced the important insight instead. The next day she made it a point to reach out to her brother and to a friend. "I do need more social support, and I felt so much better after I took the step to reach out."

By taking a positive cue from a terrible nightmare, Mia was able to convert a bad guy into a power-up. Today Mia still uses all her favorite strategies—resist, challenge, and convert—and as a result, she feels happier and braver. "When I have a nightmare, I no longer feel like I lost the battle. I may not be able to prevent a bad dream. But I'm always able to triumph, whether it's during the dream or after. And best of all, I can share what I learned about my bad guys with others who are facing them, too. That's truly been the best part of getting superbetter."

Now that you know all five potential ways to engage a bad guy, let's put that knowledge into action.

## QUEST 24: Develop a Battle Plan

Let's see how far you can stretch your psychological flexibility.

**What to do:** Pick one of your bad guys. Got it? Good.

Let's **develop a battle plan** for your bad guy that includes all five potential strategies: Avoid, Resist, Adapt, Challenge, Convert.

For each strategy, try to **think of just one thing** you could do to prevent this bad guy from ruining your day or blocking your progress.

If you find yourself stuck on a strategy, don't worry. Just do your best. If you need ideas, ask a friend or family member for their advice. You can also come back later and add more strategies. You'll have more success with this quest if you keep thinking about it, mulling it over in the back of your mind for a day or so.

**Examples:** To help you out, I've included responses from another SuperBetter player who successfully completed this quest. Liz is a thirty-two-year-old teacher whose challenge is defeating insomnia. The bad guy she chose for this quest is the White Night, or as she describes it: "A long, endless night where I lie sleepless in bed until morning."

## STRATEGY 1: AVOID

What one thing could you do to prevent this bad guy from making an appearance in your life today? *Liz says: "To try to avoid a White Night tonight, I could have zero caffeine after nine a.m."*

## STRATEGY 2: RESIST

What one thing could you do to minimize the impact of this bad guy, once it makes an appearance? *Liz says: "I can do stretches in bed to occupy my mind and relax my body. Or, I can take extra care to support my immune system the next day, since when I miss sleep, I often get sick. I could take vitamin C and wash my hands more often."*

## STRATEGY 3: ADAPT

What one thing could you do to work around or solve the problem of this bad guy once and for all? *Liz says: "Driving while exhausted is one of my biggest concerns. I don't want to get in an accident because I can't think clearly or stay awake. Maybe a short-term solution is to take a bus part of the way to work. This would basically eliminate one of my biggest fears around not getting any sleep. I will definitely try this for at least a few days and see if it makes this problem less of an issue."*

## STRATEGY 4: CHALLENGE

What one thing could you do to prove that this bad guy has less power over you than you think? *Liz says: "I guess the best way to challenge my anxiety about not sleeping would be to have a really good and productive day, the day after not getting any sleep. The next time I have a White Night, I'll make an extra effort to activate a bunch of power-ups and get at least one important thing done off my to-do list. If I show myself I can be strong even after a sleepless night, maybe I won't panic so much next time."*

## STRATEGY 5: CONVERT

How could you turn this bad guy into a power-up? *Liz says: "I have to get really creative here, because I really hate White Nights! But let's say I start a list of things that I only do in the middle of the night. So when I can't sleep, I can get up and cross something off my middle-of-the-night to-do list. I could put reading mystery novels, organizing my closet, and doing my nails on the list, since these are things I like to do but never have time for. It's not a perfect solution, and I'd much rather sleep, but I guess using the time in the middle of the night is one way to convert it into a source of good. And I've been battling this bad guy for so long, I can definitely see the benefit in trying to think completely differently about it!"*

*Tip:* Every additional strategy increases your psychological flexibility, so keep looking for more ways to battle your bad guy.

Congratulations on developing your first battle plan! As you build awareness of your bad guys and keep trying different actions, you'll find that it becomes easier to be creative in battle.

As in any game, you won't defeat every bad guy. Learning to deal with the occasional defeat is an important part of developing psychological flexibility.

"Don't judge yourself by the moments when you're not as strong as you want to be," advises Dr. Todd Kashdan, a professor of psychology and senior scientist at the Center for the Advancement of Well-Being at George Mason University, "or even as strong as you were yesterday. Allow yourself times where you're going to have mini-breakdowns, where you're going to fail a little bit."

Dr. Kashdan is well known for his research on psychological flexibility and is also a supporter of the SuperBetter method. I recently asked him what he would say to SuperBetter players who feel overwhelmed by their bad guys. "It's not about whether you're vanquished by bad guys in the moment," he replied. "It's over the long haul, when you face a difficult situation. It doesn't matter in any given moment, or even three times in a row, if the bad guys overwhelm you, if you back away. But if you look two or three weeks in a row, and there's a willingness to approach those stressful things, and to absorb some of the stress and discomfort that come with it... that's true psychological flexibility."

Here are some final tips for battling bad guys.

> **Do battle at least once a day.** Take the time, at least once a day, to notice a thought, feeling, habit, or interaction that has the potential to interfere with your health, happiness, or resilience. If you haven't spotted any bad guys today, you're either the world champion of getting superbetter—or, more likely, you're not looking closely enough!
>
> **Always power up after battle.** Whether you've successfully battled your bad guy, or you feel like it got the best of you, make sure to activate at least one power-up to reenergize. The power-up will give you access to positive emotions that can make future battles easier.
>
> **Track your encounters.** What strategies have you tried? Which ones worked? Where and when do the bad guys show up most often? Keep notes in a journal, a spreadsheet, or whatever else comes naturally. Or borrow this creative idea from Linda, a SuperBetter player whose challenge is to become better able to handle stress: "I put sticky notes with my bad guys on the fridge at home to remind me to watch out for them. I mark them with an X whenever they get the best of me. I put a check mark when *I* get the best of *them*. I can see my win-loss record easily by comparing the Xs and the checks. When I get too many Xs, I know I need better strategies."
>
> **Make friends with the bad guys that just won't go away.** You may never completely eliminate a certain pain, anxiety, or stress from your life. If the bad guy isn't going anywhere, just keep experimenting and learn-

ing more about how the bad guys work. As one SuperBetter player, Kel, whose biggest bad guy is procrastination, puts it: "Even if you record thirty losses against a bad guy, thirty days in a row, it is still a victory, because look at you! You keep getting up and fighting again and again. You have learned to recognize that bad guy in every guise and disguise available. That is a hero."

### *Skills Unlocked: How to Spot and Battle the Bad Guys*

- Don't suppress your negative thoughts, feelings, or experiences. Accept them as part of getting stronger and achieving your goals.
- When you spot a new bad guy, consider all the ways you could battle it: avoid it, resist it, adapt to it, challenge it, or convert it into a power-up.
- Experiment with different strategies. Don't reject a possible strategy without trying it at least once. And don't beat yourself up if it doesn't work; instead, learn what you can from the experiment and try again, or move on to the next strategy.
- Use the seven statements from Quest 22 to track your psychological flexibility, and to remind yourself of exactly what it takes to develop courage in the face of bad guys.
- Remember, no day will ever be free of bad guys. Don't wait for a perfect day, or even a good day, to do the things that will make you stronger, happier, and healthier. Keep taking action and making progress toward your goals no matter how many obstacles you encounter today.

# 8

## Quests

### How to Be Gameful Rule 4

Seek out and complete quests—simple, daily
actions that help you reach your bigger goals.

Every hero's journey is made up of countless quests. This is true whether
the journey is found in literature or mythology, in sports movies or
video games. From the epic Greek hero Odysseus to the Chinese warrior Mulan, from boxing underdog Rocky Balboa to Katniss Everdeen in *The
Hunger Games*, every hero must be willing to complete many smaller feats
and missions. Each and every feat makes the hero just a little bit smarter,
stronger, or braver—and more prepared for the bigger challenges ahead.

In the SuperBetter method, a *quest* is not just another item on your to-do
list. It is a purposeful action you take because it has meaning in the context
of a bigger search. Maybe you're searching for better health, or better relationships, or a better job, or a better life for your family. Maybe you're just
searching for your next great adventure. Whatever it is, completing quests
in your everyday life will bring you one step closer to that which you seek.

You've already been tackling quests in this book. Each one has been designed to equip you with new strengths and abilities that can help you on
*your* heroic journey. Here are a few more quests you can tackle right now.
Pick at least one to complete *before* you keep reading.

## QUEST 25: Muscle Up

Need to resist an impulse? Want to steel yourself to do something difficult? Here's how to get instant mental resilience.

**What to do:** Squeeze one or more muscles as hard as you can for five seconds. Any muscle will work—your hand, your biceps, your abs, your buns, your calves. The more muscles you tense up, the more mental strength you'll summon.

**Why it works:** Researchers credit a phenomenon called "embodied cognition" for this powerful mind-body effect. The brain looks to the body for cues. A strong body cues a strong brain, making it easier to summon up more courage or stick to resolutions.[1]

If you like this quest, try it as a way to combat some of your bad guys! It's a perfect addition to any battle plan.

## QUEST 26: Dream On!

Here's an easy way to boost your social resilience—if you dare: tell someone about a dream you had last night.

**What to do:** Simply say, "I had an interesting dream last night!" Describe the dream very briefly, and then ask, "What do you think it means?"

**Why it works:** Research shows that dream sharing and discussion boost trust and increase intimacy between two people. The stranger or more intense your dream, the bigger the benefit.[2]

If you can't remember a dream you had recently, or if your most recent dream is too embarrassing or personal, tell someone about a recurring dream or any particularly memorable dream from the past.

## QUEST 27: Hum for 60 Seconds

If you want to be physically stronger, **hum for 60 seconds.** You can hum any song you want.

**Why it works:** Humming increases the level of nitric oxide in your nose and sinus cavities. The higher your nitric oxide levels, the less inflammation in your nasal cavity—and that means fewer headaches, allergies, colds, asthma attacks, and infections.[3]

It's easier to hum for a full 60 seconds if you pick a specific song—"Yankee Doodle," "I Dreamed a Dream," the *Brady Bunch* theme song. Try not to give up before an entire minute is up!

## QUEST 28: Get Lucky!

Even if you're not superstitious, go ahead and **pick a lucky charm.** Lucky socks, a lucky coin, a lucky pen, a lucky lipstick—it's up to you. When you've chosen your charm, picture it as clearly as you can in your mind—or if you can go get it right now and hold on to it, even better.

Whatever you've chosen, if you really believe that it brings you luck, it *will* make you more likely to succeed. That's because lucky charms make you mentally tougher, more determined, and more ambitious.

**Why it works:** According to scientific studies, believing in a lucky object increases self-efficacy, the feeling "I can do this" (see Chapter 3). Self-efficacy is a powerful state of mind that actually improves your odds of success. When you have more of it, you set higher goals for yourself and persevere longer when things get difficult. So don't be afraid of a little magical thinking![4]

*Tip:* Try not to think about the science behind this quest too much. Research shows that the more you remember that the real power comes from your belief in yourself, and not from the magic object, the less it works. So if you believe at all in good luck, put that belief to good work!

◄►

Why seek out and complete simple quests like these? They help you develop valuable new skills—*and* flex your heroic willpower without wearing it out.

Researchers have figured out that willpower is like a muscle. It gets stronger the more you exercise it—as long as you don't exhaust it.[5] Taking purposeful action throughout the day sparks your motivation and expands your sense of what you're capable of.

It's particularly important to flex your willpower when you're trying to make a big change, or when you're coping with chronic stress, illness, or a traumatic event. Every time you set your mind to do something—and then successfully do it—you remind yourself of the power you have over what you do, think, and feel.

Researchers call this *committed action*—taking small steps each day in accordance with your goals and values, even when it is difficult for you.[6]

Quests can help you commit time and energy to the things that matter to you and that help you most—even if you're tired, or sick, or busy, or depressed. Completing just one quest a day, according to SuperBetter research, can make a significant difference in how happy, healthy, and brave you are. And as you build your willpower muscle, well-being, and sense of purpose, you can tackle bigger quests.

So how do you pick your quests? Quest design is a skill that video game designers learn and practice constantly. Quests must always come at the right time and the right place for the player, so you're virtually guaranteed to succeed. And quests must be interesting! The best quests spark your sense of curiosity and adventure. In this chapter, I'll show you how to design quests for your own life that are as fun and easy to follow as a video game.

I know that a good quest can spark motivation and build hope in even the most difficult times, because I've been there myself.

When I was getting superbetter from my concussion, my usual everyday goals went straight out the window. Work? Exercise? Fun? Forget about it. I was on complete cognitive rest, which meant I couldn't do anything that stimulated my brain: no reading, writing, email, work, or computer time. Even just watching television, playing games, and talking with others brought on severe headaches, so they were out as well. Meanwhile, physical activity of almost any kind triggered vertigo and nausea. I found myself on bed rest, with no way to entertain myself, or be productive, or connect with the world around me. It was hard to imagine *anything* I could do to have a good day. Making things worse, there is no known effective therapy or treatment for postconcussion syndrome, no pill you can take, no therapeutic exercise you can do. "Rest and wait" is the only prescription. I *literally* had nothing to do.

Weeks passed, and nothing got better. Day after day I woke up dreading the endless stretch of time before me. I was bored and lonely. I had never felt so helpless in my life. No matter how badly I wanted to get better, the doctors could not tell me one single thing to do to help my brain heal faster. I was also incredibly anxious, because I wasn't able to work, and my husband had recently lost his job.

Pretty soon a sense of hopelessness set in. Every day was full of pain, nausea, and frustration, without one single positive accomplishment to show for it. I spent hours every day curled up in a ball, weeping—as quietly as I could, because I didn't want to make my husband worry.

Fortunately, after a month of increasing depression and suicidal ideation, my game designer instincts kicked in. I knew that I needed to find *one thing to do each day* to feel a sense of purpose and productivity. If there's nothing to do in a game, no goal to pursue, no further way to make progress, the player will quit. And no matter how strong my suicidal thoughts, I knew deep down that *I did not want to quit*. Even if I couldn't get out of bed, even if I couldn't turn on my computer, I would find *something, anything* to do. I needed a quest. I needed a way to win the day.

At the time, my thinking was quite fuzzy from the brain injury, and I was emotionally beaten down. I had to ask others to help me figure out what my quests should be. So I invited my twin sister Kelly to call me once a day and give me a quest for the next twenty-four hours.

This is the first quest she gave me: "Your bed is near a window, right? I want you to spend some time looking out the window, and tomorrow, tell me if you saw anything interesting. Try to find at least one interesting thing to tell me about." *Look out the window.* This was something I could do from bed, and it didn't require too much thinking. And there was a clear goal: *Keep looking until you see something interesting!*

I'd like to be able to tell you what I saw out my window that day, but honestly I don't remember. My memory from the first few months after my concussion is a bit spotty. What I *do* remember is that that day I felt like I had a purpose. I watched the world from my window. And I looked forward to talking to my sister and telling her that I had succeeded in my quest. And when I did, I felt fantastic. Someone had asked me to do something, and I had done it. I felt triumphant!

Now, I will be the first to admit: on the face of it, looking out the window is not a particularly noteworthy achievement. But it was incredibly meaningful to me. It was the first time in a very long while that I had set my mind to do something and *succeeded*. And I admire and love my sister so much—being able to fulfill a promise that I'd made to her felt wonderful, no matter how small the task.

I didn't know it at the time, but what I was feeling that day was the benefit of taking committed action—or more precisely, the *three* benefits of taking committed action. Taking committed action, you'll recall, means doing at least one thing every day that speaks to your most important goals and values, no matter what obstacles are in your way. Researchers have shown that every time you successfully take committed action, you increase your hope, optimism, and self-efficacy.[7]

Hope, optimism, and self-efficacy are similar strengths, but they differ in important ways.

**Hope** is what you feel when you believe that *a good outcome is possible*. A good outcome might be a positive emotion you want to feel, a goal you want to achieve, a change you want to make, a task you want to accomplish, or a benefit you want to bring to others. If you can imagine any good outcome at all, no matter how unlikely, you have hope. The more different good outcomes you can imagine, the more hope you have.

**Optimism** is what you feel when you believe that *a good outcome is not just possible, it's likely*. As a result, you're willing to set higher goals and put in greater effort to achieve them. You're also more open to trying new things and taking others' advice—two things that often lead to greater success. Of course, it's possible to be *too* optimistic. If you're blindly optimistic, you may put your efforts into a fruitless pursuit, or you may fail to take necessary precautions to prevent a negative outcome. But on the whole, optimism is a valuable source of motivation. And you can easily avoid the downsides of optimism by focusing your time and efforts on simple actions that really are likely to result in success.

**Self-efficacy** is the final piece of the motivation puzzle. Self-efficacy, you'll recall, is that "I can do this!" feeling. When you have high self-efficacy, you not only believe that a good outcome is likely, you believe that *a good outcome is in your direct control*. You have the skills and abilities you need to handle your problems and achieve your goals.

Together, hope, optimism, and self-efficacy make up the secret sauce of unstoppable motivation and willpower. Researchers call these three strengths *competence and control beliefs*.[8] How competent do you feel at generating positive emotions, experiences, and outcomes in your own life? How much control do you think you have over your health, happiness, and success? The more competence and control you believe you have, the more effort you'll make to do the things that matter most to you. That's why developing your hope, optimism, and self-efficacy is so important. And quests are an ideal way to do just that.

**Designing a quest is a way to actively imagine a good outcome.** Even before you start the quest, just by thinking about it, you're already building hope. A quest is, after all, simply a description of a specific action you can take to achieve a good outcome. Psychologists call this type of action *pathways forward*. The more pathways forward you can think of, the more hope you'll have.[9]

Every quest you accept or design for yourself gives you one more pathway forward. So don't be afraid to brainstorm lots of quests. Simply making a list of potential quests is enough to spark powerful hope. (This is why the most popular role-playing video games typically allow players to accept multiple quests at a time. A player's "quest log," or list of potential quests they are ready to tackle, might contain as many as ten or more possible pathways to pursue at any given moment. With so many options, the player never loses hope that progress in the game is possible.)

**Completing a quest is a way to experience success.** The more quests you complete, the more optimistic you'll get. That's because *increasing the frequency with which you experience good outcomes* is one of the most efficient ways to increase optimism.[10]

In fact, the research shows that frequency of success matters more than the size of the success. So it doesn't matter if your quest is small or easy. In fact, it *helps* if it's small and easy, because that increases your chances of success. With each success you achieve, you become more likely to expect success in the future. (This is why game developers make the early levels of games so easy. It's important to give players a dose of triumph early on, to build their emotional resilience ahead of the challenges to come.)

**Quests make you better.** Over time, *chains of quests*—or quests that build on one another, requiring slightly more effort, skill, or creativity—

make you objectively better. You develop useful abilities, learn important information, and expand your strategies.[11] And because with every quest you complete you are inarguably getting better in concrete and specific ways, you develop more confidence in your power to positively impact your own health, happiness, and future.

Your new skills combined with your increased confidence will allow you to tackle harder quests in the future. This creates a positive upward spiral of success. (Game designers use this same method to build player skills and create escalating challenge in the game world. Players want to feel more powerful and skillful over time, which is why quests get harder and harder the further you get in the game. But to get players ready to succeed at those ambitious goals, game designers must first give them quests that train them in the necessary skills and abilities.)

I experienced exactly that kind of upward spiral myself, starting from the moment I completed my first concussion-recovery quest. In the days and weeks that followed, my husband, my sister, and I came up with all kinds of creative quests. Completing each and every one increased my hope, optimism, and self-efficacy. One day I lay in bed and drew temporary tattoos (with Sharpie markers) on my arms, stomach, and legs. My quest that day had been suggested by my husband: *If you could have any tattoos to show the world how strong you are, what would they be*? (I wrote "Pain is inevitable" on the top of my left thigh and "Suffering is optional" on my right.) Another day my quest was: *Make a mental list of jobs you still might be able to do if your brain does not fully heal.* This was a quest I chose for myself. I was anxious about potentially never being able to research or write or design or speak in front of an audience again, and I knew the only way to deal with that fear effectively would be to accept the possible reality, then imagine a happy life anyway. So I spent the day lying in bed, imagining the best outcome I could, even if my brain never got any better. My favorite two ideas were becoming a dog walker and also becoming the queen of baking cookies and cupcakes for others. (Besides games, there is almost nothing I love more than dogs and baked goods.)

A few weeks later, when I was able to be up on my feet a bit more, I took on my most satisfying quest yet. Inspired by the idea that I might want to explore baking as a career, I decided to make chocolate chip cookies—not from scratch but from store-bought cookie dough, because I wasn't really up to following a recipe yet. (I know that sounds a little pathetic, but it actually felt amazing to me at the time to be up and around in the kitchen, greasing the pan and slicing the dough.) More important, the cookies weren't for me! They were my excuse to leave the apartment and go visit someone. I was barely seeing or speaking to anyone at the time, thanks to bed rest, the "no email" rule, and the difficulty I was having making conversation. When I thought about whom I missed talking to and seeing every day, I was surprised to realize that I really missed the baristas at the coffee shop at the corner of my block where I used to get coffee twice a day. So I made it my quest to make the cookies and bring them, fresh out of the oven, to the baristas.

I will never forget how surprised and delighted they were when I presented the plate of cookies. It made my whole week. I was thrilled to realize *I could still make someone else happy,* even in my superconcussed, depressed, and anxious state. I still had the power to do good in the world, even if only a tiny bit.

Eventually, the hope and optimism that I could keep doing good in the world led me to start sharing my *Jane the Concussion Slayer* game with others—first through videos (because I couldn't write yet), and later through blog posts. And as you know, feedback on that game eventually led me to invent SuperBetter. It's hard to believe that a quest as simple as baking cookies set me on a path to do the most meaningful and important work of my life, but that's exactly what happened.

Completing quests at my absolute physical, mental, and emotional lowest taught me something important: no matter what happens to me in the future, I will always have the power to do *one simple thing* every day that I choose for myself and that feels personally meaningful.

You have that power, too, and you increase that power with every quest. Over time, even the tiniest meaningful actions add up, each one bringing you closer to a life that is truer to your dreams and free of regret.

. . .

Up until now, you've been completing quests that I've designed for you. But the most important quests you complete will be the ones you create for yourself.

So where should you start? Let's take a cue from the world of game design.

In a game, the hero's *values* are what motivate every quest. Whether it's a desire to save the world, or to protect the innocent, or to lead a life of adventure, the hero always acts in accordance with his or her most deeply held values. Your quests—your daily, committed actions—should be driven by your most important values too.

What exactly is a value? It's a way of being that brings purpose and meaning to life. It's a strength you want to show, a virtue you want to uphold, a quality you want to embody, or a way of being in service to something bigger than yourself.

Here are some examples of values:

- To never stop learning
- To be the best parent possible
- To always challenge physical limits and be an inspiration to others
- To be a loving and caring person, and to be a good friend
- To connect with and respect nature
- To enjoy everything, and never be bored, because life is short
- To serve the Lord faithfully and, through actions, be an example to others
- To explore the whole world and understand as many different cultures as possible
- To do work that matters, even if it means earning less money

As you can see, a value is different from a goal. A value isn't something you can ever *get* or *achieve*, like a degree, a promotion, a ten-pound muscle gain, a romantic partner, or a cure for what ails you. Instead, a value is a way of describing how you want to live. It's a purpose you can bring to every single day of your life: a will to learn, to love, to be creative, to do things that scare you, to help others, or do whatever else matters to you, deep down, more than anything else.

Goals come and go. Values stay with you.

Naming your deepest values is the key to unlocking untapped sources of motivation, energy, and willpower. Research shows that when action is guided by values, it's vastly easier to accomplish feats that would seem impossible otherwise. Values can motivate and energize you even in the face of depression, grief, anxiety, addiction, hardship, and pain—not to mention boredom, frustration, exhaustion, or self-doubt.[12]

You may find it easy to identify your values. If so, that's great! But many people find it helpful to try some creative exercises. Here are three quests to help you explore your values.

I encourage you to *pick at least one* of these three quests and try it right now!

*Tip:* All these quests require you to use your imagination. Don't worry if they seem a bit farfetched—just go with it!

## QUEST 29: Value Yourself

Psychologists have identified twelve different areas of life that people tend to value most.[13] Take a look at the list below, and choose the *three* areas that are most important to you right now, at this moment.

**What to do:** Imagine that you have twenty-seven hours a day, instead of twenty-four like everyone else. Which three of these twelve life domains would you pour those extra hours into?

- Marriage, romantic partnership, or intimate relations
- Parenting

- Family (other than parenting or romantic partnership)
- Friends and social life
- Work and career
- Education, training, learning
- Recreation and fun
- Spirituality, religion
- Community life (clubs, organizations, activism, volunteering)
- Physical self-care (diet, exercise, sleep)
- The environment, caring for the planet
- Aesthetics (art, music, writing, reading, media, beauty)

Now that you've picked your three most important life domains, you can identify your first three values.

**What to do:** Simply finish the following statement with the three domains you picked.

**I want to be someone who spends time and energy each day on my:**

1.

2.

3.

For example, *I want to be someone who spends time and energy each day on my: family, spirituality, and fun.*

Identifying your most important life domains will help you figure out what kinds of quests to design for yourself.

Russ Harris, M.D., is one of the world's leading practitioners of Acceptance and Commitment Therapy (ACT)—a form of therapy that focuses on helping individuals take committed action. One of his favorite ways to ask clients about their values is to have them **consider a science fiction sce-**

**nario** that he calls the "mind-reading machine."[14] Here's a SuperBetter version of that scenario.

## QUEST 30: *The Mind-Reading Machine*

**What to do:** Imagine that **twenty years from now** a strange woman walks up to you with an amazing new technology: it's a mind-reading machine! She offers to place it on your head, and then says: "I can tune this machine into the mind of someone who is thinking about you right this instant, so you can hear their every thought."

Uh-oh! Do you really want to hear someone else's private thoughts? But it's too late—the machine is on, and she's started tuning the dials. Soon you hear exactly what she promised. Someone is thinking about you right this second—thinking about, in the words of Dr. Harris, "what you stand for, what your strengths are, what you mean to them." To your relief, the thoughts you overhear are incredibly positive. When you hear them, you think, *That describes me perfectly.*

**Remember:** It's twenty years from now, and you've lived a life true to your dreams and your most important values. With that in mind, what do you hear them saying?

*Tip:* If you'd like, let the mind-reading machine tune in to several different people, so you can hear about different sides of yourself.

## QUEST 31: Alternate Universe

This quest is particularly helpful for anyone who is currently struggling with a difficult personal challenge.

**What to do:** Imagine that you've just woken up in an alternate universe. Everything there is the same as in this universe, except for one thing: all the problems you've been worried about lately have been solved.

In this alternate universe, you are free of stress, pain, depression, anxiety, grief, self-doubt, and hardship. You feel completely unburdened of the negative thoughts, feelings, and worries that used to bother you.

In this alternate universe, what will you do with yourself today? How will you spend the next twenty-four hours? What important areas of life have you been neglecting that you can now devote more time and attention to? What dreams are you free to pursue? Spend at least one full minute **imagining your schedule for the day in this alternate universe.** The more details you imagine, the better.

**Here's the good news:** Quests let you do all these things right now, even without an alternate universe to escape to. Learning to take committed action will help you be the person you want to be, even in the face of adversity and stress.

Now that you've named your values, let's find simple ways you can live by them right now.

Dr. Harris puts it this way: "Values are here and now: in any moment you can choose to act on them or neglect them. Even if you've totally neglected a core value for years or decades, in this moment right now you can act on it."[15]

It's time to act on your values. It's time to design *your* first quest!

. . .

H ere are some of the things game designers think about when they design quests:

- Does the player know exactly what must be done in order to complete the quest? In other words, is it extremely clear and *specific*?
- Will the quest seem achievable to the player, given the skills, resources, and allies she has at this exact moment? In other words, is it *realistic*?
- Will the player feel energized by this quest? Is there something fundamentally interesting, challenging, or creative about the action the player will need to take? In other words, is it *fun*?
- Does this quest teach the player something important, or help him practice a crucial skill, so I can challenge him to do something *more* interesting and ambitious later? In other words, is it *adaptive*?
- Does this quest fit into the story of the hero's bigger purpose or journey? In other words, does it have *meaning*?

Game designers must always be able to answer yes to these questions in order to ensure that players have the necessary hope, optimism, and self-efficacy to make progress in the game. And as it turns out, good quest design has a lot in common with the kinds of daily real-life goals that psychologists say are most helpful to adopt.

In *ACT Made Simple: An Easy-to-Read Primer on Acceptance and Commitment Therapy*, Dr. Harris uses the acronym SMART to refer to the five most important criteria for taking committed action: *S*pecific, *M*eaningful, *A*daptive, *R*ealistic, and *T*ime-framed.[16] *Specific* means you are clear about exactly what action you're going to take: when, where, and who or what is involved. *Meaningful* means the action is driven by your own deeply held values. *Adaptive* means you can honestly say that achieving this goal will move you in the direction of a happier, healthier, braver, or more purposeful life. (Even if it's just a teeny, tiny step in the right direction, it's still a positive step!) *Realistic* means you already have the skills, resources, and strength you need to take this action. You don't need to solve any problems or improve your health, mood, relationships, or finances to take action right away. And *time-framed* means that you've chosen a specific day—or even better, a particular time of day—to take this positive action.

As you can see, the only difference between a SMART action and a good game quest is that the game quest also has to be fun! (We'll talk more about how to make something more fun after you complete your next quest.)

## QUEST 32: Design Your Own Quest

So far, you've completed up to thirty-one quests, just by reading this book. But the most important quests will be the ones you design for yourself. That's because only *you* know what you value most in life. So let's practice the skill of designing your own quests right now.

**What to do:** Pick one of your most important values. Remember, values are the principles that give your life meaning and purpose. They describe who you want to be, at your very core.

Got your value? Good. Now simply answer this question: What is the smallest, easiest, simplest action you could take in the next twenty-four hours that would give you a chance to live by this value?

Think of something so easy, so tiny, that you have no excuse not to do it. The simpler it is, the better. If it only takes five minutes, or even a single minute, to do it, that's not only fine—that's perfect!

**Examples:** Here are some examples from other SuperBetter players.

*My value:* "Always show my family how much I love and cherish them."

*My quest:* "Leave a surprise note under my daughter's pillow."

*My value:* "Never stop learning."

*My quest:* "Write a post on Facebook asking people to share a link to an article or video that could teach me something interesting."

*My value:* "Be true to my faith and honor God."

*My quest:* "Pray for one minute."

*My value:* "Do my part to make the world a better place, and work toward causes I believe in."

*My quest:* "Donate one dollar to a cause online. (I was thinking I should donate twenty dollars, because that feels more meaningful. But if I'm being honest I might talk myself out of that because twenty dollars could be used for so many other things. But one dollar, I know I will do that, so that's my quest!)"

*My value:* "Be a good athlete and always challenge myself physically."

*My quest:* "Instead of my normal five-mile run tomorrow, I'll run one mile as fast as I can."*

*Tip:* It's fine if your first quest is something you already do regularly, or have done in the past. You don't have to get too creative here. Any action that truly reflects your values is perfect. Defining it as a quest, even if it's something you do anyway, makes you more

---

* What is simple and easy to you may be too challenging for someone else, and vice versa. It may make more sense for your quest to be *Walk one mile as fast as I can* or *Walk one block as fast as I can.* The key to good quest design is to make sure you feel capable and optimistic on your quest, with whatever strength, skills, and resources you already have. Quests are all about setting yourself up for success.

aware of the positive actions you take that help you live a life truer to your dreams and full of purpose.

**Remember to complete the quest you've just designed sometime in the next twenty-four hours!**

Whether you call them SMART actions or quests, these simple gameful goals will help you put your time and energy toward things that matter. They aren't wild dreams or pie-in-the-sky ambitions. They are the simple stepping-stones to a better life.

There *is* a place for wild dreams and big ambitions in a gameful life— we'll talk about that more in Chapter 11. But going for an epic win, or a truly heroic goal, without a steady stream of smart quests to get you there is a fool's errand. Smart goals, or quests, ensure that every day you're making a better life for yourself, right now, in the present moment. An epic win is in the future; a quest, or smart goal, is what you do today.

## A SuperBetter Story:
## Phillip the Creative Cancer Fighter

By the time Phillip Jeffrey, thirty-one, started his journey to get superbetter, he had already been living with aggressive multiple myeloma, a rare and incurable form of blood cancer, for six years.

That's four years longer than doctors had originally told him to expect. Phillip's cancer was advanced, and he had been given a prognosis of just two to three years.

"When I was diagnosed, I had no idea what multiple myeloma was. My doctor explained that it wasn't something that could be treated with an operation, because it was in my bones, and not a body part. I was shocked. At my age, getting cancer seemed as likely as getting struck by space junk in my kitchen."

Over the next six years, Phillip underwent many rounds of chemotherapy, which he describes as "lonely, challenging, and exhausting." He hit his lowest point three years into treatment, when he developed glaucoma, from the side effects of one of his medications, and nearly went blind. Losing vision is traumatic for anyone, but it was especially so for Phillip, whose greatest passion in life is photography.

While he was trying to get his glaucoma under control, he suffered another blow: a stroke in the area of the brain responsible for vision. "Thankfully, most of the damage from the stroke was temporary, although I lost enough vision that I will never drive again."

After Phillip's stroke, he was taken off his cancer medications. "The doctors believed they were more life-threatening to me than the cancer itself." Phillip found himself in treatment limbo. For the next two and a half years, his doctors used chemotherapy as sparingly as possible to avoid the dangerous complications.

By April 2012, Phillip had been off chemotherapy for a year, and his cancer levels were rising slowly and steadily. He was looking for a way to stay optimistic and engaged with the world, even though he felt very sick and was running out of treatment options. That's when he decided to get superbetter. He transformed himself from Phillip the cancer patient to Phillip the Creative Cancer Fighter, and he vowed to not let his vision problems keep him from photography.

He started his SuperBetter journey with a simple quest: "Take a creative self-portrait, somewhere outdoors, and share it online before midnight." To keep things simple, he decided to tackle this same quest, every day, for ninety days in a row.

"I wanted to spend time being creative," Phillip explains. "But I also wanted something that would force me to leave my apartment. Some days when you're living with cancer, you just won't want to get out of bed. You think, 'I have my laptop, I have my cell phone, I can hide out from the rest of the world, never engage with life beyond the four walls of my place.' That's how I felt.

"I was exhausted from the cancer treatment. And I was depressed. Partly, it was not being happy with myself and how I looked. It was very humbling for me, how cancer changed my appearance. I got so much weaker, I lost my hair, and I just wanted to hide it from the world. I needed something to help me reengage with the world around me."

Sharing the photos online was just as important as taking them in the first place. He explains: "I have a shorter lifespan than most, so I'm thinking of a legacy. I'm taking pictures that I hope will be around online for a long time, maybe twenty, thirty years."

Over the next ninety days of his photography quest, Phillip shared many of his SuperBetter experiences publicly, through his blog and a series of online videos. Here are some of his insights, in his own words.

"The first thing I've noticed with this quest is that I'm now ending every day on a positive note. I've been taking all my self-portraits during magic hour in the evening, which is the final hour before sunset when the outdoor light is the best. So I've actually gone outside for every sunset, every day. And I've been exploring the city, to find a new interesting location each day, different spaces I've never noticed before.

"I take my shots until I find one I'm satisfied with, and then I go back home, and before midnight I upload it online. I have that sense of accomplishment in taking a picture, feeling satisfied with it, uploading it—and boom, I did something today. And that makes me happy, to have a sense of purpose and accomplishment every day. I don't think long term—I don't have illusions of retiring in the Grand Cayman Islands. Instead, I'm happy each day that I wake up in my own bed and can go through the day without feeling overly tired or sick, while making progress on my photography quests."

As the weeks passed, his creative photography inspired a new series of quests focused on physical resilience. "Because I'm taking a self-portrait every day, I'm paying more attention to how I look, and I'm wanting to look stronger in my photos. This inspired me to do something I haven't done in a long time, which is working out regularly. I'm up to five to six times a week, and I feel like I'm getting in better shape. Staying in shape is important for cancer, especially with multiple myeloma, because I need to keep my bones strong. If the bones in my legs become brittle, I can have problems walking, I can break my legs very easily. I haven't been doing as much to keep my legs strong as I should. The photography quest helped me kick-start this whole other area of my health and well-being."

The upward spiral continued with each daily quest. Weeks later Phillip reported: "Every day I'm feeling more confident about what I'm learning. I'm understanding photography better, self-portraiture better, my camera better—I realized I hadn't even used all the features before. I'm developing my skills, and it feels great." These new skills led Phillip to make what was, for him, a surprising decision. "As a direct result of getting superbetter, I've decided to restart a major photography project that I had to put aside earlier during cancer treatment. I didn't think I would ever restart it, or do something this ambitious with my photography again. But having a camera in my hand has energized me to pick it back up. It's a big project. I know that it will take me another year to complete. I'm excited that I'm now actively planning to stay creative and active past these ninety days."

Buoyed by his sense of purpose and progress, Phillip made it to his ninety-day epic win easily, without missing a single creative portrait along the way. On day ninety, he shared the following reflection: "This has been amazing. I'm not feeling depressed anymore. I have more energy. I've seen real improvement in my photography. I've used SuperBetter to understand my world better and, through that, to understand myself. It was just what I needed to kick-start my life again and to focus on remaining positive, happy, and living each day to the fullest."

Phillip continues to fight cancer creatively today. Approximately one year after reaching his goal of ninety creative self-portraits, he received a new and experimental treatment for multiple myeloma. So far the results have been outstanding. His cancer has gone into remission for stretches as long as nine months at a time—and he's still making time to be creative each and every day. He recently up-dated all his SuperBetter allies: "I'm feeling great and enjoying life. I have blood tests every five weeks, and my cancer levels are still low. I feel so alive every day, focused on extending my 'between chemotherapy' periods of life for as long as possible. And I'm con-tinuing to use photography quests as therapy for health and heal-ing. Every day I enjoy chatting with people around Vancouver, taking photos, and just stopping and reflecting on how amazing my life is." (You can find Phillip's photography at www.flickr.com/photos/tyfn.)

There's one other important quest-related trick you can learn from games. It's the art of fun framing, and it can help you increase your willpower—and even procrastinate less.

*Fun framing* is what happens when you decide to do something for the pure pleasure, excitement, or enjoyment of it. Ask any kid why they play their favorite game, and the first response you'll usually get is "Because it's fun!" But what does that really mean? Fun is not a discrete positive emotion, like joy or gratitude or curiosity or pride. Fun, instead, is a state of mind. Fun is how we describe an activity that we enjoy for its own sake. Studies show that if we get paid or praised or otherwise rewarded for doing some-thing, we're less likely to describe it as fun—even if it's the exact same activ-ity.[17] That's because fun happens when we focus only on the intrinsic pleasure, excitement, and enjoyment we feel—not when we think about the extrinsic rewards we might get out of it.

It turns out that planning to have fun—instead of trying to seek re-wards—is actually a very powerful state of mind. Consider this fascinating scientific study on the benefits of fun framing.

A team of researchers from Cornell University, New Mexico State University, and the Grenoble School of Management in France decided to investigate a well-known but poorly understood phenomenon: why so many people *gain weight* during exercise programs, even if they started exercising specifically to try to lose weight. And here's what they discovered: there is a very strong link between how people think about physical activity and what they eat afterward. People who think of physical activity as "exercise" typically have more dessert later in the day and eat more high-calorie snacks. That's because they typically think of exercise as hard work, which we do to improve our health, rather than as something fun or pleasurable for its own sake. Therefore exercise deserves a "reward." (And the calories contained in the reward often exceed the calories burned during exercise, leading to weight gain.)

People who think of physical activity primarily *as a way to have fun*, however, are much less likely to "reward" themselves with food later. That's because they already feel rewarded by the excitement and enjoyment of the physical activity itself. They don't need a cookie or a bag of chips. They already had fun, and that was reward enough!

Here's the good news: the Cornell study showed that changing someone's mental framework for thinking about physical activity is not hard. Even people who think they don't like exercise are able to reframe it as a fun activity. Simply calling the activity a "scenic walk," for example—emphasizing the opportunity to enjoy pleasurable sights—rather than an "exercise walk" made all the difference. This tiny change in state of mind led people to eat fewer rewards and successfully lose more weight.[18]

What does this research mean for you? If you're trying to increase your willpower as part of your journey to get superbetter, make sure that you adopt a fun frame every time you tackle a quest.

One way to adopt a fun frame is just to say to yourself, "This is going to be fun." (This cognitive priming is similar to the *Get excited!* technique you learned about in Chapter 5.) Just telling yourself you're going to have fun is half the battle.

It will also help if you think of your daily quests as opportunities for pleasure and excitement. Before you complete a quest, ask yourself, "What's enjoyable about this?" or "What's exciting about this?" Try to find at least one aspect of each quest that you would enjoy for its own sake, whether it's learning something new or spending time on yourself, and focus on that.

Whatever you do, *don't* think of quests as difficult tasks that you need to use a ton of willpower to tackle. Otherwise you're more likely to compromise your willpower later in the day and "reward" yourself with treats that may actually make it harder to achieve your SuperBetter goals.

F un framing has another benefit: it can help you break the habit of procrastinating.

A team of psychologists at DePaul University and Case Western University decided to investigate the reasons some people chronically procrastinate—and what techniques would help them procrastinate less. So they set up an experiment in which half the participants were invited to "take a math test," while the other half were invited to "play a math game." In reality, the test and the game were the exact same activity; the only difference was in the framing.

Both sets of participants were given an hour to prepare by practicing the same kind of math problems that they would have to solve in the test or the game. They didn't *have* to practice and prepare. They were free to procrastinate—that is, to ignore the practice problems and distract themselves with any enjoyable activity they preferred.

So what happened? The participants who thought they were preparing for a test were far more likely to procrastinate. They waited, on average, until 60 percent of the practice period had passed to get started. But participants who thought they were preparing for a game were much more likely to dive in right away and take every opportunity to get better. They hardly procrastinated at all. Why? Because they didn't consider the activity to be something they wanted to avoid. It was going to be fun, so they got started right away.

*Even though it was the exact same activity,* the "game players" jumped in with more enthusiasm and motivation than the "test takers." For this reason, the researchers describe chronic procrastination as a "self-handicap" that can be eliminated by simply labeling more activities as "fun" or "pleasurable."

Both of these studies show that what makes an activity fun is not the nature of the activity but how you approach it—with a focus on the potential pleasure, excitement, and enjoyment. The same exact activity can be fun or work, something to avoid or something to dive right into, simply because of the way you describe it to yourself.

Whatever your challenge or goal is, fun framing can help you do more of what will truly help you get superbetter—and less of what might make it harder. Just remember to think of each and every quest that you accept or design for yourself as a chance to have a little fun.

Here are a few more tips for designing your quests:

**Ask your friends and family for quests.** Ask them to suggest one tiny thing you could do in the next twenty-four hours to be happier, healthier, stronger, or braver—or more of *any* value that you're comfortable sharing with them. Friends and family are a great source of new and interesting ideas. Plus, you'll get bonus motivation and satisfaction from completing a quest that someone you care about personally challenged you to do!

**If you like a quest and want to do it often, turn it into a power-up!** Quests are a way to explore different actions and see what brings you genuine strength, happiness, and health. If you really enjoy a quest, turn it into a power-up so you'll be able to make it a habit.

**To really create momentum, design a quest chain.** A quest chain, in video games, is a series of quests that all focus on the same activity or skill. Each one requires just a little more effort, ability, or creativity. To design a quest chain, start with a basic quest: *What's the smallest, tiniest committed action I'm confident I can take in the next twenty-four hours?* Then once you've done that successfully, just keep asking follow-up questions: *What's the next easy action I can take?* or *If I do that again, how can I make it more challenging or more interesting?* A quest chain can have anywhere from three to a dozen quests. Eventually, as you build momentum and learn more about what you're capable of, the tiny steps you're taking will turn into leaps and bounds.

### Skills Unlocked: How to Tap the Power of Quests

- A quest is anything you can do in the next twenty-four hours to bring about a good outcome or a positive result for yourself.
- The most powerful quests are those driven by your values—whatever brings a sense of vitality and purpose to your life.
- Completing at least one quest a day will build your hope, optimism, and self-efficacy—the three building blocks of extreme motivation and willpower.
- Make sure your quests are SMART, like a game designer's: Specific, Meaningful, Adaptive, Realistic, and Time-framed.
- You can *always* complete at least one quest a day, even when you are busy, sick, exhausted, stressed, in pain, or otherwise distressed. Take committed action: commit to finding at least one tiny way every day to focus fully on the things that matter most to you.
- Quests create an upward spiral. The more quests you complete, the more time and energy you'll find to invest in your most important goals and values.
- Approach every quest as an opportunity to have fun. You'll procrastinate less and enjoy more willpower as a result.

# 9

## Allies

### How to Be Gameful Rule 5

•————————•

Recruit your allies—friends and family members
who will help you along the way.

The advice in this chapter is based on a simple "aha!" moment I had when I was recovering from my concussion: *It's hard to be vulnerable and ask for help with a serious problem. But it's easy to invite someone else to play a game.*

After all, we do it all the time. Collectively, we spend more than a billion hours a week playing video games with our friends and family.[1] We spend even more hours playing cards, board games, and sports together.[2]

The ease with which we invite each other to play is the key to feeling more connected and getting more social support when we need it most.

Having social support makes it easier for us to achieve our goals. It's not just that our friends and family help us directly by offering their time, advice, or resources. Medical research shows that our bodies respond to social support in dramatic ways, getting stronger and more resilient every time someone helps us.

Every time you get support from someone—an encouraging word, a shared laugh, a hug, a satisfying conversation, a gesture of kindness, a few minutes of fun together—the following things happen:

- Your stress levels go down, as measured by a drop in cortisol, the stress hormone.
- Your immune system is bolstered. Wounds heal faster, you catch fewer colds, and you even fight diseases like cancer more effectively.
- Your heart literally gets stronger. In fact, your whole cardiovascular system works more efficiently, with lower blood pressure and a decreased heart rate.[3]

No matter what challenge you're facing, this kind of physical resilience helps you have more strength and energy to achieve your goals.

And let's not forget the immediate and very practical benefits of social support: the resources your allies can provide, whether it's words of wisdom, ideas, information, supplies, introductions, a spare hand, a fresh perspective, or just good company.

Social support also potentially gives you more time on this planet to pursue your biggest dreams. A meta-review of 163 different studies of social support and mortality found that increasing the number of positive social interactions you have each day extends your life expectancy as much as giving up a pack-a-day cigarette habit or reaching a healthy weight.[4] (That is, on average, it adds just over six years to your life expectancy.)

But what if you're naturally introverted or a very private person? What if you have fewer close friends and family than you'd like? The good news is that you don't need an extroverted or outgoing personality to achieve a strong sense of social support. And you don't need a large group of friends who you feel comfortable sharing your problems with. Having just one or two allies makes a huge difference. Scientists define a true *ally*, or strong social tie, as *someone you can speak to honestly about your stress and challenges* and *whom you believe you could ask for help with a serious problem*.[5]

Of course, knowing how beneficial it can be to ask for help and to speak honestly about your challenges doesn't necessarily make it easy to do. I know this firsthand. When I was dealing with my biggest personal challenge, the long recovery from concussion, I was scared to tell others how much I was hurting. And I didn't want to be a burden to anyone by asking for help. I felt this way even about the people closest to me, like my husband and my twin sister. So how did I do it?

In this chapter, you'll learn to share your challenge and ask for support gamefully. You'll discover how the seven gameful rules actually make it easier for friends and family members to know exactly what to do to help you—by bringing you a power-up, helping you resist a bad guy, or completing a quest with you. You'll develop the skills to cultivate connectedness when you need it most—not by asking for help, but by inviting others to play and to team up with you on cooperative missions and adventures.

It's not just easier to recruit allies this way. It actually makes your relationships stronger. As we've seen in countless studies in this book already, when you play a game with someone, you build the positive emotions, the mirror neurons, and the lasting trust necessary to truly be there for each other. You'll be surprised how much positive impact this will have not just on you but also on the people you invite to be your allies.

As one SuperBetter player, who was invited to help his brother play for depression, explains: "We talk in SuperBetter-ese now. We say things like 'That sounds like a bad guy' or 'You should add that as a power-up.' We didn't have words to talk about this stuff before. Now I have words to put to goals he has. It makes a big difference. I honestly had no idea before what I could say or do to help him. Now I do."

When it comes to social support, I often think of the wisdom of one of my favorite storytellers, G. K. Chesterton: "There are no words to express the abyss between isolation and having one ally. It may be conceded to the mathematician that four is twice two. But two is not twice one; two is two thousand times one." Even if you think you're not the kind of person who can ask for help, you *can* make an ally. This chapter will show you how.

But first let's take a quick look at the top five reasons why it's so much easier to get superbetter with at least one ally by your side.

## The Top Five Ways Your Allies Can Help

Our SuperBetter players have teamed up with allies all over the world. They've joined forces with friends and family, coworkers and coaches, doctors and therapists, teachers and online buddies.

I asked them what their allies do for them that helps the most. Here are the top five ways they say their allies give them extra strength and motivation, week in and week out.

**1. My ally suggests a quest.**

"Sometimes I get stuck thinking up my own quests, so I ask my allies, including my kids, for new ideas. Plus, if my allies tell me to do something, I always make more of an effort. I don't want to let them down." —Mark, forty-nine, whose challenge is getting fit for fifty

**2. We activate a power-up together.**

"My allies know what all my power-ups are, and they've been conspiring behind my back to make sure that at least one of them activates a power-up with me every day. Literally, they made a schedule. It's really sweet." —Sarah, nineteen, whose challenge is discovering life after soccer (and dealing with postconcussion syndrome)

**3. We brainstorm strategies for a bad guy.**

"There are days where I feel like there is no possible way I can win against the bad guys. If I'm having one of those days, I can just say to my favorite ally, my sister, 'I'm stuck in the Void of Guilt. Help!'" —Regina, thirty, whose challenge is overcoming the working mom blues

**4. We have a daily or weekly "debrief" or check-in.**

"Every day I look forward to telling my boyfriend what I've done to get superbetter. I tell him which quests I completed, which power-ups I activated, and which bad guys I battled. It motivates me to do more and try harder, because I know he wants to hear good news. But if I tell him I did zero quests, activated zero power-ups, and spent all day getting beat up by the bad guys, I know he'll give me a little extra attention and care that night. He seems to have a much easier time understanding what I'm feeling when I put it in simple game terms." —Maisie, twenty-eight, whose challenge is finishing her Ph.D.

**5. We celebrate an epic win together.**
"Most of my allies are online friends. They helped me plan a Day of Chris celebration for after I achieved my first big goal, which was to walk one hundred miles total. I've been adding up fifteen-minute walks after each meal, which is a big part of managing my blood sugar and staying healthy with diabetes. It took me three months to reach my epic win. As I got closer, my allies started encouraging me to spend a whole day celebrating my hard work by doing just things I love. I took photos of how I spent the Day of Chris to share with them." —Chris, thirty-one, whose challenge is having a strong mind and body

You're starting to get a better idea of just how allies can help you get superbetter. Before you start recruiting your own, let's warm up your social muscles.

It turns out that just *thinking* about getting help or giving help can give your social resilience a boost. To find out how, try this quest!

## QUEST 33: Imagine That!

It's time to tap the power of your imagination.

**What to do:** Take a minute right now to consider three fictional scenarios. Each one asks you to imagine yourself facing a very unusual challenge. You'll need to pick one person who you would join forces with as you tackle each hypothetical challenge. The scenarios are fictional, but the person you pick should be real, someone you already know and are close to in everyday life.

There's just one rule for this quest: you must pick a different person for each scenario. It's no fair calling on the same ally for all three crazy challenges! At the end of this quest, you should have a total of three different people in mind.

What if you draw a blank and can't think of anyone you could ask for help in these situations? That's okay—just flip the scenarios around. Imagine that *someone you know*—someone specific—is facing the crazy challenge, then think about what *you* would do to help. (When it comes to boosting social resilience, thinking about how *you* could become an ally for someone else is as beneficial as imagining someone else being an ally for you!)

These scenarios are silly on purpose, so don't take them too seriously. Just pretend for a moment, and let your imagination take hold! (A special thanks to game designer Chelsea Howe, currently creative director for Electronic Arts Mobile, for creating these crazy scenarios with me.)

**Scenario 1:** Oh no! A meteor struck planet Earth, and its cosmic rays have turned millions of people into mutants with unpredictable superpowers. Guess what? *You* are now one of those mutants with superpowers. You're pretty sure you can figure out a way to use them for good. But in the meantime the government is after you.

Who can you trust with your secret? Who will you tell the truth to about your superpowers? Who can help you figure out what to do with them?

**Pick one Mutant Superpower ally now.**

**Scenario 2:** Uh-oh! The local chocolate factory exploded! A raging river of delicious chocolate has covered your home and everything in it. Fortunately, the elves who run the factory have a plan to clean up the mess: they're going to eat all the chocolate themselves—yum! Unfortunately, it will take them at least a week to eat it all.

Who is the person geographically closest to you who you could stay with, or at least borrow clothes and other useful things from, until all the chocolate is cleaned up? Or, if your house is the first to be cleaned up, who is the *first* person who lives near you, who you will offer clothes or a place to stay?

**Pick one Chocolate Mudslide ally now.**

**Scenario 3:** Whoa! Your eccentric, long-lost aunt Zelda just left you one million dollars in her will. If you spend it all by next Tuesday, you'll inherit a *billion* dollars. But there's a catch: you have to spend the first million without accumulating a single worldly possession, and you can't give the money away or donate it to charity.

Aunt Zelda's will stipulates that you can enlist only one person's help in spending the first million. If you tell anyone else what you're up to, the money goes to her cat. Who do you enlist as your coconspirator, as you try to unlock the billion dollars? Who would be able to help you come up with a winning strategy? Who would you have the most fun with as you blow through the first million dollars?

**Pick one Million Dollar Spree ally now.**

**Why it works:** When you vividly imagine fictional scenarios like the ones in this quest, you activate important social emotions like gratitude, empathy, trust, and compassion—all emotions that make you more likely to get and give support in the future.

Now that you've completed this quest, you've not only sparked some helpful social emotions, you've also identified three potential allies to recruit for your game. (Or perhaps, you've identified three people you'd like to become an ally to!) So let's talk more about exactly what an ally does.

This SuperBetter story captures the ally experience perfectly—much to the surprise of its hero, Alex, who never wanted any allies in the first place.

## A SuperBetter Story: The Reluctant Hero

Alex Goldman, thirty, a public radio show producer who lives in New York City, is the last person you'd ever expect to recruit allies. "There's nothing in the world I hate more than asking for help," he told me on the air, when we chatted on his radio show in late 2011.

Alex is an avid bike rider, but in the summer of 2011, he suffered a terrible accident when he was knocked off his bike and run over by a car. "I had multiple fractures in my leg," he recounted, "and I needed two surgeries to fix them. After my first surgery, I spent three weeks with rods and clamps drilled into the bones in my leg. I had a second surgery to remove them, and then I spent six weeks on crutches."[6]

Even after he started walking again, Alex faced a long road to recovery. "I walk with a limp now, and every step is pretty painful," he said. "My leg swells up in the afternoons. I can't do any of the exercise I used to do, especially riding my bike. The medical professionals looking at my injury have not been all that clear about whether this is permanent or not. As you can imagine, this has left me incredibly depressed."

Alex turned to SuperBetter during this difficult time. I spoke with him on air before he started playing, to go over the rules. He was convinced that recruiting allies would be the toughest part of the game for him, harder even than running a marathon on his broken leg! But when we spoke again, six weeks later, he had not only achieved his first epic win—a three-mile bike ride around Brooklyn's Prospect Park—but to his great surprise, he also had a whopping eleven allies by his side when he did it.

How did he get from refusing to ask anyone for help, ever, to being surrounded by friends and coworkers cheering him on?

It started slowly, with just two allies—his wife, Sarah, and his colleague PJ. He told them about his goal and asked them to spend the next six weeks helping him achieve it. To break the ice, he showed Sarah and PJ his list of bad guys: "Stuff like not socializing, staying up really late but not getting anything done, junk food, generally things that kept me sedentary and lethargic and unhappy." Then he shared his power-up list: "Anything that would get me physically moving or interacting with other people." With PJ at work and Sarah at home, he had someone around essentially 24/7 to help him keep moving and avoid succumbing to the bad guys.

Alex admitted that he never would have asked for this much help on his own. "To be quite honest, the process was hard for me," he said, "even though the game rules made it easier. But the flip side of it being really difficult was that it was also really nice to have people hold me accountable. The behavior I'd developed after the accident was just to sit around feeling sorry for myself. Having people trying to push me to behavior that would make me feel better was superhelpful."

Once Alex saw the advantages of having allies, he decided to expand his circle of support. But he didn't feel comfortable talking to other friends or colleagues yet about his challenges. So he turned to online discussion forums and social media. As an avid player of *Team Fortress 2*, a popular online team-based shooter game, Alex felt comfortable recruiting allies from a pool of strangers online. Soon a dozen allies he'd never met in real life were sending him ideas for power-ups, bad guy strategies, and quests. They also helped him decide on the epic win he would try to achieve: getting back on his bicycle and riding one lap (or three miles) around Brooklyn's Prospect Park.

"I suppose this is a bit of a no-brainer, but I was shocked at how motivating it is to have other people designing quests for me," Alex said. "The quests my allies have given me have been much more interesting and enlightening than anything I've come up with myself." His favorite one required him to buy his wife a flower and purchase two new toys for his cats. The twist: he had to travel to the flower shop and pet store on foot, ensuring he would get some physical exercise. "This suggestion was very smart, because I'm much more motivated to make my wife and cats happier than I am to do my own physical therapy," he said. He reported it "a huge success—I not only achieved my physical activity goal for the day, my cats and wife are looking at me like I'm their hero."

Alex also appreciated an ally who sent him a fifteen-dollar gift certificate to a bar near Prospect Park, with instructions to enjoy a beer—but only *if* he completed a lap of the park on foot first. It was more great motivation to get out and work toward his epic win.

Having allies and completing quests started to make a real difference in how Alex was feeling every day. As he described in *The SuperBetter Diaries*, a blog he kept during his eight weeks of play: "I'm now in my fourth week using SuperBetter, and my coworkers have been talking about how uncharacteristically sunny my disposition is."[7] This gave him the perfect opportunity to talk more openly about his rehabilitation and to recruit even more allies.

These friends and coworkers turned out to be just as supportive and helpful as his online allies—giving quests, sending power-up reminders, and rooting against the bad guys. More important, they were there in person for Alex's attempt at an epic win. On a cool morning in November, eleven allies showed up bright and early to complete a lap of Prospect Park with him.

"Even though I usually hate this kind of cheer 'em on, rah-rah type of attention, which is why everyone thinks I'm a selfish, ungrateful curmudgeon, it was very flattering and encouraging that a lot of my coworkers and friends came by to show their support," he said afterward—clearly still a bit wary of social support but just as clearly happy to receive it.

So how did his attempt at an epic win go? "The ride was a victory. It was the first time in six months I'd gotten back on my bike, which has been really difficult and terrifying for me. It was a big step. And yes, it definitely felt epic!"

To help him celebrate and remember the feeling of victory, one of Alex's allies made a video of the bike ride and set it to the theme from *Chariots of Fire*. Alex proudly shared the video online. And when I talked to him on the radio after six weeks of play, he admitted how surprised he was that recruiting and collaborating with allies turned out—shockingly, for a self-described curmudgeon!—to be his favorite part of the experience.

Three years later I touched base with Alex to see how he's doing. He still credits SuperBetter with helping him bounce back faster and stronger from his traumatic injury. He's an active athlete again, with a newfound ability to ask for help. "I healed up really, really well. SuperBetter definitely helped," he told me. But for Alex, a speedier physical recovery wasn't the biggest benefit of getting gameful. "In the end," he said, "getting superbetter for me was actually much more about emotional and mental health than just a physical recovery."

There are lots of ways to seek and offer social support, but as Alex's story shows, social support in SuperBetter has a structure—to make it easier to ask for help and easier to give it.

The structure is simple. In SuperBetter an ally is someone who:

- Knows what challenge you're tackling
- Has a good sense of your favorite power-ups and biggest bad guys
- Is game to check in with you periodically to hear how your Super-Better efforts are going (in person, on the phone, by email, by video chat, on a social network, or however you feel most comfortable communicating)

That's it. There are lots of other incredibly helpful things your allies can do for you once they're on board—and we'll talk about that in just a bit. But to make someone an ally, all it takes is for you to share your game and for them to accept the invitation to play.

It helps if your ally understands a little bit about SuperBetter. But most SuperBetter players I've interviewed have found it very easy to explain the concept of real-life power-ups, bad guys, and quests—it only takes a minute. And if you'd like to give your allies a chance to dig deeper, sharing this book is one way to get them up to speed; a faster way is to send them a link to the video of the TED talk I gave on SuperBetter (search online for "The game that can give you 10 extra years of life").

Here are some tips for talking to potential allies about SuperBetter:

- **Start by sharing your challenge**. "I'm playing a game to help me [your challenge here]. If you're up for it, I'd love to have you as my ally in the game."
- **Explain what it means to be an ally**: "You'll give me advice and en-couragement and let me tell you about all my adventures."
- **Set some time boundaries for the game**. For example, "I'd love for you to be my ally for the next thirty days," or "Would you be willing to play with me until I go back to school?" or just "Let's try this together

for a week!" Providing clear boundaries makes it easier for your ally to accept the invitation.

- **Give each ally a quest of their own to help them get started.** Tell them, for example, "The best thing you could do for me this week is to just text me once a day to remind me to not give in to the bad guys." Or "Your first mission as my ally is to think of a new power-up for me. Preferably one I can do in bed." Or "I have a quest to pick a new mantra. Will you send me some of your favorite inspirational quotes?" Giving your ally quests is a way to tell them exactly what you need—and solves the problem of them wondering on their own what they can do to help. Once they get the hang of the SuperBetter rules, most allies have little difficulty coming up with their own quests.

Once your ally accepts the invitation to play, there's no limit to what they might dream up to do to help! For example, when Jens, a player in the Netherlands, made it his SuperBetter challenge to quit smoking, his ally surprised him with an extra source of motivation: a friendly bet. "He proposed that if I went one hundred days without smoking, he'd turn over all the soil in my garden and prepare it for planting. If I failed, I'd have to clean his house all winter." Jens won the bet.

If your allies would like some ideas about how to help you get superbetter, share the following advice with them. (You'll notice that the advice describes SuperBetter players as "heroes." So if someone is your ally, *you* are that person's hero!)

## HOW TO BE AN AWESOME ALLY

If someone in your life is tackling a tough challenge or trying to make a positive change, you can help them. With your support and encouragement, they're much more likely to achieve their goals.

You'll benefit, too. Being a good ally means practicing and mastering important skills that make you a better friend, parent, coach, or partner.

Plus, every time you take action as an ally, you increase your own social resilience—the strength that makes *you* more likely to get support in the future when you need it most.

Here are the top ten ways to be a powerful ally.

1. **Know your hero.** Being an ally always starts with getting to know your hero's current challenge, power-ups, and bad guys. (And their secret identity, if they've chosen to adopt one!) Ask your hero to give you a quick rundown.

2. **Bring your hero power-ups.** Now that you know your hero's power-ups, offer to activate one together. For example, if your hero has a five-minute dance party as a power-up, invite them to throw a dance party in person or over video chat with you. Or send favorite power-ups your hero's way. If your hero has dark green veggies as a power-up, bake your hero some cheesy kale chips. If one of their favorite power-ups is looking at photos of baby animals, share one by email or social media. And if you have an idea for a new power-up, suggest it—and ask your hero to let you know if it helped!

3. **Help your hero battle a bad guy.** Pick a bad guy on your hero's list, and try to think of a strategy to help him or her successfully battle it. Do some research online to find tips and tricks that have worked for others facing a similar bad guy. Or use your creativity! Whatever strategies you suggest, ask your hero to report back on how well they worked.

4. **Give your hero a quest.** It's not always easy to see the path forward. You can help your hero by challenging him or her to accomplish a task of your choosing in the next twenty-four hours. Remember, a quest is any tiny way your hero can get stronger, happier, healthier, or closer to a big goal. Be sure the quests you give him or her are realistic—and it's always more fun when you offer to go on a quest together! (If you're stuck for ideas, just give your favorite quests from this book, including the adventures at the back!)

5. **Get a report.** Ask the simple question "How is your SuperBetter journey going?" You can spark conversation by asking specifically about different things. "What's your favorite power-up so far?" "Is there a bad

guy you feel you've made a lot of progress with?" "Have you done any interesting quests lately?" "What quest is coming up next for you?" You can get a report by phone, email, video chat, in person—whatever feels natural. If you're really close with your hero, you can ask for a daily report. It can give him or her a huge emotional and motivational boost to know that every day will end with the chance to connect and reflect. Otherwise, just reach out and ask for a report whenever you can. Many allies find that touching base once or twice a week is plenty.

6. **Hunt the good stuff.** One of the most important things you can do is to shine a light on your hero's hard work and accomplishments. Think of yourself as a detective—your mission is to hunt the good stuff they're doing, then make a big deal out of it. You'll want to do more than just say "Good job." When he or she makes a heroic effort or accomplishes a tough goal, ask questions about how they did it. What were their strategies? Where did they find the strength? Ask how it feels now that they've done it. Ask what it inspires them to do next. Or tell them what it inspires *you* to do!

Psychologists call this *active constructive responding*. It means taking someone's good news or success and helping them really savor and celebrate it. Active constructive responding is a skill—the more you practice it, the more naturally it will come to you. Just remember, it's not about over-the-top praise or positive feedback. Just try to ask three questions about any good thing that happens. Then reflect back to them what you've heard!

7. **Celebrate their secret identity.** If your hero has adopted a secret identity, find out the inspiration behind it. Were they inspired by a character from a book, a movie, a comic, a play, mythology, or history? Or is there another story behind its creation? Asking your hero to tell you how they came up with their secret identity is a great way to learn more about what they value and the strengths they want to develop.

Once you know more about their inspiration, see if you can have fun with it. Look for a digital image online that relates to their secret identity, and share it with your hero. Dig up some quotes from the book, movie, or story that inspired them, and deliver one each week—

by email or text if you're long distance, or you can handwrite the quotes and slip them somewhere to surprise your hero! If you're artistic, draw a doodle of your hero in their new secret identity. There are infinite ways to show your hero that you truly see them as the powerful, awesome person they want to be.

8. **Stay tuned.** Sometimes the best way to show support for someone is just to pay attention to what they're doing and saying. It's kind of like when you're having a conversation with someone. When they're talking, you want to nod your head and say "Mmm-hmm" occasionally—so they know you're still with them. It's good to develop the same kind of habit the rest of the time, too—little cues that let your friend know you're paying attention. This is thankfully made easier if your hero is active on social media or has a blog. If so, like, favorite, or comment on your hero's posts often—especially ones about getting superbetter! Think of your likes, favorites, and comments as virtual nods and "mmm-hmms!" They let your friend know they're not alone—and that you're with them every step of the way.

9. **When the going gets really tough, have a heart-to-heart.** Scientists have found that when it comes to feeling deeply supported, three kinds of social interaction build those bonds best: voice, face to face, and touch. So when your hero really needs a boost, you have three options. First, you can *speak up*. Research shows that when it comes to expressing support, a phone call is more powerful than the written word. Second, you can *show your face!* It turns out that we convey friendship, love, and encouragement through our facial expressions more than any other way. So when it's time to connect, how about a video chat? Finally, you can *reach out—literally*. Scientists have shown that physical touch— like a hug or a high-five—boosts confidence, eases pain, reduces stress, and strengthens relationships. In order to give this kind of support, you'll want to actually see your friend in person whenever possible.[8]

10. **Be a rock.** This is the toughest ally skill to cultivate. It means that even when you're busy, you take the time to touch base with your hero, every single day you can. Touching base can be as simple as sending a text message, or posting a comment on their social media feed, or asking a

single question about their SuperBetter day when you see them. Studies show that when it comes to social support, *quantity counts as much as quality*.[9] So don't wait until you can devote a lot of time to your hero. Just take thirty seconds out of your day to give support, and it will add up to a huge positive impact, one day at a time.

◄►

Remember, forging a powerful alliance doesn't benefit only you—it helps your friends and family better understand what you're going through. It lets them discover concrete ways to give you support that will actually make a difference.

This is especially important if you're facing a huge obstacle or going through a really tough time. Your loved ones can feel powerless to help in the face of your challenge—even though they desperately want to. But it doesn't have to be that way. A meta-analysis of seventy different psychology and medical studies revealed that when the friends and family members of someone going through an illness, injury, or tough crisis are given suggestions for improving communication and support with their loved one, the friends and family experience less stress and less anxiety, report happier moods, and have more physical energy.[10]

One SuperBetter player, Joe, a senior advertising executive who lives near Tampa, saw this benefit himself when he started a familywide Super-Better game. "We've started a SuperBetter Great-Grandmother Program for my mother, who has two children, five grandchildren, and thirteen great-grandchildren," he told me recently. "The two aims of the program are, one, to support and comfort her with loving messages and phone calls as she adjusts to assisted living, and two, to teach the extended family how to set up their own SuperBetter games, to help them build their own healthy networks of friends and family. It's been a huge blessing so far." Twenty-seven family members in total joined up as allies for Super Great-Grandmother Jeanette, and they are all working together to make sure she receives one phone call, letter, or photo every single day. More important, Joe told me, "everyone in the family is now thinking about their own power-ups, bad guys, and how they can help each other. It's been a great bonding and learning experience for all."

Joe's game isn't just multiplayer—it's practically massively multiplayer! You don't need to be so ambitious yourself. But when it comes to games, the more the merrier—and social resilience can ripple through your entire social network. Inviting allies to play isn't good just for you—it's good for them, too.

Joe's experience is not unique. As you'll see in the next story, a gameful approach to social support can give your allies more power, courage, and optimism—and as a result, you get stronger, not only individually but also together.

## A SuperBetter Story: Long-Distance Allies

It took three months of collecting power-ups, battling bad guys, and completing quests for Kate, twenty-six, to finally feel superbetter from her latest battle with depression. But for Kate to experience a major breakthrough in her relationship with her girlfriend, Laura, it took only three *days* of playing.

Kate and Laura have a long-distance relationship. Kate lives in Columbus, Ohio, where she works in IT support at a small nonprofit. Laura lives a three-hour drive away in Ann Arbor, Michigan. The couple met on a popular online dating site and felt such a strong connection, they decided to try to make it work, even though they could see each other only on weekends.

"I was honest with Laura about my struggles with depression and anxiety, right from the beginning," Kate told me when I interviewed her about her SuperBetter experience. "But telling someone you struggle with depression doesn't mean they'll really understand what you're going through. Even though Laura knew about it, I think my depression was like a black box to her. She couldn't see inside. She never really knew how it was affecting me day to day."

Laura's distance made it hard for her to know when Kate was having a particularly tough day. But SuperBetter changed that, almost overnight—as soon as Kate decided to show Laura her lists of power-ups, bad guys, and quests. "I was a little embarrassed to ask my Laura to be my ally and play with me," Kate said, "but she was excited to play. She told me she was happy to have a concrete way to help."

What kind of help did Kate ask for? She kept it simple: she wanted to talk with Laura every night for a couple of minutes about which bad guys she had battled, which power-ups had helped, and what quest she was hoping to tackle next. They were already video chatting every night, so checking in about the game was an easy ritual to introduce.

It took a few days for Laura to pick up the lingo of SuperBetter, but once she caught on, it was easy for them to start talking for the first time in detail about Kate's mental and emotional challenges. "The game talk let her see all the specific ways I was struggling," Kate said. "I could say, well, 'I'm having a tough time with the Self-Critic today, because I look in the mirror and only see flaws.' Or I could say, 'Help me put down the Warped Magnifying Glass, because I'm beating myself up about a small thing that happened about work.'"

This kind of conversation was new to the couple, even though they were already quite close. "I have all this negative self-talk inside my head that doesn't really come up in conversation, despite the fact that I struggle with it daily. The daily game check-ins gave me a way to share it."

As Laura started to understand the daily effects of Kate's depression better, questing became an important part of their alliance. "She could see exactly what I was struggling with, and she would give me quests that encouraged me in the right direction." Laura gave Kate, for example, a List Your Best Attributes quest that challenged her to list as many good qualities about herself in one minute as she could. She also gave Kate a You Are Beautiful quest, which required her to allow Laura to tell her "You are beautiful" for a full minute without any interruptions or negative self-talk.

Kate looks back now at the three months that she and Laura had daily SuperBetter check-ins as a crucial growth period for their relationship. "No one wants the world to see their weaknesses, struggles, and dark places. But the SuperBetter rules let me put these issues on display in a safe, constructive, and positive way. They let me show myself that I'm working to move past struggles and to improve myself, and for my girlfriend to see that as well."

"There's no question, as a result of playing together, we got so much stronger. There was so much more emotional intimacy. I think it's because the SuperBetter rules reward emotional honesty and vulnerability—something the world as a whole does not often do."

With Laura as her closest ally, Kate made so much progress that she no longer considers depression the primary challenge in her life. "It's something I'll always have to deal with, but it doesn't have to define or limit me." So she is turning her gameful superpowers toward new goals. "SuperBetter has been such a positive way of looking at things that I've started tackling a whole other set of changes I want to make in my life," she told me. Her current SuperBetter challenge is to jump-start her career: She wants to learn more computer programming so she can move out of her current role in IT support to become a systems administrator. And, she is happy to report, Laura is still a powerful ally, encouraging her every step of the way.

***

If you're still feeling unsure about inviting someone you know to be your ally, let me leave you with one final piece of encouraging data.

Our SuperBetter players have invited many thousands of allies to play with them online. And our data show that these friends and family absolutely relish the opportunity to help. How do we know? People who initially joined SuperBetter as allies logged in, on average, *twice as often* as people who signed up to play for their own challenge! And they took more game actions, on average, every time they logged in than did players working on their own challenges—leaving supportive comments, suggesting quests, and so on. In other words, most allies are more than just willing to play along—they are excited to be a part of your journey. As one SuperBetter ally put it, "It means a lot when a friend or family member asks for help, and it means a lot to be recognized for the support you give."

I don't want to paint an overly rosy picture. There's always the chance that you'll invite someone to play who will be too busy right now, or too focused on tackling their own challenges, to fully embrace the experience. Or someone you invite may be biased against games and not bring enough enthusiasm to the occasion. It's natural to feel hurt or disappointed if this happens. But the potential benefits of social support are so enormous, I encourage you to be willing to risk a little disappointment in order to pursue something that will truly make you stronger. (If you're unsure who to recruit as your first ally, it certainly doesn't hurt to invite someone who already plays a lot of games—or someone who has offered to help or expressed their support for you in the past.)

And remember, you don't need a lifetime commitment from your allies. Interviews with SuperBetter players have shown that even if your ally fully engages with you around the game for only *as little as one week*, you will still both reap significant benefits. It takes only a little bit of play to spark feelings of closeness, improve communication, and strengthen your mutual understanding.

## AN ALTERNATE STRATEGY: RECRUITING ALLIES ONLINE

As important as it is to have at least one ally whom you can see in person, that may not be the best way for you to start your game. In fact, roughly one in five new SuperBetter players says they would rather start their game with *virtual allies* than with everyday friends and family.

If you're a very private or introverted person, you may feel this way, too.

Or you may have a very practical reason for not wanting to recruit close friends and family. As one player explained on the SuperBetter discussion forum: "I'm working through painful feelings about some of the people in my life, and it would be really awkward for me to say to someone, 'Hey, I think *you* are one of my bad guys!' So for now, I think it's better to share this stuff with strangers."

Virtual allies are particularly helpful if you're looking to connect with someone who has already been through the same challenge you're tackling right now.

Or you may simply be one of the 25 percent of Americans who say they have no confidants with whom they feel comfortable discussing important personal matters.[11] (This number has more than doubled over the past two decades—so if you don't have any obvious candidates for allies, don't worry. You're not alone.)

If you fall into any of these boats, you can start recruiting allies today— online. There are discussion forums and social media groups online for just about any challenge you can imagine. Not sure where to start? At Areyougameful.com, I've gathered links to popular forums and groups for the most common SuperBetter challenges. You can also discover fellow players by searching for the hashtag #superbetter on social media networks, like Instagram, Twitter, and Pinterest. (I've made a surprising number of virtual allies doing that!)

Experienced SuperBetter players frequently rave about their virtual allies. As one player puts it, "I could never have guessed that I would start to feel so close to my allies—people that I've never met in real life, who I don't even know what they look like—and really care about them, about their dreams and their struggles, and feel happy and proud when they do well. The ally experience has been far more personal, invigorating, and valuable than I had ever guessed when I started. I love my allies! We are a family of sorts—the good kind."

Better yet, research suggests that virtual allies can increase your social resilience, even if you only ever communicate by screen. As one meta-analysis of forty-five different scientific studies shows, most people experience a genuine increase in perceived social support by participating in online communities dedicated to giving one another advice and encouragement.

As your social resilience increases, you may find yourself more comfortable with the idea of recruiting allies from your everyday life. Think of online allies not as a *substitute* for everyday allies but rather as a *springboard* for you to eventually create more powerful alliances in the rest of your life.

I hope you're convinced, and now it's time to take this game from single-player to multiplayer. Let's make that happen right now—with a very important quest.

## QUEST 34: Recruit Your First Ally

**What to do:** Pick one person in your life to invite to be your first SuperBetter ally.

If you're not sure who, these brainstorming questions can help:

- Who do you feel you can really be yourself around?
- Who can you ask for help if you really need it?
- Who do you have great conversations with?
- Who do you play games with?
- Who makes you smile whenever you see or talk to them?
- Who gives you good advice?
- Who do you admire and would love as a coach or mentor?
- Who makes things more fun when they're around?

When you've picked your first ally, all you need to do to complete this quest is to reach out.

"I'm playing a game to help me [name your challenge]. I'd like you to play the game with me. It will only take a few minutes a week, and we can play over the phone, by email, online, by video chat, or in person."

**Alternative quest:** Post a message on any online forum or social media group introducing yourself and your challenge.

Good luck—and may your allies always have your back!

### *Skills Unlocked: How to Supercharge Your Social Support*

- Instead of asking someone for help with a problem, invite someone to play a game with you.
- Explain how the game works. Share your challenge, power-ups, and bad guys. This is all it takes to turn any friend or family member into an ally.
- Be sure to report to your allies often about your progress in the game, so you can get tons of advice, encouragement, and support.
- Give your allies their own specific quests to keep them motivated and inspired. Remember, a quest is a teeny-tiny task they can accomplish in the next twenty-four hours—like sending you an inspirational quote by text message or choosing one power-up from your list to do together.
- If you're not comfortable inviting friends or family to play with you yet, start with virtual allies. Online discussion forums and social media support groups are the perfect place to make new friends who'll understand exactly what you're going through.
- Remember, just a week of gameful interaction is enough to reap huge benefits in your relationships and boost your social resilience. So don't worry if one of your allies gets busy and forgets to play, or if a long time passes between SuperBetter check-ins. Just keep living gamefully, and try to share your adventures with many different allies along the way.

# 10

# Secret Identity

## How to Be Gameful Rule 6

Adopt a secret identity. Pick a heroic nickname that
highlights your unique personal strengths.

This is the most playful of all the rules for gameful living. It requires
you to have a sense of humor, and not take yourself too seriously. It
also involves a bit of creativity and self-reflection to pick the right heroic nickname.

What is a secret identity? Think of it as an avatar for the real world. In
video games, avatars are the heroic characters we play as. We see the virtual
world through their eyes, and we draw on their special strengths.

As we saw in Chapter 3, playing a video game with a heroic avatar can
bring out your heroic qualities in real life. But you don't need a video game
or a 3-D character to maximize your heroic potential. Your own imagination
and creativity are strong enough to do the trick. Simply by adopting a heroic
nickname, or secret identity, you can bring out some of your most important
challenge-facing attributes, like determination, courage, and compassion.

Your heroic nickname could be inspired by fiction, myth, history, or even
family legend. Here are some of my favorite secret identities from successful
SuperBetter players. As you can see, they all highlight different strengths
and struggles unique to the player.

"I'm going to be the Dread Pirate Rosie, after the Dread Pirate Roberts from my favorite movie *The Princess Bride*. I've always been secretly a swashbuckler at heart, but too shy and unfit to do much in real life. When I'm more secure about my physical fitness and self-confidence, I plan to learn to fence and sail."

"My secret identity is Rodger Cole because it is the English version of my father's name. This name gives me strength because my father always stayed calm, simple, and generous in any situation. I want to honor him and be strong like him."

"I'm Psyonic Girl, like a comic book superhero. Sometimes negative emotions overwhelm me. But not Psyonic Girl! She is able to control her psyche at all times and can conjure her own feelings of well-being, happiness, and love."

"I've gone with Dunky Dory—which sounds silly and makes me smile! Dunky, because my real name is Duncan. Dory, after Dory from *Finding Nemo*—I love this character because that fish takes everything in stride, doesn't worry about any personal shortcomings, 'just keep swimming.'"

"I've chosen Kingfisher Fire as my secret identity. It's from a poem by my favorite poet, Gerard Manley Hopkins, which includes the line 'What I do is me, for that I came.' I'm using SuperBetter to get better from a lot of different things, but I feel like all of them are barriers that get in the way of my being able to say, 'What I do is me.'"

"I'm Mary Fuckin' Poppins. As that genius woman once said, 'Just a spoon full of sugar helps the medicine go down!' These days I've got a hell of a lot of medicine to swallow. This nickname also shows I have a strong sense of humor, which I think will be really important to me for not giving up and reaching my goals."

"My secret identity is Sergeant Self-Care. Self-care is my focus on my way to becoming SuperBetter from PTSD. I've always put helping others at the top of my life's to-do list. But I'm finding out that if I don't love and care for myself first, I can't do that for anyone else. I picked the title Sergeant because one of the most inspiring characters I've ever encountered is Sgt. Carwood Lipton from the *Band of Brothers* series. Sergeant Lipton was an actual soldier who fought as a US paratrooper in World War II. He was courageous even when put in terrifying situations and did his job to the best of his ability at all times. His ability to be humble and have a positive attitude while providing life-saving compassion for his fellow soldiers is truly an inspiration."

◀▶

Why adopt a secret identity? Although this rule seems quite playful, it has a surprisingly powerful impact.

A secret identity helps you focus on what researchers call your *signature character strengths*—the heroic qualities that are core to who you are.

Signature character strengths are different from one person to the next: determination, kindness, humor, spirituality, a sense of adventure, or love of learning. Figuring out *your* strengths will help you develop new strategies for reaching your goals—strategies that are customized for you and therefore more likely to work.

As you tackle different challenges, you might decide to draw on different strengths. Switching up your secret identity can help you do just that. When I was battling mild traumatic brain injury, I became Jane the Concussion Slayer—inspired by the fictional Buffy the Vampire Slayer—to bring out my courage and determination. When I was trying to get pregnant with my husband, I became Jane of Willendorf—inspired by the thirty-thousand-year-old curvaceous stone figure known as the Venus of Willendorf, presumed to be a fertility good luck charm. Becoming Jane of Willendorf helped me focus on different strengths: my ability to love and be loved. As your challenges and goals change, you may find it helpful to don a new heroic persona.

A secret identity has another surprising effect: it brings your allies closer—*if* you reveal the secret. Some SuperBetter players keep their secret identities to themselves. (After all, how many years did it take for Clark Kent to reveal he was Superman to Lois Lane?) But if you *do* choose to share your heroic persona, you will find that it's a powerful way to communicate to friends and family who you want to become—as well as the strengths and powers that are essential to your journey.

Perhaps most important, a secret identity is the first step toward telling a heroic story about yourself. Researchers who specialize in post-traumatic and post-ecstatic growth have discovered that telling a heroic story about your struggles is one of the most important triggers for unlocking growth from challenge. It helps you discover not just your strengths but also your purpose: ways you can use your strengths to help others.

As the behavioral scientist Steve Maraboli once said, "If you are not the hero of your own story, then you're missing the whole point of your humanity."

In this chapter, I'll teach you several fun ways to explore your heroic qualities and invent a secret identity. By discovering your signature character strengths and telling your own heroic story, you'll not only get stronger yourself—you'll inspire others to become happier, healthier, and braver, too.

Let's start with a quick quest.

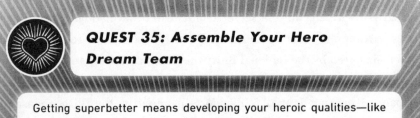

### QUEST 35: Assemble Your Hero Dream Team

Getting superbetter means developing your heroic qualities—like bravery, kindness, humor, appreciation of beauty, leadership, or love of learning.

You can find these qualities in any heroic narrative, real or fictional—film, comics, TV, mythology, video games, literature, history, religion, social activism, or sports (to name some of the most likely places you might look for heroic inspiration).

Everyone is drawn to different heroic stories. Picking your favorite heroes reveals a lot about *your* character. Why? Because we're usually drawn to heroes who embody the strengths we already have inside us and that we have the potential to develop even further. In other words, your favorite heroes are like a mirror for your own heroic qualities. This is true even if you feel like you haven't done anything heroic in your life yet, or lately.

To find out more about *your* signature character strengths, let's **assemble your hero dream team.**

A hero dream team is simply three or more heroes assembled to work together to achieve a common goal. Each one usually has a different strength or ability. You can find examples of dream teams everywhere in culture, from comic books to music to sports. Think of the Avengers, made up of the diverse superheroes Captain America, Iron Man, the Hulk, Thor, Black Widow, and Hawkeye. Or the Traveling Wilburys, a superband that included the Beatles' George Harrison, Bob Dylan, Roy Orbison, and Tom Petty. Or the teams that play in the World Cup, when a country's best soccer players join forces to face off against the rest of the world.

*Your* hero dream team could span every category of hero you can think of. Be as creative as you like. Why not have a hero dream team made up of Spiderman, the Buddha, Serena Williams, Sherlock Holmes, and your mom? (Can you imagine the adventures those five could get up to?!)

**What to do:** To perform this quest, pick at least three heroes. Whose character makes you feel like you could do anything, if you were more like them? Whose story inspires you to strive harder? Whose adventures embody the kind of life you want to lead? Here are some more brainstorming questions to help you assemble your unique dream team.

- Who is your favorite TV character?
- Who is your favorite movie character?
- What book character do you identify with?
- Who is your favorite professional athlete?
- Who is your most inspiring hero from history?
- Who fascinates you from mythology?
- Who is your favorite musician or band?
- Who is your favorite character from video games?
- What artist or creator inspires you?
- Whose life story intrigues you?
- Who do you think is the most interesting comic book super-hero?
- Who in real life or fiction has overcome a challenge similar to yours?
- What spiritual figure exemplifies the kind of person you'd like to be?
- Who is your modern-day (real-life) hero?
- Who else—famous or not—do you admire?

*Tip:* If you're stuck, do an Internet search for "top heroes in [your favorite medium—literature, film, comics, mythology, video games, history, the Bible, etc.]." There are inspiring "all-time great" lists for just about any kind of hero you can imagine.

**My hero dream team is made up of:**

1.

2.

3.

*Tip:* If you have more ideas, don't hold back! You can add as many heroes to your dream team as you want. The more, the merrier.

**There's one more superimportant step to this quest.** For each hero you've picked, identify at least one skill, power, virtue, or character strength that you admire. If you picked Boston Marathon champion Meb Keflezighi, for example, you might say "grit" or "competitive drive." If you picked Queen Elsa from the Disney movie *Frozen*, you might say "the ability to embrace her own power and use it without fear" or "the courage to celebrate who she is." Whatever you do, **don't skip this step!** The more clearly you can articulate the strengths in your heroes, the better picture you'll have of your own heroic qualities—whether they're already in full force in your life or simply waiting to be developed and unleashed.

Now that you've identified a few of your favorite heroes and gotten a glimpse into your own heroic potential, you're ready to hone in on just what makes *you* uniquely heroic.

Let's not waste any time. It's on to the next quest! (And a quick heads-up: this chapter is *full* of quests—more quests than any other chapter in this book. That's because *you* are the true expert on your own identity. *You* are the best source of knowledge about your own heroic strengths. So instead of me giving *you* information, for most of this chapter, you'll be tapping your own insight—with the help of some gameful guidance.)

## QUEST 36: *Spot Your Strengths*

You have at least five powerful resources that can help you be resilient in the face of any obstacle.

These five powerful resources are your **signature character strengths**—the virtues that come easily to you and that bring you tremendous satisfaction when you exercise them. And according to two of the most important and widely cited researchers of happiness and well-being, Dr. Martin Seligman and Dr. Christopher Petersen, these strengths determine how you will best cope with adversity—and what will bring you the greatest joy and satisfaction in life.

Dr. Seligman and Dr. Petersen oversaw a team of forty researchers to identify these strengths. Together they studied nearly one hundred cultures around the world and tested 150,000 subjects in order to determine the full range of virtues that both bring happiness and increase our resilience every time we use them. They identified twenty-four different character strengths in total—now known as the Values in Action (VIA) strengths—and they are listed for you below.

**What to do:** I want you to read through the list, and **pick the five strengths that stand out as describing *you* best.** Don't overthink it. If you prefer, there is a fancy 120-question online test you can take to figure out your top five strengths (and I'll tell you how to do that in a minute). But in experiments I've conducted, most people can simply look at a list and pick out at least four of their top five strengths, compared with the results from a more formal test. So go ahead.

**Which *Five* Describe You Best?**

- Creativity: You show great imagination and originality of thought; you always go beyond traditional thinking.

- Curiosity: You love to explore and discover; you have an eager desire to know about new things.
- Open-mindedness: You are always receptive to new ideas or arguments and think things through carefully from all sides.
- Love of learning: You naturally seek out new knowledge, and mastering new skills is a passion.
- Perspective and wisdom: You have a talent for advising others and for making sense of the world around you.
- Bravery: You don't shrink from challenge, threat, difficulty, or pain; opposition will not stop you from doing what is right.
- Persistence: You take pleasure in finishing what you start, and you follow through no matter what obstacles you face.
- Integrity: You strive to be authentic and genuine and are true to yourself no matter what.
- Vitality and zest: You live as if life were an adventure; you bring energy to everything you do.
- The ability to love and be loved: You are a caring person who creates very close relationships with others.
- Kindness: You take the time to do for others; helping comes naturally to you.
- Social intelligence: You understand other people, and can anticipate their feelings; you fit in naturally in many different social situations.
- Active citizenship and teamwork: You have a strong sense of social responsibility; you do your share and give back.
- Fairness: You treat others equally and fight for justice when necessary.
- Leadership: You inspire and motivate others; you are an effective organizer who makes things happen.

- Forgiveness and mercy: You give others a second chance and accept their shortcomings with grace.
- Humility and modesty: You value others as highly as yourself and don't seek the spotlight; you let your accomplishments speak for themselves.
- Prudence: You are a careful, thoughtful person and rarely do things you regret.
- Self-regulation and control: You have tremendous willpower; you are able to control your thoughts and feelings.
- Appreciation of beauty: You notice what is excellent and beautiful all around you; you often feel awe and wonder.
- Gratitude: You express your thanks often; you appreciate the good in life and others.
- Hope: You expect good things to happen in your future, and you work to make your dreams come true.
- Humor and playfulness: You see the lighter side of life; you are always making others smile.
- Spirituality: You seek a higher purpose in life and meaning in all you do.

As you've probably already figured out from this list, a signature character strength is not just any skill or talent, like being bilingual, athletic, or a good computer programmer. The difference between an ordinary talent and a signature character strength is that your signature strengths speak to your deepest values, to what you cherish most, to what brings meaning and purpose to your life.

**Example:** You might be very good at cooking, for example, but psychologists would not consider that one of your signature character strengths. However, it could be a *clue* to them. If you feel incredibly satisfied whenever you cook for your family, one of your top strengths

could very well be "the ability to love and be loved." If you enjoy in-
venting new recipes, your probably have the strength of creativity.
And if you find great pleasure in watching cooking shows and discovering new techniques, "love of learning" might be one of your
strengths. Any of these deeper strengths would help explain why you
derive so much pleasure from and devote so much energy to cooking.

Now that you know what a signature character strength is, have you
got your top five? Good! If it's not too tricky, try to rank them in order,
with number one being the absolutely most essential to who you are.

**Next step:** Now write down your top five strengths and put the
list someplace where you'll see it often over the coming days and
weeks. This list is a reminder that you have a unique combination of
strengths that can and *will* aid you in any challenge.

**Bonus mission:** If you're looking at your list and are not sure
you've really captured your signature strengths, here's a bonus
quest that will also build your social resilience. Show the complete
list of twenty-four strengths to a friend or family member, and ask
him or her to pick your top five for you. To make it more fun, offer to
do the same for them. Compare your lists and see if you agree with
each other's choices. If they pick totally different strengths for you
than you picked for yourself, you might just have an abundance of
strengths to work with. Nothing wrong with that!

*Tip:* If you want cold, hard scientific evidence of the fact that you
do indeed have five of these strengths, there's a special bonus
quest just for you. Go to www.viacharacter.org/Survey, and take the
scientifically validated strengths survey. This online survey contains 120 questions and takes ten to fifteen minutes to complete. It
will give you a detailed explanation of your top five strengths—and
even more confidence in the fact that you can effectively use them
to solve problems and pursue your dreams.

You've completed two incredibly important quests already in this chapter. You've assembled a hero dream team and you've identified your own signature character strengths. Now it's time to combine all this inspiration and self-knowledge... into a secret identity.

## QUEST 37: Adopt a Secret Identity

Your next mission is to pick a heroic nickname that will inspire your SuperBetter journey and highlight your unique strengths.

There's no wrong way to invent a secret identity. Here are some of the most common approaches taken by SuperBetter players. Try one, or try a few, and see which secret identity fits you best!

- **Pick one of the heroes from your dream team list**—and give yourself a heroic nickname inspired by their character and strengths. You can simply adopt their identity just the way it is ("I'm Iron Man," "I'm the goddess of love, Aphrodite"), but I encourage you to customize or personalize it ("I'm Iron Man Casey," "I'm Kelly, the Goddess of Love").
- **Combine two or more heroes from your dream team list into a unique new identity.** Here's how one SuperBetter player did it: "My secret identity is Captain Wonder. It's a combination of two of my favorite heroes: Captain Picard from *Star Trek*, and Wonder Woman."
- **Give yourself an honorific** and become the Queen of, King of, President of, High Priestess of, Sheriff of, or Princess of your favorite signature strength or unique trait. For example: Roger, the King of Curiosity; Mary, the Queen of Reinvention; or Jim, the High Priest of Rock 'n' Roll Cooking.

- **Pick a new middle nickname**, like Jane "Adventure" McGonigal or Harry "The Bear" Smith.
- **Try an online name generator** that can create thousands of customized or randomized heroic names for you. You could become Valentine Dragonhowl, Tsunami Heartwarrior, or even Pudding Pathfinder. (Yes, that is a real suggestion!) I've included URLs for some fun fantasy and superhero name generators in this endnote.[1]
- **Pick a fun adjective or title** you could combine with your first name, like Chelsea the Great (inspired by Catherine the Great) or SuperTony (inspired by Super Mario).

**One more idea:** Scramble the letters in your name to make a new name. (My name anagrams to Ace Longing Jam, for example!) This idea is inspired by what a SuperBetter player, Meike from the Netherlands, decided to do: "My secret identity is Ekiem. I just used my real name backward. I am here to become a better version of myself, and I think we all have deep down in ourselves the abilities and power to do so. I am here to bring the hero that already lies inside of me to life . . . so, Ekiem!" Although this method may not explicitly call out your signature strengths, it does help remind you of your power for self-transformation. You can get help with anagrams using an online anagram server at http://wordsmith.org/anagram. It's your turn. What hero best represents *your* superbetter self?

**My secret identity is:** _____.

**This hero's strengths, superpowers, virtues, and special abilities are:**

1.

2.

3.

Now that you have a secret identity, what should you do with it? Here are the top ways to celebrate your secret identity, as chosen by SuperBetter players:

**Create a visual clue**. Find an image that reminds you of your secret identity, and put it in a place where you can see it often. It might be on your refrigerator, by your mirror, or in your wallet. Or keep it digital: change your computer desktop image or phone background image to something that reminds you of your secret identity.

**Adopt a mantra or call to action.** Choose a short, powerful phrase that will remind you of your secret identity's strengths and inspire you to leap into action.

**Wear it with pride.** You don't need to wear a giant Superman "S" under your button-down shirt, but do consider picking out something small—a wristband, shoelaces, sunglasses, a piece of jewelry, socks— that represents your secret identity. Wear this item on days you really need to draw on your heroic strengths.

**Pick a theme song.** In TV and movies, heroes have a song or instrumental score that plays whenever they swoop in to save the day. Pick one for yourself. (Hint: Soundtracks are a great place to find dramatic music!) Listen to your song whenever your heroic powers need a boost.

**Sneakily show it off.** Hide your secret identity in plain sight. Take a new profile photo for a social media account that hints at your secret identity without giving it away.

**Collect heroic quotes.** If your secret identity is inspired by an existing character or real historic figure, collect a few favorite quotes from them. If your secret identity is completely original, collect quotes from the members of your hero dream team (from Quest 35), or anyone else you think your original hero would be pals with. Put your quotes in a journal, a quick-access file on your phone or computer, or on sticky notes you can hide around your house. You can even write your heroic quotes on tiny slips of paper, put them all in a jar, and use them as daily fortunes.

**Immerse yourself in the world of your hero.** If you're inspired by a film or TV character, hold a movie night or rewatch your favorite season. If you're inspired by a book character, reread your favorite book or read it out loud to someone else. If your secret identity is informed by a real-life hero, see if you can find a memoir by, biography about, interview with, or speech by them. Just make some time to truly enjoy the story that inspires you.

**Reveal your secret identity to someone you trust.** Share your alter ego with one of your allies, so they can see your heroic strengths and celebrate them with you.

Whatever you decide to do with your secret identity, remember that it's an opportunity to be playful and creative, to honor the stories and heroes that really speak to you, and most of all, to find new ways to express and celebrate the best version of yourself—your superbetter self.

## A SuperBetter Story: The Next Doctor

Josué Cardona, also known (to a select few) as the Next Doctor, is someone who can attest to the power of a good secret identity.

Originally from Puerto Rico, Josué, thirty, now lives in North Carolina, where he has his own psychotherapy practice. But when he started playing SuperBetter two years ago, he was still in school, trying to earn his counseling license and deciding what career step to take next.

"Taking on the secret identity had a huge effect on me," he told me recently—before admitting that I was only the second person he had ever shared his secret identity with. (His girlfriend was the first.)

Josué's SuperBetter nickname is a reference to the long-running British science fiction television series *Doctor Who*. "I adopted the identity 'the Next Doctor' because I wanted to get my counseling license"—or literally, to become the next psychotherapy doctor in the town where he lives. "But it was also more than that. I relate greatly to the character of the Doctor," meaning the time-traveling hero known for saving civilizations while also helping ordinary people. "The name represented for me both the path toward completing my training and also taking on more of the heroic qualities of the character, including helping others, curiosity, love of learning, and integrity."

Josué told me that adopting a fictional secret identity felt, surprisingly, like revealing his true self. "I saw the Next Doctor as an ideal self, what I wanted to become. But I also felt he was exactly me, just more. When I embraced the secret identity, it was like 'coming out of the closet' in a way about my own strengths. I suppose I was building up to it already. I was slowly becoming more comfortable with outwardly and actively displaying those strengths. Taking on the identity, it took it to a new level."

As the Next Doctor, Josué went on to earn his license as a mental health counselor. He then decided to start his own private practice, even though it was financially risky. The risk has paid off so far, as he reports that his practice is successful.

I was most struck in talking with Josué by how much his secret identity has helped him cultivate the virtues he values most. He clearly is inspired by his secret identity to become a better counselor to others, in very specific ways. "On the television series, the Doctor has seen a lot and knows a lot. He's traveled to every corner of the universe and through every moment in time," he said. "And yet he sees each person as something new and special. He is infinitely curious about them and admires them. Whenever I see the Doctor talk about how great each and every person he's ever met is, I remind myself that I want to make sure I make my clients feel the same way."

Like many successful SuperBetter players I've spoken to, Josué has transitioned from formally playing the game to just living more gamefully. "I haven't officially logged my quests or power-ups or bad guys in almost a year," he said. "But those concepts are still with me. They are now a part of how I think. I use them with clients, too. They're a part of my everyday vocabulary." He has held on to his secret identity, too. Today he still keeps a miniature TARDIS, the Doctor's time-traveling machine, on his desk at work as a reminder of the person he has committed himself to being. "I think about the Doctor all the time," he said. "I'm still the Next Doctor, more and more every day."

◄►

As you're starting to see, adopting a secret identity can be a lot of fun. But it also comes with some serious benefits.

Now that you know your signature character strengths, and you have a heroic nickname to remind you of them, you can start to use these strengths to your advantage.

Over the past decade, researchers have shown that people who *make it a daily habit* to think about their character strengths experience three key benefits.

First, they're more successful. People who are more aware of their strengths experience greater goal progress and achievement. (Remember, when scientists study the benefits of strengths, they aren't talking about ordinary skills or talents. They're looking at the twenty-four Values in Action strengths—the virtues you read about in Quest 36.) One study found, for example, that after selecting their own three-month goals, individuals were significantly more likely to achieve them if they first made a list of their character strengths, then purposefully applied them to the challenge.[2] In fact, not only did they achieve more, they were also happier and more satisfied with their lives at each check-in over the course of the three-month-long study.

Knowing and practicing your strengths daily not only makes you more successful, it also makes you happier. One randomized, controlled study examined six different methods for improving overall well-being, including keeping a gratitude journal and communicating positive feelings to a loved one, among others. The single most effective intervention, it found, was creating a list of signature character strengths. Six months later individuals who had listed their strengths were significantly happier than they had been at the start of the study. Moreover, they were happier than anyone else in the study. And the more they continued to think about and practice their strengths daily over the six-month period, the happier they were.[3]

Finally, focusing on your strengths can help you cope more effectively with any illness, injury, or disability—from arthritis, cancer, chronic pain, and infertility to substance abuse, eating disorders, and PTSD.[4] Studies have found that the more we think about and use our strengths during treatment or recovery, the more social, productive, and satisfied with our lives we are, even while experiencing significant health challenges. (All the signature character strengths deliver real benefit, but the strengths that seem to help *most* with this kind of coping are bravery, kindness, humor, appreciation of beauty, and love of learning. For that reason, some psychologists suggest cultivating these strengths in particular if you're facing a period of treatment or recovery.)[5]

That people who know their strengths and use them effectively are happier and more successful may seem obvious to you. But the reality is that all too often, especially when we're facing tough challenges, we focus on our weaknesses instead of our strengths. Many of us find it easier to list a dozen personal flaws than to name a handful of character strengths. This is particularly true for anyone who deals with anxiety, depression, or self-doubt.

Of course, it's important not to completely ignore our weaknesses. After all, that's why we battle bad guys! But to get the full benefits of your character strengths, you have to think about them and use them daily. This is one of the best reasons to adopt a secret identity. Whenever you use your heroic nickname, you'll be actively reminding yourself of your strengths.

It's easy to start using your strengths with greater purpose. Your next quest will show you how.

# QUEST 38: Seven Ways to Be Strong

**What to do:** Take a few minutes right now to brainstorm seven ways to practice your character strengths—and embody your secret identity—in daily life.

**Examples:** Here are some examples of how to practice a strength in new and different ways. (They're inspired by the excellent resource "340 Ways to Use VIA Character Strengths" by clinical psychologists Dr. Tayyab Rashid and Dr. Afroze Anjum. Check out the complete list online—you'll find the URL in the endnote.)[6]

If one of your strengths is *love of learning*, try learning a new word or phrase in a foreign language and using it in conversation today.

If one of your strengths is *vitality/zest*, try doing something that you already do ordinarily (like putting away laundry or walking the dog), but bring more physical energy to it, and notice how it feels.

If one of your strengths is *social intelligence*, try watching a TV show or film with the sound off, and see what emotions you can observe just through facial expressions and body language.

If one of your strengths is *justice/citizenship*, try spending fifteen minutes this week cleaning, decorating, or caring for a communal place like a park or a shared kitchen.

If one of your strengths is *forgiveness/mercy*, try planning out what your response should be the next time someone offends you. Remind yourself of your plan (rehearse it if possible), and periodically affirm, "No matter how he or she offends me, I will respond as I have planned."

If one of your strengths is *spirituality*, try spending a few minutes today reading from a spiritual text, then discuss the ideas in it with someone you trust and respect.

**Now it's your turn:** Pick seven ways of using your strengths and embodying your secret identity. (Be sure to base this list on *your* top five signature character strengths that you identified in Quest 36.)

1.
2.
3.
4.
5.
6.
7.

**Why it works:** This is the same kind of intervention studied by researchers at the University of Pennsylvania and the University of Michigan. In their study, participants identified their signature character strengths and then brainstormed seven different ways of using them over the next week. After using their strengths seven different ways in seven days, participants were happier and more satisfied with their lives—not just during that week but for six months after as well.

You are now set up for *exactly* the same success. You have a list of seven concrete actions you can take to use your strengths with more awareness and purpose. Try to do one of these things every day, for the next seven days, until you've done them all. If you get distracted, or if you forget to use a strength one day, don't worry— just pick the quest back up where you left off!

## A SuperBetter Story:
## The Family That Plays Together

Aaron Winborn, a web developer and father of two young girls, started playing SuperBetter a few months after his diagnosis at age forty-four with the neurodegenerative disease ALS, also commonly known as Lou Gehrig's disease. By the time he decided to adopt a secret identity (Aaron Skywalker, after *Star Wars'* Jedi fighter Luke Skywalker), he had already lost all manual dexterity in his hands. Using voice-recognition software, he wrote me to say that he had just achieved his first epic win: moving into a wheelchair-accessible house so that he would be better able to navigate life with ALS.

Although he suspected that some people might not understand how a game could help with such a serious diagnosis, Aaron wanted to spread the word to other ALS patients about the difference a gameful approach could make. "I am under no illusions that positive thinking will do much for the outcome of my disease. Stephen Hawking aside, virtually no one survives more than a few years with this disease. But what SuperBetter can do, I believe, is to increase one's quality of life, one day at a time."

SuperBetter gave Aaron and his wife a concrete and positive way to help his two daughters, ages five and eight, adjust to the family's new difficult reality. The girls were given special ally duties, such as helping him activate his most important daily power-ups—a series of "Superman flying poses" and "Jedi fighter training maneuvers" that were really stretching exercises designed to move his muscles and joints through their full range of motion. Adopting a superhero identity also let Aaron project an image of strength to his daughters, even in the face of a weakening physical body—which was very important to him, as a father, to do.

Aaron also invited a wider circle of family and friends to play, using power-ups and bad guys to communicate with family and friends about the progression of the disease, and to let them know exactly how they could help. He gave his closest allies roles inspired by the same *Star Wars* universe. One friend, Liane, became Liane-Wan Kenobi, Spiritual Adviser—a role inspired by Obi-Wan Kenobi, the mentor who trains Luke Skywalker in the ways of the Jedi. "As my spiritual adviser," Aaron explained to me, "her special power is *Cut to the chase*." In other words, she would be an honest, direct, and supportive partner in conversations about mortality and meaning of life that Aaron wanted to have. "She also has her own important quest: Assign weekly readings." Each week she would share a reading from a different philosophical or spiritual tradition, which they would then discuss together.

Eventually, Aaron decided he didn't need a secret identity anymore. He had become a real-life hero to many thanks to the incredible determination and love for his family that he continued to show as his ALS progressed. Sadly, Aaron passed away three years after his diagnosis, at the age of forty-seven. But the gameful approach was an important part of his coming to terms with the reality of ALS. "When someone has received a diagnosis of the ultimate incurable terminal illness, what they need more than anything else are superpowers. I want to thank you for reminding me of mine," he wrote me. And then encouraged me to share his story: "I want to help other people to discover theirs."

Adopting a secret identity has one more benefit that you need to know about, because it can transform the way you think and feel during the most stressful times of your life.

A secret identity can help you solve a problem that scientists call the *self-reflection paradox*.

When you're facing a tough challenge, it's natural to spend a lot of time thinking about it. But is it helpful or harmful to do so? Paradoxically, it's both.

Psychologists Ethan Kross, a professor at the University of Michigan, and Özlem Ayduk, at the University of California at Berkeley, explain the paradox like this: "On one hand, countless studies indicate that encouraging people to reflect on negative feelings or stressful experiences leads to important physical and mental health benefits. On the other hand, an equally large body of research indicates that people's attempts to understand their feelings or make meaning out of stressful experiences often backfire, entangling them in ruminations [or compulsive thought cycles] that make them feel worse."[7]

Kross and Ayduk have been researching the self-reflection paradox for years, attempting to answer this question: "Why do people's attempts to make sense of their negative experiences sometimes succeed, and at other times fail?" Their research findings reveal a surprising answer: *to benefit from thinking deeply about your own personal challenges, think about your challenges as if they were happening to someone else.*

The technique is called *self-distancing*, and Kross and Ayduk have completed several of the most important studies of it. "Self-distancing," they explain, "is what happens when you take a step back when thinking about your own experiences and reason about them from the perspective of a distanced observer, like a fly on the wall." Instead of getting caught up in your own intense feelings and the details of your experience, you look at the bigger picture.

According to their research, the most common sign of successful self-distancing is using "third-person" language. Instead of asking myself, "Why do *I* feel sad about the news I found out today?" I would ask myself, "Why does *Jane* feel sad about the news she found out today?"

Thinking about our own experiences in the third person can feel strange or awkward. If you heard someone else talking about him- or herself in the third person, you might think it the sign of a raging egomaniac, or at the very least a touch of eccentricity. (As Kross and Ayduk point out, the NBA superstar basketball player LeBron James famously talks about himself in the third person, as in "I want to do what's best for LeBron James.")

Fortunately, the experts don't recommend that you talk or think about yourself in the third person all the time—far from it. You should use the self-distancing technique only when you need to get perspective on a very big challenge, a stressful situation, or a traumatic experience.

If you master the technique, you'll experience a range of physical, mental, and emotional benefits. You'll have less cardiovascular reactivity when you think about challenges, stresses, and traumas—meaning your blood pressure will be less likely to go up, and your heart rate will return to normal faster. And brain scans show that self-distanced thinking involves less activity in the subgenual cingulate cortex—the region of the brain that lights up when depressed individuals get stuck in negative thought patterns. In other words, self-distancing strengthens your body *and* reinforces a more positive neural circuitry.

A review of studies from the past thirty years shows that self-distancing works equally well whether you're thinking about the past, the present, or the future.

*The past:* People who practice self-distancing experience less anxiety and distress when they recall painful memories or traumatic experiences.[8]

*The present:* Self-distancing enhances willpower.[9] If you face a temptation, you'll be better able to exert self-control if you take a moment to think about the situation from a third-person point of view. Instead of asking yourself, *Do I want that candy bar?*, ask yourself, *Does Jane want that candy bar?* It sounds like an absurdly simple trick, but it works. When you think of yourself in the first person, you're more easily caught up in your momen ary feelings and cravings. But when you think of yourself in the third person, you're more likely to see the bigger picture, remembering your long-term goals and most important motivations (like being healthy for your loved ones, or having more energy later to work on your novel, instead of feeling sugar-crashed and guilty). Getting self-distance allows you to focus on the big picture, which helps you stick to your goals.

Self-distancing has another benefit in the present: it leads to *greater engagement in constructive problem solving*—which means getting less wrapped up in thoughts and being better able to focus on taking helpful action.[10]

*The future:* Self-distancing makes you more likely to adopt a challenge mindset, instead of a threat mindset, when you face new obstacles. As you'll recall from Chapter 5, having a challenge mindset means feeling realistically optimistic that you have a chance to succeed, learn, or get stronger from a stressful situation, whereas having a threat mindset means focusing only on the potential risks and harms. People with a challenge mindset are, overall, happier, healthier, and more successful in achieving their goals than people with a threat mindset.[11]

The benefits of thinking about the future with some self-distance continue even after you've faced your obstacle head-on. In laboratory and real-world studies, immediately after tackling a stressful task, people who adopted a third-person perspective beforehand spent significantly less time doing negative *postevent processing*—or stewing on something that didn't go well, blaming yourself, and just generally beating yourself up for not doing better.[12]

Finally, self-distancing dramatically improves psychological flexibility. You'll remember from Chapter 7 that psychological flexibility is the willingness to do things that are difficult for you, in the service of your goals. When you think about your situation with self-distance, you are more likely to act according to your deepest values, even if you risk negative feelings, pain, rejection, or failure. In other words, self-distancing makes you braver.[13]

N ow that you know all the benefits of self-distancing, you might be wondering how adopting a secret identity helps you practice and master this powerful technique.

A secret identity makes it easier to create self-distance when you need it most. Because you don't normally identify yourself with the heroic nickname, using it creates just enough mental distance to get a better perspective about the challenge and stresses you face. See for yourself how it works—in the next quest!

## QUEST 39: What Would a Hero Do?

**What to do:** Think about something specific that's causing you stress, worry, or excitement. It could be something you are doing later today, or something that is far in the future. Whatever it is, make sure it provokes a strong emotional reaction (positive or negative) when you think about it.

Got it? Good. Now ask yourself: *What would a hero do?*

Not just any hero. Think about **the hero you've already adopted as your secret identity.** (If you haven't figured out your secret identity yet, come back to this quest later!)

Recall the **strengths, superpowers, virtues, and special abilities** you've already associated with your secret identity—from creativity, courage, and kindness, to humor, justice seeking, or imperviousness to physical pain. How would your hero use these specific strengths to prepare for or deal with the challenge or obstacle at hand?

In other words, ask yourself: *What would [your secret identity] do?*

When you consider this question, be sure to use third-person language. Don't say (or think, or write), "I would . . ." Instead, say (or think, or write) "Jane the Concussion Slayer would . . . ," "Sergeant Self-Care would . . . ," or "Mary the Queen of Reinvention would . . ."

**Why it works:** Asking "What would [your secret identity] do?" is a great way to get a little self-distance—and in doing so, give yourself smarter, more motivating advice.

Experts explain: "Small shifts in the language you use to refer to yourself—specifically, using your own name and other non-first-person pronouns like 'she' or 'he'—enhances your ability to regulate your thoughts, feelings and behavior under stress."[14]

Incorporating your secret identity into the process (instead of using your regular name) provides an added benefit: you'll be able to focus on your signature strengths as a way to solve problems and take action more effectively and with greater joy. Dig deep into the strengths and powers you've identified as being important to your hero—they can be a springboard to a thousand different strategies.

I've used this quest effectively in my own life, so I know how powerful it can be. Earlier this year, when I was making purchases for our twins' nursery, I was wracked with the kind of self-doubt and anxiety that is quite common in first-time parents. I worried constantly: *Is this crib safe enough? Will my babies develop asthma or allergies if I don't buy organic? And holy moly, there are five million different strollers to choose from! How in the world do I pick one?* Every purchase left me feeling more *insecure* instead of more prepared! It was crazy-making. So I thought back to the secret identity I'd adopted while undergoing IVF treatment: Jane of Willendorf, inspired by the ancient fertility goddess the Venus of Willendorf. And I asked myself, *What would Jane the fertility goddess do?*

And then I thought: *Every time Jane of Willendorf picks something out for the twins, she feels happy, because this is exactly what she hoped for! How could something she wanted so very much become a source of constant anxiety instead of a source of constant joy? She won't let it. She is a fertility goddess! She is confident and her love conquers all.* Just by stepping back and looking at the situation with a bit of distance, I realized that I was letting myself turn what should have been a joyful experience into a stressful one. But I could choose to celebrate every moment of preparation, just by summoning up my own superpower: the ability to love and be loved. From that moment forward, whenever I felt a twinge of worry, I relabeled it a "twinge of love"—and I enjoyed it!

**Quest complete:** By completing this quest, *you* will be able to get the same kind of fresh perspective on your own source of stress or worry. Good luck!

Now that you know how self-distancing works, let's keep practicing.

Quest 39 was designed to help you think about your future. The next quest will teach you a powerful way to reflect on *past* stressful or upsetting events—without falling into the dark side of the self-reflection paradox.

## QUEST 40: Tell a Hero's Story

Your goal in this quest is to tell a quick story about a hero—you.

**What to do:** Every hero faces obstacles and setbacks. Think about **something that sparked a negative thought or feeling in you,** sometime in the past few days. It might be a moment when you were frustrated or disappointed with yourself, an argument you had with your romantic partner, an unpleasant conversation at school or work, a moment you found yourself annoyed or angry with someone else, when your feelings were hurt, or an experience that provoked some anxiety or self-doubt.

Do you have an experience in mind? Good.

Now tell **a quick story reflecting on this experience.** The purpose is to figure out *Why did the hero feel or react that way?*

You can think through your story in your head right now, or write it down, or talk it out with an ally.

Start with **what happened** and **how the hero reacted**. Then spend some time reflecting on **the reasons for that reaction**, as if it were a mystery you're trying to solve.

Your story may also celebrate things the hero did to make the situation better—or notice things he or she did to make things worse. It may be a story of the hero's strengths *or* vulnerabilities (or both!), because even superheroes always have at least one vulnerability.

Be sure to tell this story **as if it happened to someone else— specifically, to your secret identity.** As you think up your story, use third-person (self-distancing) language, like *Why did Iron Man John react this way?* or *What might be an underlying cause for Dread Pirate Rosie's feelings?*

**Quest complete:** You've completed this quest successfully when you've told *your* hero's story!

**Why it works:** Self-distancing shortly after a difficult experience helps you feel better and think more clearly about it for days afterward. In fact, research shows that the benefits of just one quick self-distancing quest should last at least one full week. During that time, you're less likely to get caught up in negative memories. And if you do think about the experience, you'll feel less distress and more acceptance. Over time the more you practice this technique, the less time you'll spend caught up in unhelpful thought patterns that drain your energy, tax your body, and distract you from making progress toward your goals.

Eventually this technique of reflecting on daily events can help you tell the story of your entire SuperBetter journey. It's a story you'll want to tell and retell often, as you make sense of all the ways your life, and your sense of what is possible in your future, is changing.

Barbara Abernathy, Ph.D., has seen the power of heroic narrative up close in her own work. She is the head of the Pediatric Oncology Support Team, a nonprofit organization that provides free psychological support to children with cancer and their families. She is also an expert in post-traumatic growth. Based on her own work with patients and their families, she believes that storytelling and role-playing potential new identities are the cornerstone of post-traumatic growth.

"We learn about ourselves by the stories that we tell," she explains. "In fact, we create ourselves through conforming to our own mythic story."[15]

Crucially, Dr. Abernathy argues, our stories are not an outcome of the challenges we face or the lives we've already led. Rather, they are "a powerful, global coping strategy" that can actually transform the trajectory of our lives while we are still facing our toughest challenges. In other words, the stories we tell about ourselves can change what we think we're capable of—and therefore what we do each day.

One SuperBetter player, Shelley, a forty-nine-year-old entrepreneur in Houston, says that changing her story was a key personal breakthrough. "While I endured chronic fatigue syndrome, I learned this story: 'I am weakened, fragile, vulnerable to exhaustion and environmental overload.' I hated that story. With my whole being, I hated it." She knew she needed to write a new, more heroic story for herself. So instead of letting her illness wear her down and force her to stay in bed constantly and lead a smaller and smaller life, she became Big Life Shelley. With this secret identity, she told a very different story about herself. "'I am capable, creative, giving, growing, unstoppable! I can lead a Big Life, even if I feel sick.' I tell myself this story even when I am feeling grindingly slow instead of sleek, fast, and amazing. *Especially* when I feel crummy, I need to remember this story."

A major life challenge of any kind—positive or negative—provides the opportunity for adopting a new role identity and creating a new mythic story. Dr. Abernathy frequently encourages the children and families she works with to consider the question: *Who am I now?* This is a good question for you to ask yourself, too—by way of adopting a new secret identity whenever you need one.

*Who am I now?* Your answer may change once, twice, or many times over the course of your SuperBetter journey. Allow yourself to become someone different, someone new, whenever you need to. Experiment with becoming someone stronger, wiser, braver, calmer, or sillier, someone with a higher purpose or with a laser focus, someone open to whatever the future holds. Telling a new heroic story is one of the best predictors of post-traumatic and post-ecstatic growth.[16]

So play with your identity. Tell new stories. Re-create the myth of who you are.

Let your secret identity be a powerful tool for you not only to practice your signature strengths and master the art of critical self-distance but also to reinvent yourself—again and again—and explore *all* possible best versions of yourself.

### *Skills Unlocked: How to Adopt a Secret Identity*

- Pick a heroic nickname that conjures your signature strengths.
- Your signature strengths are the virtues and abilities that make you uniquely you. Use them to tackle your challenges, and you will not only be more successful, you'll be happier along the way.
- Let your secret identity remind you to practice your signature strengths on a daily basis, and to keep exploring new and different ways to use your strengths.
- Use your heroic nickname to practice self-distancing, the powerful technique of reflecting on your own problems as if they were happening to someone else.
- Reveal your secret identity to people you trust. Tell your allies your hero's story so far.
- Tell a new heroic story, or adopt a new secret identity, whenever you want to focus on a different set of strengths. Re-create your personal mythology to represent the stronger, braver, and happier person you're becoming.

# 11

## Epic Wins

### How to Be Gameful Rule 7

Go for an epic win—an awe-inspiring outcome that
helps you be more motivated and less afraid of failure.

An epic win is a special kind of goal. It's designed to be more like *game* goals than ordinary self-improvement goals.

Here are some examples of epic wins from successful Super-Better players:

- Go twenty-four hours without being bored. (Challenge: depression)
- Sleep one night without my iPod. (Challenge: insomnia)
- Keep up with my husband on a walk around the lake. (Challenge: getting in shape)
- Dance in public. (Challenge: social anxiety, low self-esteem)
- Go one week without using my inhaler. (Challenge: asthma)
- Meditate for thirty minutes in a row. (Challenge: anxiety)
- Take my kids to the movies—and be able to sit with them the entire time. (Challenge: back pain)
- Fix up three broken bikes from the thrift shop and donate them back, ready to ride. (Challenge: rehabilitating from knee surgery after a bike accident)

- Complete a twenty-mile fundraising walk. (Challenge: find a new, more fulfilling job)

These goals—like the goals of all good games, from golf to sudoku to *Super Mario*—have four things in common: they're realistic, challenging, energizing, and forgiving.

A gameful goal is *realistic* if you have reason to believe you'll successfully achieve it if you make your best effort. After all, games are designed to be winnable.

A gameful goal is *challenging* if, in order to achieve it, you have to learn a new skill or draw on strengths like creativity, cleverness, and grit. A goal without an interesting challenge is just work!

A gameful goal is *energizing* if just thinking about it fires you up. You know you'll feel fantastic if you achieve it. Game goals are usually quite energizing—which is why, whether it's a sport or a video game, players often throw their arms up in the air and roar with pride after they achieve a victory.

Most important, a gameful goal is *forgiving*. If you don't achieve success on your first try, all is not lost. Nothing terrible will happen to you or others. In fact, even if you fail, something good will happen—you'll learn strategies and ideas for doing better on your next attempt or on your next goal.

◄►

Why aim for an epic win? When you're going through a difficult change or a tough life challenge, it's important to be able to find opportunities for success and breakthroughs.

Researchers call this powerful skill *positive reappraisal*, or benefit finding.[1] It means being aware of good outcomes that can come even from stress, trauma, or a major life change. Positive reappraisal is a powerful source of mental, emotional, social, and physical resilience: it lowers stress hormones, improves mood, leads to greater relationship satisfaction, *and* boosts immune function.[2] But you don't develop it by chance. The best way to get good at positive reappraisal is to set yourself up for regular epic wins or positive breakthroughs.

As the legendary football coach Vince Lombardi famously said: "Winning isn't everything. But *making the effort* to win is."*

Your epic wins may seem minor to someone else. They probably won't be breaking news or Nobel Prize–worthy. But the key to a good epic win is that it feels like a huge leap forward to *you*, while still being totally achievable. As one player, Sam, put it after he achieved his first epic win:

> Going without my inhaler for six days maybe sounds like no big deal. But when I chose my epic win, I thought it was a real long shot. I accomplished it quicker than I thought was possible. Six days I have been free of the asthma pump! After six months of wheezing, coughing and all kinds of medications, I am breathing just fine on my own. Feel like I do have some power over my health, after all.

As Sam discovered, one of the key benefits of an epic win is that it can change what you think you're capable of. It can reveal that you have more control over your life than you'd thought. And once you know that, you can aim for more ambitious epic wins.

Designing gameful goals for yourself is a skill, one you'll get better at with practice. This chapter will teach you the techniques of gameful goal setting and positive reappraisal—and help you plan your own exhilarating course of epic wins for the future.

L et's start by talking about the simplest version of an epic win: the measurable win.

A *measurable win* is a very clear goal, with progress you can objectively track and an obvious way to know when you've achieved it. Here are some examples:

---

* You may be more familiar with the quotation "Winning isn't everything, it's the only thing," which is also attributed to Vince Lombardi. However, Lombardi spent the last few years of his life claiming he was misquoted and insisting he had said "making the effort" to win was everything. Interestingly, interview transcripts show that he did, in fact, say *both* versions of the quotation at various times in his life—but that over the years, he increasingly insisted that "wanting to win," "the will to win," or "making the effort to win," rather than winning itself, is what matters most. See Steven J. Overman, "'Winning Isn't Everything. It's the Only Thing': The Origin, Attributions and Influence of a Famous Football Quote," *Football Studies* 2, no. 2 (1999): 77–99.

- Get eight hours of sleep every night for one week.
- Lose five pounds.
- Put $250 in savings this month toward a dream trip.
- Go twenty-four hours without needing pain medication.
- Send a thank-you message to a different friend every day for twenty-one days.
- Finish a 5K charity run.
- At a networking event, introduce yourself to ten people.

As you can see, every measurable win has a number involved. There's no room for error or subjectivity—you either achieve it or you don't.

By way of contrast, here are some *nonmeasurable* versions of the same goals that would make for absolutely terrible epic wins: *Get more sleep. Lose weight. Save money. Be less dependent on pain medication. Feel more gratitude. Start a running routine. Be more confident in social settings.*

All these goals are worthy endeavors! But they are basically useless when it comes to being gameful, because they establish no clear win condition. How will you know for sure when you've achieved one? You won't—not unless you have a way to measure it!

It's quite easy to create a measurable win for yourself. Think of a habit or activity you'd like to do often, an ability you'd like to improve, or a milestone you'd like to reach. Then pick a target number that feels *interesting* to you—interesting, because it's challenging, and because you're not 100 percent sure you can do it. Then create a goal around that number.

Remember, it's essential, for an epic win, that you *not* be completely confident that you can achieve this goal. If you are 100 percent confident, then it's probably a *quest* and not an epic win. Quests are about making steady progress. An epic win should feel like a major breakthrough—like you've just found out something new and awesome about yourself when you achieve it.

Measurable wins are the building blocks of getting superbetter, especially in the early days. They help you tackle your biggest challenges and take purposeful strides toward your most important goals. Just be sure to start small—the smallest leap you can make *without being 100 percent sure you can do it*. Because you're going for breakthroughs, you may have to try more than once. This is perfectly normal—and perfectly gameful. (Remember, video games are designed to help players get better by continually requiring them to aim for goals just beyond their current ability—goals they are almost never expected to achieve on the first try.)

Whenever you achieve a win, set your eyes on a bigger one. Before you know it, you'll be achieving wins that truly change your perception of what you're capable of.

Let's brainstorm some possible measurable wins right now—with a quest.

## QUEST 41: Plan a Measurable Win

A measurable win is a great way to stretch your limits and inspire extra effort. What will *your* first measurable win be?

Here are some brainstorming questions to inspire you:

- What would you feel really proud to do for seven days in a row?
- What do you want to go an entire twenty-four hours *without* doing?
- What's a "personal best" record you could aspire to set? In other words, what's the "most" you've ever done something? Can you beat that number?
- If you're working toward a big milestone—an amount of money you want to save, a number of pounds of muscle you want to gain, a word count for a book you want to write—what mini-milestone could you get to in the next thirty days?
- What number just *feels* epic to you? For example: *Read 1,001 stories to my kids. Walk 500 miles. Take 365 creative self-portraits.* Just pick a number that feels huge and worth celebrating— then challenge yourself to get there. (Just be sure if you pick a

truly epic number that you have an easy way to tally! I prefer to use a tiny notebook or a sheet of paper taped to the wall.)

**Why it works:** The key to the power of measurable wins is that they are goals you choose for yourself, based on the skills, abilities, and habits *you* want to develop. Research shows that choosing your own goals leads to better health and happiness, faster. In fact, every time you achieve a goal of your own choosing, you improve your odds of achieving the *next* goal. (Even if the next goal is much more ambitious!) Scientists call this the *upward spiral of positive outcomes*— and it happens only when *you* are in charge of the goals you pursue.[3]

**What to do:** List at least one measurable win for yourself here.

1.

You're not committing to any epic wins yet—so feel free to give yourself a few options to choose from.

*Tip:* Remember, it's not a measurable quest if it doesn't have a number in it!

Not all triumphs come with numbers attached. Let's talk about another popular type of epic win: the breakthrough moment.

A *breakthrough moment* is a major, positive turning point in your efforts to get superbetter. It's an event you can aspire to and plan to do that will show off your strength and resilience. It can also be a way to demonstrate and celebrate your commitment to your goals.

In Chapter 9, you read about Alex Goldman's epic win, getting back on his bicycle to ride for the first time, six months after he was hit by a car while riding. This is the perfect example of a breakthrough moment. Alex not only had to summon up his courage to ride again; he also had to complete enough physical rehabilitation to be able to ride the three-mile loop. His Prospect Park ride was both a physical and a mental breakthrough.

Sometimes a breakthrough moment will happen when you least expect it, and that doesn't make it any less worth celebrating. But actively planning for and vividly imagining your next breakthrough moment—just as Alex did, preparing for and envisioning his Prospect Park ride over a six-week period—has two major advantages.

First, when you *purposefully* set out to achieve a breakthrough moment, you'll reflect on your own strengths, values, and goals as you decide what you want your moment to be. This reflection can lead to important self-insight. What counts as success to *you*? Second, keeping a breakthrough moment firmly in mind can become a powerful source of motivation, as you visualize your future success and what it will feel like to achieve it.

Here are some additional examples of planned breakthrough moments, in the words of the SuperBetter players who achieved them:

"I want to be self-employed, but I need to save more money and make more contacts before I can quit my current job. My first epic win was to put myself out there with my own official website. I've let the world know who I am and what my talents are."

> —Darren, thirty-eight, whose challenge is to work for himself

"One of my allies suggested that my first epic win should be to un-friend my ex-girlfriend on Facebook and delete her as a contact on my phone. Honestly, I was shaking while I did it. But now it's like two tons of weight have been lifted off my shoulders."

> —J.T., twenty-five, whose challenge is
> getting over his ex

"As planned, I went to Cheesecake Factory *and did not order cheesecake* (or any dessert for that matter). I feel like I've earned a black belt in will-power."

> —Melissa, forty-two, whose challenge is getting
> healthy and feeling beautiful

Some breakthroughs are bigger than others. Some take weeks of effort to achieve, while others happen in an instant. But they all represent a kind of personal leveling-up in real life. Each breakthrough is a celebration of strength and shows a commitment to positive transformation.

What will *your* next breakthrough moment look like? Try this next quest to find out.

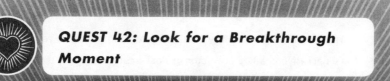

## QUEST 42: Look for a Breakthrough Moment

A breakthrough moment is a positive turning point in your Super-Better journey. Once you achieve it, you can be confident that you're making real progress and developing powerful new strengths.

Here are some brainstorming questions to guide you:

- What big step could you take in the next week that would signify a major commitment to your goals?
- What is one thing that you've been unable to do due to injury, illness, or extreme stress that you would like to be able to do again soon? Could doing it for the first time again be a breakthrough moment?
- What's something that scares you but that you could reasonably do in the next thirty days?
- How could you show off a new skill or strength you've been developing—in public, or to friends and family?
- What have you been procrastinating about, or avoiding doing, that you really want to get done once and for all?
- What good news would you want to yell from a mountaintop?

- Could you do something to honor, remember, or commemorate an important event in your past, or a person who influenced your decision to get superbetter?
- Can you think of any other major leveling-up moment for you in real life? What could you accomplish in the next ninety days that would tell the world (or even just yourself), *I am so much stronger than you had any idea!*

**Why it works:** The ability to identify turning points in your own life's narrative is a key predictor of post-ecstatic or post-traumatic growth.[4] Every breakthrough moment, or turning point, you achieve helps you tell a new story about yourself and the powerful strengths you're discovering.

**What to do:** List at least one potential breakthrough moment for yourself here.

1.

*Tip:* You're not committing to any epic wins yet—so feel free to give yourself more than one option to choose from.

## A SuperBetter Story: The One Who Didn't Quit

"I hardly recognize myself. And that's a good thing." Those were the first words Meg shared with her allies two years ago, after achieving her breakthrough moment: finishing a twenty-mile fund-raising walk to help end hunger.

At the time Meg was twenty-six, living in a suburb of Boston and working for a major corporation whose values did not reflect her own. "It was a really difficult time for me," she told me recently, looking back on the experience. "I hated my job, and I saw little hope of anything in the future. So I took the chance to sign up for SuperBetter."

At first, Meg was unsure what to tackle as an epic win. But when a coworker told her about an upcoming charity walk, it seemed like the perfect opportunity to take a step in the right direction. She might not feel that her employer was a force for good, but she could do something individually to make the world a better place.

Before the charity walk, Meg had only ever walked as far as six miles. "My goal was to get as far as possible before my legs simply gave up and detached themselves from my body," Meg said. "I figured on that happening at roughly Mile 10."

She started the walk on a small team, made up of coworkers and acquaintances, all cheering each other on. At Mile 10 most of them called it a day. But Meg wanted to keep pushing. At Mile 12 her final remaining teammate decided to go home. "It was the most demoralizing moment of the entire day," she said.

But she decided to keep walking—despite a calf cramp, a sore knee, and blisters forming on her feet. "By Mile 18, the aches in my body were breathtaking," she recalled. "I was sunburned and exhausted to the point of tears." She still can't say for sure what compelled her to keep going and to push through the pain. Part of it was wanting to do as much as she could for a good cause. Part of it was a growing curiosity. Had she completely underestimated what she was capable of?

Despite her pain and exhaustion, she eventually crossed the finish line onto the Boston Common, hobbling and elated. "I distinctly recall shrieking, through my tears, 'I did it! I walked twenty miles! I [effing] did it!!'"

"Even now I remember every sympathetic and amazed expression I encountered at work the next day. No one, including myself, seemed to believe that I had managed to make it. That *I* was the one who went the distance, who didn't quit."

Four months later Meg wrote down her reflections about the epic win that she achieved, despite not truly believing it was possible.

"Every ache in my body that day filled me with fiery joy. A twenty-mile walk? I did it because I could. And no one can take that away from me. Now when my old inadequacies rear their heads, I find myself hitting back rather than shrinking from my fears. *I'm going to look silly, and people are going to laugh at me*, the negative thoughts come. Then my victory crows, *This?! This is a body that has walked twenty miles! Let them look!*

"I'm still overweight, out of shape, asthmatic, and given to bouts of lethargy, but I no longer care so much about how I measure up in comparison to other people on the street. The walk has devoured my doubts. Now I'm likely to look at a challenge, whether physical or emotional, and decide that I have the endurance, determination, and motivation to succeed.

"Since the walk, life has brought its usual bevy of strife and disappointment. The difference now is that when I falter and sulk and feel gloomy, I can look up at my bedroom wall to my framed Walk for Hunger completion certificate—and remember that I can, in fact, do the impossible."

Meg still comes alive when she talks about that day. "I am not exaggerating when I say that walking twenty miles and achieving that epic win changed my life," she told me more than two years after the charity walk. "My entire self-concept had to be rewritten to acknowledge that I could meet that kind of challenge."

She used that momentum to make other changes in her life, including finding her way into a career where she can be a force for good not just one day but every single day: "The Walk for Hunger fed my desire to do more good, to participate in my community." Today she works in Boston at a job she is extremely proud of: as a department coordinator in the health care oversight field, where she ensures that people get the health care they need, when they need it most. "I'm loving every minute of it," she said.

Although Meg doesn't battle the same bad guys she used to, she has made her two favorite SuperBetter quests a part of her regular routine. "I still set myself up weekly for a *Do something that scares you* quest, and I complete a *Take pride in something about yourself* quest every single day," she told me. She keeps up these gameful habits because you never know when life will throw an unexpected obstacle your way. "I will always be the superbetter version of myself," she said, "no matter what obstacles come."

---

Measurable wins and breakthrough moments help you tackle your challenge directly. But there's one more way you can go for an epic win—sideways.

For the past three years players have been reporting their epic wins via SuperBetter online. My analysis shows that roughly one in four have been "sneak-up sideways" wins. This term is inspired by John Stuart Mill, an early nineteenth-century British philosopher, who once said, "Happiness should be approached sideways, like a crab."

In other words, instead of trying to be happier, aim for more concrete goals, like learning something new, helping others, or using your creative talents to make something. Happiness is more likely to be created as a by-product of these meaningful goals than by trying to be happier.

Likewise, when it comes to getting superbetter, it sometimes helps to take a sideways approach. Instead of trying to solve your problems directly, you can focus on a goal that is tangential or even (seemingly) unrelated to your primary challenge. The nonprofit organization Soldiers to Summits, for example, takes U.S. soldiers and veterans on expeditions to some of the highest mountain peaks in the world. Many of the trips are designed to take a sideways approach to treating post-traumatic stress disorder. Many participants find tackling the gameful goal of summiting a mountain more energizing and easier to measure than trying to heal from PTSD. (Helpfully, making a difficult mountain climb is also a known path to post-ecstatic growth—which would ultimately help combat symptoms of PTSD.)

Laura, thirty-three, started playing SuperBetter while pregnant. "I'm getting SuperBetter because my second baby is due any day now," she wrote at the time, "and as all parents know, the first three months or so are pretty rough. I figure something that encourages me to take care of myself is a good thing."

But Laura struggled to find an epic win that felt both realistic and inspiring. "*Make it through the next three months* is going to happen whether I get stronger or not, since I can't stop the flow of time. *Avoid depression* seems unrealistic, since I have a history of depression, and it sometimes hits despite my best efforts. *Have a happy family* is way too dependent on factors outside my control. As you can see, I just can't find an epic win that I like!"

Laura turned to her allies for ideas and wound up adopting an unlikely goal for someone whose challenge was to make more time for her own needs. Her epic win: *Help other new moms*. More precisely, she decided to create a *power pack*, a customized set of power-ups, bad guys, and quests, that she could share with other new parents.

Whenever Laura found a power-up that worked well for her, spotted a particularly tricky bad guy, or completed a satisfying quest, she would add it to the power pack. Eventually she published her pack online, with power-ups like "*Sunlight!* Get outside, even just by sitting on your front steps for a few minutes" and quests like "*I feel pretty*: take time to do one thing that makes you feel pretty today. Put up your hair, put on earrings, or just put on a pretty lip gloss. It doesn't matter if nobody will see it. You know you're beautiful!"

Afterward Laura reflected, "This was the perfect epic win for me. As a stay-at-home mother, you don't get much sleep, your brain is awash with hormones, you don't get much adult interaction, and to top it all off there aren't any concrete goals or projects to work toward. Creating my own power pack gave me a sense of daily purpose and progress. And it felt meaningful, because I knew it would help others."

Laura's story is the perfect illustration of how personal well-being is sometimes better achieved by finding a slightly higher purpose. Your purpose doesn't have to be world-changing or Nobel Prize–worthy! Turning your focus outward even a little bit can help you tap into a more authentic motivation and achieve something that brings a powerful sense of pride. In short, *your* perfect epic win may not be something that you do for yourself—it may be something you do for others.

Consider the experience of Dylan, forty-one, who had lots of goals when he started getting superbetter: eat more healthfully, get fit, lose weight. There were plenty of obvious measurable wins that Dylan could have chosen related to these goals, but he was tired of counting calories and clocking workouts. So after a few weeks, he decided to reframe his challenge with a very creative twist. "I'm getting SuperBetter so I can be a better human to my dog," he announced. He felt that getting off the couch, having more energy, and being physically fit would ultimately benefit not just him but also his six-year-old mutt, Cody, who loved long walks and always wanted to play.

But how was he to measure success in making *his dog* happier? An ally on an online discussion forum inspired him with the following idea: celebrate more frequent dog birthdays. The ally wrote: "My own beloved dog died in May, and it didn't occur to me until she was dying that I should have given her more birthdays. Since a dog's year is one-seventh of ours, that means they should have a birthday once every fifty-two days. A dog birthday is a day in which you do all the things that dogs love: walks, throwing sticks, playing. It's also, like any birthday, a way of facing mortality, which means cherishing what we have when we have it."

And just like that, Dylan knew what his first epic win would be: to celebrate a year's worth of dog birthdays with Cody, one every fifty-two days, full of long walks and epic play sessions. "The weight off my mind is incredible," he said after picking the new win. "I feel like I can be successful now, instead of feeling like a failure that the progress is so slow."

Dylan's choice reveals one of the main benefits of sneaking up sideways on your win: a sideways goal is often more *forgiving*. Like many people who struggle to achieve health goals, Dylan was used to beating himself up for not reaching his quickly. Every setback became a reason to doubt himself more. Focusing on something so joyful and not directly related to his health challenges helped him drop the baggage of self-doubt and negative thinking—which also allowed him, slowly but surely, to drop some extra weight.

Crucially, what Dylan celebrated as an epic win *wasn't* the thirty pounds that he ultimately lost. It was the seventh dog-birthday that marked his true moment of triumph.

Both Laura and Dylan benefited from pursuing epic wins that weren't obvious at the outset.

Should you consider going this counterintuitive route? Here are some of the most common obstacles that players face when trying to pick an epic win. If *you're* hitting any of these roadblocks when you try to brainstorm a win, sneaking up sideways may be right for you.

- **Your goal doesn't inspire you**. "I decided my first epic win would be to exercise five times a week for an entire month. But I'm just not excited about it. It feels like something I *should* do, not something I want to do."

- Achieving your goal depends on too many factors **not in your control**. "I'd like to say my epic win would be to find a loving partner and start a family. But I know that's not really in my control. I can't make someone magically appear and fall in love with me. So what can I do to win in the meantime?"

- Achieving your goal is **simply not possible**—and you're not sure where else to look for one. "My reality is that my symptoms are not going away, and they are going to get worse over time," wrote a player living with the progressive neurodegenerative disease ALS. "That doesn't make me want to give up—far from it! But it does make it hard for me to figure out what to pick as an epic win, since a cure is not a possibility for me."

- You have no goal. **You cannot imagine anything that would make you feel happy or successful**. As one player put it, "My problem is, I cannot think of anything, even something small, that would give me joy." This problem is surprisingly common. The neurochemistry of depression, anxiety, PTSD, traumatic brain injury, chronic pain, and many other illnesses can make it extremely difficult for sufferers to anticipate positive future outcomes.[5] (A dopamine imbalance is often to blame.) If this is true for you, you are far from alone. But know that even if you can't imagine an epic win for yourself yet, *you can still achieve one*. Try Quest 43 below, or ask your allies for suggestions.

Sneaking up sideways on your challenge can help you leapfrog right past any of these obstacles and achieve an epic win sooner than you think. You don't have to pick a goal that directly solves your problems. It's okay to have fun with it and aspire to *any* kind of accomplishment that appeals to you.

To give sneaking up sideways a chance right now, try the next quest!

---

### QUEST 43: *Sneak Up Sideways*

The rules for sneaking up sideways on a win are simple. Just think of a goal that gives you a spark of joy, curiosity, purpose, or meaning. It can be big or small, silly or serious; as long as going for it sounds like *fun*, it will make a great epic win.

Here are some brainstorming questions to help you sneak your way to a happier, healthier, braver you. Remember, just for the moment, forget your practical goals. It's perfectly okay if your answers to the questions have *nothing to do* (at least on the surface!) with the challenge you've chosen for yourself.

- *What's the most fun thing you can imagine doing thirty days from now?* Whatever it is, announce to yourself that *doing that thing* is going to be your first epic win. Now go try to plan it and make it happen!
- *What's an activity that you've always wanted to explore but never felt like you had time?* Pick an amount of time to commit to it over the next ninety days. If you spend at least that much time doing it, you win.

- *What's a cause or charity you care about?* Pick a way to show your support, whether it's raising money or volunteering a set number of hours, over the next ninety days.

- *How could you express yourself creatively?* Choose to make a video, write a song, self-publish a book, create a photo gallery, sculpt something, paint a mural, write an epic poem, or otherwise share a vision and make your voice heard.

- *Where would you like to go that you've never been before?* Plan a trip or a local adventure someplace new. It's a great way to motivate yourself sneakily to do all kinds of other worthy things, whether it's get in shape, save money, make more time for friends and family, finish that thing you've been procrastinating on, or even just get out of bed when that's difficult.

- *Who is a person you care about deeply?* Choose to do something special for that person, such as throwing a gratitude party for him or her. (Invite all the guests to bring a thank-you letter or other expression of gratitude for the guest of honor. You can do a gratitude party online as a virtual party, or in person.)

- *What's a new skill you could learn in the next six months?* Make a plan for how you'll learn it. Then pick a way to show off your new skill in a big way. That demonstration is your epic win.

- *What challenge have you always wondered if you were up for?* Whether it's running a marathon or taking an online course, finally give it a shot once and for all.

- *What do you already know that you could teach others?* Decide to pay it forward by sharing your wisdom and expertise with someone who could really benefit. It could be anything that shares knowledge: editing twenty Wikipedia articles on a topic you care about, giving a demonstration at your workplace, starting a blog or podcast, volunteering at a local school, self-publishing a self-help manual, or even starting a group to teach people how to get superbetter!

**Why it works:** When people pursue goals that match their core values, they put in more effort and are therefore more likely to achieve them. Moreover, when they do achieve their goals, they reap greater benefits: more happiness and a sense of personal satisfaction that lasts longer.[6] Sneaking up sideways will help you focus on *your* core values—not what you think you *should* be doing but what you really want to do.

**What to do:** List at least one surprising idea for an epic win here.
1.

*Tips:* You're not committing to any epic wins yet—so feel free to give yourself more than one option to choose from.

Even if you decide to tackle a measurable win or a breakthrough moment first, keep these sneaky wins in mind for the future!

## A SuperBetter Story:
## The Master of Sneaky Wins

You truly never know where your epic wins will take you. Andrew Johnston, forty-five years old and a father of three, is living proof of that.

Five years ago he hit rock bottom. Laid off from his job as an executive recruiter, he was unable to find work, despite having an MBA and spending hours a day on the search. After a year of fruitless efforts, his family's savings were gone, and their home in the Denver suburbs was nearing foreclosure.

Andrew seemed to be failing at everything, no matter how hard he tried. He needed to succeed at something, anything. So in the midst of this difficult time, he started devoting a few hours each day to something he'd had personal success with in the past: running.

Andrew was an experienced marathoner, and he picked up the hobby again—this time with more intensity. "I poured all my energy into it. I cranked it up to extremes," he told me. He got faster, he ran longer, and he started competing in local races. He mastered grueling mountain terrain, tackling runs with thousands of feet of elevation gain. He finished ultramarathons, races at least fifty kilometers long. Every running goal he set for himself he achieved, even as he continued to struggle to find work.

It was a paradox. He could see his strengths so clearly when it came to running—commitment, determination, planning, and perseverance. He knew from over a decade of experience in recruiting and financial management that these character strengths are essential to success in the business world. So why, in his own life, weren't they translating into better career resilience?

Finally he got a break, teaching business courses at a local community college. Soon afterward he had an epiphany. Maybe running, which had seemed like a distraction during his long period of unemployment, was in fact a path toward a career breakthrough.

Andrew went to the dean of the college and proposed an unusual course. It would be based on the idea that distance running builds the skills needed for success in business. He would call it "Change Through Challenge," and—the craziest idea of all—the final exam would be to run a full marathon, all 26.2 miles.

It took some convincing, but Andrew won the dean over. The class filled up completely—and to make it more challenging, nearly every student in the course was brand-new to running. Over the sixteen-week course, they read business books and did two training runs together each week. Everyone in the course finished at

least one race, and more than 70 percent of the students successfully completed the full marathon. (Others whose fitness hadn't
quite progressed far enough by the end of the course had the option
to run a 10K or half-marathon as their "final exam.")

What started as an experiment is now an unqualified success.
Andrew has taught the "Change Through Challenge" course three
times so far. And he is full of pride when he tells me that it is now
officially approved as a credit-earning business course across the
entire Colorado community college system. This year the program
is expanding to Denver high schools. Meanwhile, his innovation has
not gone unnoticed. Since starting his course, he has been pro-
moted to associate dean of instruction.

Andrew believes that every victory he achieved running during
that difficult time boosted his confidence and determination, which
gave him the strength to keep looking for career wins. Without the
athletic wins, he doesn't think he would have had the optimism and
creativity to imagine a marathon-based business course.

Today Andrew brings the philosophy of epic wins into his class-
room, where the SuperBetter method is now a part of the official
curriculum. "Not one person walks into the first class thinking they
can run a marathon," he told me. "When they see the training
schedule, they all freak out. The numbers look impossible. They
just can't picture themselves being successful." But for most students, belief kicks in very early in the process—usually, Andrew
says, after they achieve their first breakthrough moment. "Running
five miles is the real turning point for most students. It's longer
than any of them have ever run in their lives. Suddenly they say,
'I've never done that before, but I just did it.' Something clicks for
them. A goal that used to seem impossible is now suddenly possible. It changes their whole mindset: *What else that seems impossible
now could become possible in just a few weeks?* They become curious
and want to find out."

This curiosity about what's possible is the quintessential
experience of pursuing epic wins. And as Andrew's journey reveals,

*any* effort to achieve a personal breakthrough—even one that
seems unrelated to your most pressing challenges—can lead you
to the most wonderful and unexpected outcomes.

"I almost lost everything," Andrew said. "But look where it led—
to the most meaningful work of my life. I never expected to be here.
But now I know. A real terrible thing can be a godsend."

Like many of the epic wins described in this chapter, Andrew's involved
a *physical* triumph, something athletic in nature—walking, bicycling, running, summiting a mountain, or dancing in public. This isn't just a feature of
the particular stories I've selected. In fact, if you search the SuperBetter da-
tabase for all the epic wins from more than 400,000 players, four of the ten
most commonly appearing verbs are *walk, run, exercise,* and *dance.* (Other
top epic win verbs include *finish, find,* and *create.*)

What's perhaps surprising is that these athletic verbs are commonly
found as epic wins for *every possible challenge* you can imagine, not just fitness or weight loss challenges. Physical and athletic epic wins are extremely
popular among people tackling obstacles as diverse as overcoming depression or anxiety, recovering from concussion, coping with diabetes or PTSD,
becoming a better parent, finding a romantic partner, and even finding a
new job.

Why? Based on the stories I've heard and the data I've seen, I would have
to say that athletic triumphs make for particularly motivating and compelling epic wins—meaning, if you're still not sure what kind of epic win to go
for, *you cannot go wrong with a walk, run, swim, cycle, or dance epic win.*
Here's why:

Physical activity is a known mood booster, which helps with almost any
challenge. And exercise is one of the most effective treatments for depression, something that can often stand in between you and your nonathletic
goals.[7]

Exercise changes your perception of pain, making you tougher and *less*
sensitive to painful stimuli. (Scientists say this is because exercise puts physical, often painful, stress on your body; the more you exercise, the more

"normal" your brain interprets pain signals, and therefore it pays less attention to them.)[8] Being less vulnerable to physical pain is a type of resilience that can help you feel stronger in all areas of your life.

Athletic goals typically require a commitment to training, which builds determination and willpower—two strengths that benefit you in any challenge.

An athletic epic win—like completing a charity walk, running a 5K, finishing a yoga boot camp, earning your first belt in a new martial art, or participating in a fund-raising dance-a-thon—also gives your social resilience a huge lift, by connecting you to a much bigger community. If you have friends, family, or coworkers who participate with you, which is often the case, all the better for increasing your social strengths!

Finally, athletic wins often have a built-in sense of meaning and purpose, because so many walks, races, and athletic events are organized to raise money and awareness for a good cause. More meaning and purpose means more motivation, plus more positive emotions like gratitude, compassion, spiritual connection, awe, and wonder.

For all these reasons, at some point in your SuperBetter journey, you may find that an epic physical activity goal is the kind of triumph you want to pursue. Even if you're not looking at improved fitness or weight loss as a goal, the unique combination of mental, emotional, social, and physical strengths you'll gain by pursuing an athletic breakthrough makes it among the most transformative wins you can aspire to.

◄►

You've brainstormed at least a few epic wins for yourself. Now it's time to pick the one you want to aim for first.

I recommend giving yourself a chance to achieve your first epic win quickly—if not in the next week, then at least in the next month.

As you consider which epic win to aspire to first, you might find it useful to check out the Epic Win Possibility Scale—a thirty-second tool you can use whenever you set your mind on a new potential win. Try it out, in your next quest!

## QUEST 44: The Epic Win Possibility Scale

Have you chosen a smart epic win? Here's one way to find out.

**What to do:** Rate your potential epic wins on the Possibility Scale!

*What will it take for you to achieve your epic win?*

0—You could accomplish your epic in win in the next hour without breaking a sweat.

1—You could do it in a day, any day.

2—Give it a good week, and there's at least a 50/50 chance you'll be there.

3—It'll take a couple of weeks and a strong effort.

4—You could accomplish it in thirty days, if you make a heroic effort.

5—Six weeks should do the trick.

6—A few months and real commitment, and you'll get there.

7—It might take six months, but it's worth it.

8—With heroic focus, and some help from the most important people in your life, you could do it in a year.

9—If you're being honest, it takes a pretty wild imagination to picture yourself achieving this goal at all.

10—Someone would win a Nobel Prize if they achieved this epic win. Maybe *two* Nobel Prizes.

**Scoring:**

0–1: Dream bigger! You're stronger than you think.

2–5: Congratulations! You're perfectly on target for your first epic win.

6–8: You've got a great epic win, and you're superambitious! Here's a gameful tip: If you ever start to feel frustrated that you're still far away from your goal, break it up into two or three smaller epic wins (somewhere in the 2–5 range) that you can tackle one at a time.

9–10: Good for you for being fearless—but getting superbetter will be more fun if you aim for something in the 2–8 range. And who knows? Rack up a few smaller epic wins, and you might become more likely to achieve your totally fearless goal!

*Tip:* Now that you've got the hang of it, use this chart whenever you decide to set out toward a new epic win. And don't be afraid to imagine wins with a rating of 9 or 10 for yourself—just make sure to line up some more quickly achievable ones along the way.

Here are some final tips for pursuing your epic wins with a gameful mindset.

**Tell your allies about the epic wins you plan to pursue.** Making a public commitment to a goal increases your odds of achieving it.[9]

**Be open to trying again**. You'll achieve greater triumphs if you're open to failing the first time. (Imagine how boring games would be if we played only games that were so easy, we were assured of winning.) Thirty-five years' worth of goal-setting research shows that *harder goals inspire greater effort*, as long as the goal is not absolutely and obviously beyond a person's control or ability.[10]

**Go only for wins that genuinely matter to you**. This is the most important rule of all. When it comes to personal growth, success, and happiness, it's not *how much* motivation you have that matters—it's what *kind* of motivation. If your main motivation is to please someone else, or to live up to some external standard, you won't be very happy, even if you do reach your goals. But if you pursue goals of your own choosing, you're likely to be happier and healthier, whether or not you ever achieve them. (Fortunately, when you pursue goals of your own choosing, you *are* more likely to be success-ful.)[11] Just remember, epic wins are a place to proudly—and if necessary, defiantly—proclaim what *you* want to be able to do.

### Skills Unlocked: How to Achieve an Epic Win

- An epic win is a gameful goal: it's realistic but challenging; energiz-ing but forgiving. Every epic win you go for should provoke at least a little bit of curiosity and wonder: *Can I really do this?*

- Going for a measurable win is the easiest way to stretch your abilities and make leaps forward. Pick an improvement you'd like to make, and stick a number to it.

- Plan a breakthrough moment. Imagine the single action you could take that would show off your commitment to be stronger.

- You can also sneak up sideways on success, by going for an epic win that seems to have very little to do with your primary challenge. Just pick any goal that truly energizes you. This is a good strategy if you're having a hard time finding a goal you feel truly optimistic or excited about.

- Consider a physical feat for a future epic win, no matter what your challenge. Physical feats have provided some of the most meaningful transformations in SuperBetter history.

- Always share and celebrate your wins with allies. No matter how or-dinary your win might seem to someone else, relish it as if you just climbed Mount Everest. Celebrating positive achievements is a piv-otal step toward post-ecstatic and post-traumatic growth.

# 12

## Keeping Score

The art of keeping score isn't practiced very often in the digital age. Today most games are scored automatically. At the bowling alley, computers tally points. Online Scrabble calculates your word scores for you. Video games track your experience points and level you up without any effort on your part.

But when it comes to getting superbetter, you might want to keep your own customized, personal game score. *Keeping your own score is the best way to really internalize the rules of a game—and to get a deeper understanding of your own play.*

This has been true of games as long as humans have played them. In fact, my favorite argument in favor of personal scorekeeping was written over one hundred years ago, in a 1914 issue of *Baseball Magazine*. "The Pleasure and Profit of Keeping Score" was an editorial that strongly encouraged baseball fans to fill out their own scorecards during professional games. Track every run, hit, and error, it argued, in order to better understand, remember, and enjoy the game. Here's how sportswriter C. P. Stack made his case:

> Most spectators watch a great play with an interest, which, however intense, is forgotten in the thriller of the next inning. They leave the grounds with a hazy idea of a rather enjoyable afternoon, whose main features are

scarce refreshed by reading press accounts of them some hours later. Keeping score remedies all this. It burns the play into memory. It greatly increases the spectator's knowledge of the game.... And, best of all, it is a pleasure in itself. A few simple rules, practice—and keeping score becomes second nature.[1]

This recommendation makes just as much sense for the SuperBetter method today as it did for baseball then. By keeping a close record of your own gameful efforts, especially during the first days and weeks of play, you'll develop a much deeper understanding of the seven gameful rules. And by keeping score during the most important periods of challenge and growth in your life, you'll better remember exactly what you did to get stronger— making it more likely you'll do it again in the future.

There are lots of ways to keep score in SuperBetter. You can tally power-ups activated and bad guys battled. You can count quests completed and epic wins achieved. Use these numbers to motivate yourself. Can you set a new record? (Ten power-ups in a single day!) What's your longest streak? (Thirty days in a row of completing at least one quest!) Keeping a notebook, journal, spreadsheet, or blog is an easy way to track your successes.

Besides these simple tallies, something bigger is at stake. The true measure of a gameful life is your growing resilience—your physical, mental, emotional, and social strengths. So how will you know you're truly increasing your resilience? In this chapter, I will suggest easy scoring techniques to help you measure the powerful difference that gameful thinking and acting are making in your life—including how to set a new high score that represents your overall gameful skills and newfound resilience in one simple number. The higher your high score, the more likely you are to lead a life that is not just longer but also truer to your dreams—happier, healthier, and braver—and most important, a life with no regrets.

Let's start with the simplest way to keep track of your SuperBetter progress—a *daily score*. As one SuperBetter player puts it, "An epic win may be far away, but you can always win the day." Just aim to get your daily dose of SuperBetter:

### *3 power-ups + 1 bad guy battle + 1 quest = a daily win*

This SuperBetter dose was tested by both the University of Pennsylvania and Ohio State University Wexner Medical Center, and it's what I recommend to all SuperBetter players. *Every day try to activate at least three power-ups. Do battle with at least one bad guy. And complete at least one quest.* This is just enough gameful activity to help you develop significant resilience, while still fitting easily into your daily routine.

Some players incorporate their daily dose into their regular to-do list. Just add "Power-up 1, Power-up 2, Power-up 3, Battle, Quest," and cross each item off as you complete it.

Other players keep a journal of their SuperBetter adventures so they can look back and see just how far they've come. If you'd like to try it, the daily dose makes for a perfect structure for journal entries. Every day write down which three power-ups you activated, which bad guy you battled (and which strategy you used), and which quest you completed. The daily dose format makes it quick and easy to keep a compelling record of your gameful journey.

Keeping a daily score can help you build a sense of momentum as you try to rack up daily wins. Can you go for four, five, six, or even seven wins (a perfect score!) in one week?

A daily score can also help you learn something useful about your Super-Better habits. As one player explained it to me, "I noticed that I never get my daily dose on Sundays. The day slips by, and despite having all this free time, I've done nothing to get SuperBetter." Fortunately, spotting this pattern helped him adopt a new strategy. "I officially declared all Sundays 'Super-Sundays.' I make it a special challenge to get my daily dose."

This is what I recommend for you: *Track your daily dose for two weeks.* Once you've tried it, you'll always be able to use this scoring method again when you need it—for example, if you're facing a new challenge, experiencing a time crunch, or just want to renew your commitment to getting superbetter.

*Three power-ups, one battle, and one quest.* This is all you need to do to ensure that you've done everything you can today to keep getting stronger, happier, braver, and more resilient.

Another easy way to build momentum and get some personal insight is to go for a *personal record*.

A personal record, or PR for short, is your all-time best result at any given challenge. Athletes and game players of all kinds track their PRs, whether it's the farthest they've ever run, the most assists they've made in a single game, the fewest moves it's taken them to win a chess match, or the fastest time they've been able to play through an entire video game from start to finish (also called a "speed run"). Setting PRs like these can inspire you to try harder, be more ambitious, and get more creative. It's an excellent way to playfully explore the limits of your own potential.

After you've gotten the hang of a daily score, I encourage you to try to set a SuperBetter PR or two of your own. Here are some ideas to get you started.

- Your **most powerful hour**: How many different power-ups can you activate in a single hour?*
- Your **most powerful day**: How many different power-ups can you activate in a single day?
- Your **most epic battle day:** What's the greatest number of bad guys you've ever survived in a single day? (It may have been a truly terrible day, but it's also a measure of just how strong you are to get through it.)
- Your **longest daily win streak:** How many days in a row can you get your daily dose of SuperBetter without missing a single day? (Remember, the daily dose is at least three power-ups, one bad guy battle, and one quest!)

These four PRs are the most popular to go for among SuperBetter players. Feel free to invent your own new categories for records.

---

* As far as I know, the world record for most powerful hour is twenty-three different power-ups in a single hour. Feel free to try to break that record if you dare. I imagine it would take a lot of careful planning, and the help of an ally or two!

You can also go for personal records that are more customized to your challenge. For example, if your challenge is to finish your first novel, you might want to set a PR for the most days in a row you've written at least one hundred words. If your challenge is to get fit, your PR could be for the most steps taken in a single day (measured with the help of a pedometer!). If your challenge is to conquer anxiety, you could set a PR for the longest you've been able to spend time somewhere, or do something, that ordinarily makes you anxious. Look for the little things you can track and measure that will be a real indicator of progress for *you*. (A personal record also makes for an excellent epic win.)

If these scoring techniques seem too simple to make a significant difference in your life, let me give you an example of how keeping a tally can transform your behavior in surprising and profound ways—an example from my own SuperBetter journey.

## A SuperBetter Story: My Story, or 154 Good Days

Back in 2010, six months into life with postconcussion syndrome, I was still struggling with migraine headaches on a daily basis. They were bad enough that I was taking the maximum safe dosage of pain relievers almost every day—sometime three different medications a day. I knew I was getting better in some ways—I could think clearly at last, and I could work for several hours a day. But I was still spending way too many daylight hours resting in bed, nauseated and half-blind from the headaches. I felt far from back to normal.

I didn't have unrealistic expectations. But I needed to have hope that not *every* day would feel like a bad day. What would be good enough for me? I decided that if I could have just two good days a week—two days where my headaches were mild enough that I could skip pain relievers completely—I could be happy. I could live with five bad days a week, as long as I knew I could have two good ones.

But at the time, I honestly had no idea how many good days I was having. The days all blurred together into one long lousy week, one terrible month. So on January 1, 2010, I started keeping track. I taped a plain piece of white 8.5"-by-11" paper by my bedside and started a tally. Every night before I went to sleep, if I'd gone medication-free, I gave myself a check mark. My hope was that I would have a hundred check marks by the end of the year.

The next few weeks were hit or miss. The first week I had only one good day, but the next I had two. The third week I didn't have any good days. But the fourth week I had three!

Just keeping score this way had a very interesting effect on me. Whenever I had a miserable migraine day, instead of slipping into depression and despair, I could look at the growing tally next to my bed and say, "Look at all those good days you've had. Statistically speaking, you *are* going to feel better tomorrow or at the very least the day after. This pain is not forever. Hang in there." The tally turned into objective evidence that gave me hope for the future.

I also started craving a check mark at the end of the day. I wanted the feeling of pride and accomplishment I got when I added a new notch to the tally. When a migraine hit, instead of reaching for a pill right away, I would lie in the dark for an hour, in hopes that I could still earn a check mark for the day, waiting to see if the headache would pass on its own. And sometimes, to my great surprise, it did! It was a revelation to me. *Sometimes the headaches got better on their own.* If not for my extra motivation to bump up my score, I'm not sure I ever would have realized that sometimes my migraines actually went away without any pills.

Soon my score was no longer just an objective record of my behavior. It was motivating new, healthier, and more empowered behavior. I practiced the "power breath" (exhale twice as long as you inhale) as a first response to headaches, instead of medication. Sometimes it worked, sometimes it didn't. When it did, I felt powerful. But even when I decided I needed pain relievers after all, the result was still positive: I'd waited so long before taking any medicine that I often wound up taking a much lower dosage for the day. This triggered an upward spiral. Not only did I start earning more check marks, and counting more good days, but the medication actually started working better when I took it. (I had been decreasing my tolerance to it by taking it less often.)

This gave me more confidence that I was really getting better, and the newfound confidence led me to spend more time out in the world and less in bed. And so the upward spiral continued: the more I was out in the world, the less attention I paid to the migraines. (It turns out that being active and busy reduces pain perception!)[2] Less pain perception meant I racked up more good days and a higher score. A higher score meant more confidence and therefore more daily activity. It was a virtuous cycle, all kicked off by the simple act of keeping a tally.

By the end of the year, I had 154 check marks—on average, *three* good days a week, not two. I set a much higher score than I thought possible. And my high score was reflected in the fact that I felt much more in control of my life.

And that's when I stopped keeping score. I didn't need an objective tally anymore to tell me I was getting better. I was confident that my health was strong enough that I could enjoy my life, do important work, and be there for my family.

Ideally, this is how keeping score should work for you, too. It's not a habit you have to keep up forever. Keep score only until you internalize the sense of progress and accomplishment that you crave. Keep score until you know for sure that you've achieved real growth—just as I did.

Now that you've got a few basic ways to keep score under your belt, let's talk about some more creative options.

One of the signature benefits of the SuperBetter method is developing a clearer sense of your personal strengths and capabilities. Hopefully, you already feel more in touch with your heroic qualities just by getting this far.

As you go forward, you may discover that friends and family are also able to see your strengths growing—in fact, they may be able to see it more clearly than you can! Particularly during times of extreme stress, you may need an outside perspective on what you're doing right. (This is especially true if you have a tendency to be humble, or if you often experience self-doubt.) That's why I suggest that you consider enlisting your allies in helping you track your heroic strengths.

I call it *leveling up with allies*, and here's how it works.

First, remember the list of top five heroic strengths that you identified in Quest 36? Whatever's on that list—whether it's love of learning, spirituality, creativity, fairness, or zest for adventure—*that*'s what you're going to try to level up. In video games, leveling up means increasing your character strengths point by point until you reach specific score milestones. These milestones typically come with new powers and opportunities.

Next, if you haven't shared your strengths list with anyone yet, do that now—because you're going to need someone to award you strengths points! Pick at least one trusted ally, and share your top five strengths with them.

From here on out, your scoring job is over. You only need to focus on using your strengths as much as possible in daily life. It's your ally's mission now to look for opportunities to award you strengths points.

Let me give you an example. When I was Jane the Concussion Slayer, my husband and I kept a notebook with a list of my top five strengths—including creativity, love of learning, and determination. At the end of each night, when we would check in about the day, he would pull out the notebook and give me points for my achievements, like this:

- +5 creativity, for making a YouTube video explaining why you're designing a game to heal from a concussion
- +10 love of learning, for using your fifteen minutes of clearheaded thinking today to find a scientific paper about how to heal from post-concussion syndrome

- +20 determination, for making it to the doctor's appointment even though you felt dizzy

The actual points didn't really matter so much; they could have been +500 or +.00001 for all I cared. What really helped was being seen as strong, instead of weak, by someone I cared about. And let's face it, it feels good to be celebrated by others.

As Jess, thirty-one, a marketing director who played SuperBetter through several hospital stays and surgeries, put it:

> Getting points from my allies totally boosted my feeling of accomplishment. I would get really frustrated and downtrodden over having eleven million doctors' appointments every week. I felt like I was going nowhere. The points system helped me to see just how every appointment, every hour spent at work, even every load of laundry was an accomplishment for which I should be proud. I couldn't view my own situation objectively. Having someone step in and say, "Man, that was really awesome, and I think you should win +10 Courage for that" gave me a better perspective on my achievements.

Make sure you pick an ally who will have lots of chances to spot you showing off your strengths—whether it's because they live with you or see you every day or talk to you frequently.

Although you might feel a little embarrassed about asking someone to give you this kind of explicit positive feedback (and you wouldn't be alone!), consider this: when we surveyed SuperBetter allies about which activities they most enjoyed doing for their heroes, they rated "Giving +1 achievements" as their second-favorite activity. (The top-rated activity was sending general messages of encouragement and support.) Remember, people who care about you are hungry for concrete things they can do to help and support you. By asking them to give you strengths points, you're giving *them* the chance to do something that feels good and makes a difference. It's win-win.

Now for practicalities. You can collect points from your allies verbally, by email, or by text message. If you're sharing your SuperBetter journey publicly, you can collect them from readers or viewers in comments on your photos, videos, blog posts, or other social media. (Hope you're not shy about people telling you how amazing you are in front of others!)

If you want to keep a formal score, you can choose to add up the points in a notebook or on a spreadsheet. Or you can simply treat each +1 as a high five and not bother with any math. (This is what nearly half of all players do.) If you *do* add the points up over time, give yourself a reward when you reach major milestones, like +50 curiosity or +100 courage.

Leveling up points does not have to be complex or even a particularly formal practice. Here's what I suggest: Ask at least one ally to give you strengths points over the course of one or two weeks. After that, take a more informal approach. Plus-ones can become a shorthand you use to congratulate and encourage each other. Don't feel limited to the twenty-four signature character strengths; you can recognize any positive quality you want. And feel free to give allies their own +1s, whenever they're being strong for you or facing their own challenges! You'll find that looking for strengths in others is a remarkably rewarding way to show them love or understand them even better.

◄►

There's one more kind of score you may want to keep track of: your results on a measurement tool called an inventory.

An *inventory* is a survey that has been designed to measure a specific psychological trait or experience, such as optimism, anxiety, courage, depression, or life satisfaction. Inventories are typically subject to rigorous scientific testing, to ensure that they effectively measure what they claim to be measuring.

Throughout this book, you have taken informal versions of scientifically validated inventories to measure your own psychological strengths, such as your ability to adopt a challenge mindset in the face of stress (Chapter 5) and your willingness to take committed action toward your goals (Chapter 8). Similar inventories were used by researchers at the University of Pennsylvania and Ohio State University Wexner Medical Center to determine the effects of playing SuperBetter. Through these inventories, the researchers determined that playing SuperBetter for six weeks significantly decreases depression and anxiety and significantly increases self-efficacy and life satisfaction.

As you tackle your challenges gamefully and build up your strengths, you may wish to have access to some of these same powerful measurement tools. Typically, the most rigorously tested inventories are not easily available outside scientific journals. However, to help *you* get access to these important resources, I've gathered up all the inventories that will be most potentially useful to you on your SuperBetter journey—and I've made them freely available at Areyougameful.com.

Some of these inventories include:

- The Optimism Test
- The Meaning in Life Questionnaire
- The Gratitude Survey
- The Close Relationships Questionnaire
- The Silver Linings Questionnaire
- The Health-Related Quality of Life Questionnaire
- The Reasons for Living Inventory

These five inventories were used by the UP and OSU researchers to study SuperBetter's effects:

- The Center for Epidemiological Studies Depression Scale
- The Generalized Anxiety Disorder Scale
- The New General Self-Efficacy Scale
- The Satisfaction with Life Scale
- The Measure of Perceived Social Support

You can decide for yourself which traits or experiences *you* want to track over time as you play. If you're experiencing a particular problem, such as depression, anxiety, or PTSD, the inventories that measure their specific symptoms can help you more objectively see if and how you're improving. If you're trying to increase character strengths, such as curiosity or grit, you'll be able to demonstrate concrete growth by taking the relevant inventories periodically through your journey.

There is one special inventory that I encourage *everyone* to take: the Gameful Strengths Inventory, or GSI. It's a custom inventory that I designed, with the assistance of science advisers at UC Berkeley and Stanford University, specifically to measure the benefits associated with adopting a gameful mindset: increased creativity, optimism, courage, hope, determination, social connection, and self-efficacy.

You've read about these gameful strengths throughout this book—and completed quests to develop them. They make you resilient in the face of any challenge and can help you unlock the benefits of post-ecstatic or post-traumatic growth.

If you want to check in on the development of *your* gameful strengths, this inventory can help. Take it periodically—once a month is plenty. You may want to take it whenever you achieve an epic win or choose a new challenge, to set a new baseline score. (You'll find a downloadable and printable copy of the GSI at Areyougameful.com, and I encourage you to save a copy each time you complete it so you can look back at your specific score changes.)

Whenever you take the GSI, you'll get a score that not only reveals changes in your mindset; it will also tell you exactly which gameful rules you will want to devote more time and attention to in the future, if you want to experience more benefits and growth.

Taking the GSI for the first time is your final quest for this part of the book. Ready? (And congratulations on getting this far!)

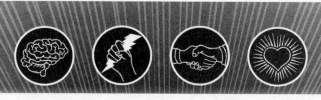

## QUEST 45: How Gameful Are You?

**What to do:** Answer each question on a scale of 0–5 points. Give yourself 0 points for "No way!" (you completely disagree with the statement), 5 points for "Heck, yeah!" (you completely, wholeheartedly agree with it), and points in between if you agree a little bit, somewhat, or a lot.

1. I'm optimistic about my future.
2. I frequently look for new things to learn or new experiences to try.
3. Every challenge I face is an opportunity to learn or to grow.
4. I can think of at least one thing I could do in the next hour to feel happy, strong, or productive.
5. I do what matters most to me, even if it's hard, painful, or scary.
6. I can do things in a new way. I'm not limited to the way things have always been done.
7. I have faith in my ability to accomplish whatever I set my heart to.
8. I feel grateful to many different people.
9. This week I was able to overcome an obstacle.
10. Setbacks don't discourage me.
11. I feel a strong bond with other people who are going through the same challenge I face or who have already been through it.
12. When I face a problem, I can usually find a way to solve it.

13. I can think of at least one goal I would like to accomplish to-morrow.

14. If I'm not sure whether I can do something successfully, I feel motivated to try and find out.

15. I have something specific to look forward to.

16. If I don't like how I feel, I can change it.

17. I often lose track of time, because I get so immersed in an activity I enjoy.

18. I enjoy coming up with new, creative strategies.

19. I can think of at least one other person who really wants me to succeed.

20. I have the courage to face life and whatever challenges and complications it brings.

**Scoring:** Add up your points for a gameful score that should fall somewhere between 0 and 100. Keep reading to find out what your score means!

Your Gameful Strengths Inventory score is a way for you to compare how your mindset is changing from time to time. There's no score that means "gameful enough" or "not gameful enough." Instead of focusing on the specific number, focus on whether your number goes up or down over time—and keep trying to set a new high score.

*If your score goes up*, it means you're able to draw on your natural, gameful strengths more effectively than in the past. You should feel a sense of confidence in your growing gameful abilities, and satisfaction that you've successfully cultivated such powerful ways of thinking.

*If your score goes down*, it means your gameful strengths may need a bit of bolstering or just reawakening. If so, there are two things you can do to reengage a gameful mindset.

First, make it a point to spend more time in the next few weeks *playing games*. This is the fastest and surest way to boost your gameful strengths—just play. It sounds obvious, but it is a too-often-overlooked strategy. Why? Because we're culturally biased to think about games as "time wasters" instead of "strength builders." Basketball, sudoku, *Super Mario*, *Settlers of Catan*, crossword puzzles, *The Sims*, hide-and-seek, bridge—really, any game at all will do. If you normally spend no time at all playing games, spend thirty minutes this week playing. If you normally spend ten hours a week playing games, play with a bit more purpose this week: play something that is particularly challenging, and if possible, spend more time on multiplayer games.

If you want to be even more strategic about upping your score, you have a second option. Identify the questions that you have the lowest scores for, or any questions that you scored lower on this time than the last time you took the inventory. Then use this information as a reminder to practice the gameful rules that will help you exactly where you need it most. Here's how:

*If you have a lower score for question 3 or 12:* Your challenge mindset needs strengthening. Revisit the quests and advice in Chapter 5.

*If you have a lower score for question 4, 16, or 17:* Focus on collecting and activating new power-ups over the next week (Chapter 6).

*If you have a lower score for question 6, 9, 10, 12, or 18:* Take a look at your list of bad guys, and spend time this week coming up with and testing as many new strategies and battle plans as you can (Chapter 7).

*If you have a lower score for question 2, 5, or 13:* Focus on completing quests this week (Chapter 8)—as many as you can!

*If you have a lower score for question 8, 11, or 19:* Make an effort this week to connect with at least one ally or to recruit a new one (Chapter 9).

*If you have a lower score for question 7 or 20:* It's a good time to pay extra attention to your secret identity (Chapter 10). Try using your strengths in a new way this week, or telling a new heroic story about yourself.

*If you have a lower score for question 1, 14, or 15:* Spend some time thinking about your epic win this week (Chapter 11). If the win you're aiming for doesn't feel realistic anymore, come up with a new one. Or if it just doesn't inspire and energize you right now, replace it with one that does.

◄►

Finally, just for fun and a bit of extra motivation, I want to leave you with a few mini-games—timed ways of keeping score, competitively and cooperatively, with friends, family, and other SuperBetter allies.

When I was designing interactive experiences for the Nike Digital Sport team, mini-games were a core component of our motivational strategy. How could we keep competitive athletes inspired during training, week after week, season after season? How could we inspire someone with an already hectic schedule to squeeze in an extra thirty minutes of life-changing physical activity in the evening, so they were more likely to achieve their health and fitness goals? Personal records helped a great deal, but of all the strategies we tested, mini-games sparked the biggest surge in activity and effort. There's just something about making a challenge social that brings out the best in us.

To help *you* get a surge in your gameful efforts when you need it most, I've created seven social mini-games you can try. Whether you play them competitively or cooperatively, they'll not only give you a motivational lift—they'll also help you discover new ways to get stronger, even after you're already a total pro at getting superbetter.

## COMPETITIVE MINI-GAMES: CHALLENGE A FRIEND!

If you have a competitive spirit, you might find it fun to compare your gameful efforts against one or more friends. Here are a few ways to bring on the competition.

## First Power-up of the Day

Whoever power-ups first, wins. Send a message by text, email, or social media to claim your victory. (Include a photo of the power-up as proof!) This mini-game is more fun when you go for best of three days, best of five days, or even best of thirty days! *You decide if staying up until 12:01 a.m. counts, or if you want the competition to start at sunrise.*

## The Quest Race

Whoever completes a list of quests first, wins. Here's how it works: Each player must contribute one quest to the race. If there are four players, you'll be racing to complete four quests total. Before the start, all players must agree that all quests are reasonable; it's no fair creating a quest to run 10 miles or donate $100 to charity if you are the only person in the group who can realistically do that! Once you have your quest list, it's ready, set—go! The first person to successfully complete all the quests wins. Photo and video proof is encouraged. This mini-game gets more fun the more players you invite to compete.

## Battle Report

Pick a common bad guy that you share. This week you'll all pay special attention to battling this bad guy. Come up with as many different strategies as you can. Creativity counts! At the end of the week, compare your lists of strategies. Each player gets one point for every strategy he or she comes up with that isn't on anyone else's list! The player with the most points wins. Bonus: At the end of the week, you'll all have a heap of strategies to try against one of your most annoying bad guys!

### SuperBetter Survivor

You can try this challenge by yourself, but it's more fun with a friend or two. Here's how it works: On day one, you activate at least one power-up. On day two, you activate two different power-ups. On day three, three different power-ups... and so on, increasing your goal by one more every day. If you don't hit your daily goal, you're out of the challenge. The last survivor standing wins!

*Tip:* With any of these competitions, you'll want to challenge someone who is already playing SuperBetter, whether it's someone you know in daily life or someone you meet online. You might also consider challenging an ally or two, even if they're not trying to get SuperBetter themselves. After a day of activating power-ups and completing quests with you, who knows? They might be inspired to choose their own challenge—and go for their own epic win!

# COOPERATIVE MINI-GAMES: TEAM UP FOR A MISSION!

Perhaps you'd rather join forces than compete. If so, you can keep a multiplayer score that emphasizes teamwork. Here are a few cooperative high scores you can try to achieve.

### The Dirty Dozen Mission

Together, you must successfully battle a total of at least twelve different bad guys this week. (You might battle five and your partner seven; or if there are three of you, you could battle four bad guys each. You get the idea.) Let each other know every time you log a successful battle. If you reach a dozen before the week runs out, mission accomplished!

## The Power 100 Mission

Together, your team must try to activate one hundred different power-ups. Set a target time: If there are two of you, it might take you thirty days. If there are ten of you, you can try to do it in a week. Try to hit one hundred before time runs out—and keep a shared list of power-ups to make sure you don't count the same power-up twice! Bonus: At the end of this mini-game, you'll have a custom list of one hundred power-ups that you can use in the future—and share with others, if you choose!

## Team Streak

How many days in a row can your team of two or more get your daily dose of SuperBetter? (That's at least three power-ups, one bad guy battle, and one quest a day.) The more people you team up with, the harder it is to keep a streak going—but the more people you'll have cheering you on and encouraging you to win the day! You can turn this into a team-based competition, too: each team tries to outlast all the others by keeping their streak alive the longest.

◄►

As you can see, you have myriad ways to set a new high score. But if there's anything more satisfying than setting a new high score, it's this: keeping the game going.

The philosopher and religious studies professor James Carse once wrote that there are two kinds of games: finite and infinite.[3] A *finite* game is played for the purpose of finding out who wins. An *infinite* game is played for the purpose of keeping the play going as long as possible.

Chess, soccer, *League of Legends* matches, mah-jongg, political elections—these are all finite games. They drive inexorably to someone's victory and therefore an end to the game.

SuperBetter, on the other hand, is an infinite game. The better you play it, the longer you have to play.

Every time you complete a quest, battle a bad guy, or activate a power-up, you're increasing your resilience—and therefore increasing your statistical life expectancy. I call this *bonus life*, and it's inspired by the experience of earning extra lives in a video game.

If you've ever played a classic video game, you know how this works. Players start with a predetermined number of lives, or chances to win the game. Run out of lives, and it's game over. But achieve smaller goals and play consistently, and you can extend the duration of your game. Get ten thousand points in *Pac-Man*, and you earn an extra life. Collect one hundred gold coins in *Super Mario*, and they're worth an extra life. Many modern games have adapted this mechanism in new ways. For example, if you ask your friends for help in *Candy Crush Saga*, you can earn countless extra lives.

Earning more time to play and pursue your goals in real life isn't quite as exact a science as earning it in video games. But as a metaphor, it can give you incredibly valuable insight into what you can do today to give yourself the best chance for a long and happy life.

There are lots of ways to track your progress and add up your bonus life, thanks to the growing field of resilience research. Scientists is this field use the same methods and longevity models as actuaries, the professionals who depend on complex mathematical and statistical methods to calculate risks and policy prices for life insurance companies. However, in the case of resilience research, the scientists are looking for the daily habits that *extend* life rather than shorten it. I've reviewed hundreds of scientific papers on the relationship between the four types of resilience—physical, mental, emotional, and social—and longevity, and here's what I've learned:

- Every minute of leisure time physical activity that you do, whether it's walking around the block, doing push-ups, or dancing around your living room, *adds seven minutes to your life expectancy*, according to a study of more than 650,000 people.[4] This means you can add seven minutes to your life right this second just by powering up your physical resilience for a single minute. (So consider standing up while you read the next page in this book!)

- Spending more time with your friends and family increases your life expectancy as much as quitting smoking, losing weight, lowering your cholesterol, or decreasing your blood pressure, according to a study of just under 17,000 individuals.[5] That means increasing the amount of positive daily social interaction you get is worth up to *three bonus hours of life every day you give and receive social support.* (So consider sending a positive message to one of your allies right this second!)

- Optimism and self-efficacy, which you build up every time you achieve an epic win or complete a quest, are not only associated with longer life—they also predict how much you'll thrive, and how long you can ward off cognitive decline as you age. Based on the increased self-efficacy documented among SuperBetter players by the University of Pennsylvania researchers, this means if you spend the next six weeks working toward an epic win, *you are potentially gaining five days of a happy and healthy life.* (So take ten seconds right now to visualize your next epic win!)

- Even if you never increase your physical or social resilience, seeking out more positive emotions every day alone can add a full decade to your life. One major study collected seventy-five years' worth of data and found that women who felt a wider range of positive emotions (from gratitude to amusement to hope to pride) in their twenties and thirties went on to live 10.7 years longer. (The different emotions felt were tracked in journals the women kept throughout early adulthood.)[6] Numerous other studies have confirmed this benefit: every positive emotion you feel, even if it lasts only a fleeting moment, is associated with a longer life.[7] (So treat yourself to a quick power-up tonight, no matter how tired or busy you are.)

Remember, when it comes to bonus life, we're talking about statistical probabilities based on data gathered from tracking hundreds of thousands of people over decades in more than a thousand peer-reviewed scientific studies. That's a lot of evidence, but it's not a guarantee. So please don't take any of the time bonuses too literally! Bonus life is a playful framework for thinking about how the small choices you make today add up to big changes over the course of your life. You can be confident that every time you complete another quest in this book—and every time you follow one of the seven SuperBetter rules in your life—you are heading in the right direction, to a happier, healthier, longer, and more accomplished life. How much longer? When you add up the benefits of all four types of resilience, the research suggests you can live up to ten years longer.

*A full decade of bonus life.* Just imagine the dreams you can chase, and the happiness you can create, with ten extra years.

Whether being gameful ultimately gives you an extra year or an extra decade of bonus life, it's going to start changing your life immediately. Your extra resilience will increase your creativity, your courage, your curiosity, and your determination *right now*. You will have the strengths you need to experiment and challenge yourself more, to set higher goals for yourself, and to make more time for your family and all the things that matter most to you.

That's where *spending* your bonus life comes in. To benefit the most from your extra life, you can't treat it as a bonus you'll cash out when you're ninety-nine years old. You have to spend it *today*. If you wait years or decades to spend your bonus minutes, hours, or days, you'll have lost the opportunity to spend them when they can change the entire rest of your life for the better. We started this book talking about the most common regrets that people have on their deathbeds. Living gamefully means spending your bonus life long before you have the chance to develop any regrets.

This is why my very last recommendation to you is this: Do a few gameful calculations, and figure out just how much bonus life you've earned recently. It doesn't have to be exact. If you spent an hour playing SuperBetter, give yourself seven minutes. If you spent a week, give yourself three hours. If it's been six weeks and you've achieved an epic win, give yourself five days. *Then mark this amount of time somewhere on your calendar, and plan to spend it on something that will fuel your dreams.*

Spend seven minutes doing something for a loved one. Devote three hours to learning something new. Plan a five-day dream vacation or staycation (stay-at-home vacation); sign up for a five-day fitness boot camp; or set aside five Saturdays to work on a memoir or novel.

Use this playful method of tracking as a way to *give yourself permission* to do what matters most, today. The biggest benefit of getting stronger, happier, and braver is finding the courage and means to live a life truer to your dreams right now—no matter what obstacles you face along the way.

I f you spend your bonus life right away, you will recognize the signs of post-ecstatic and post-traumatic growth in your own life—the five potential positive changes that allow you to lead a life free of regret.

1. **Stronger:** You have a newfound sense of personal strength and resilience.
2. **Closer:** You enjoy more intimate relationships with loved ones, and more compassion for others.
3. **Clearer:** You've changed or strengthened your priorities about what is important in life. You have a willingness to spend more time on the things that matter most.
4. **Braver:** You feel empowered to pursue new dreams, change your life plan, and take advantage of new opportunities.
5. **Greater:** You have a stronger sense of purpose, a changed philosophy of life, renewed spirituality, or deeper wisdom.

Pay special attention to each of these areas of potential growth. Some of the changes may happen quickly; others may unfold more slowly over time. Periodically ask yourself, *Have I changed in any of these ways since facing my challenge? Do I feel stronger, closer, clearer, braver, or greater?*

When I look back at my own SuperBetter journey as Jane the Concussion Slayer, I *do* see growth in myself in all five areas. I know I'm stronger because after facing and recovering from suicidal thoughts, I have not had a single day of even mild depression since. I believe something has permanently shifted in how I process failure, disappointment, and adversity. (And I better understand now how play can help me change my brain chemistry when I need it most.) I'm closer, because I not only feel gratitude to the friends and family who helped me through my darkest hour; I also have a level of deep empathy I'd never felt before, a personal connection with, and a desire to help, all others who have experienced their own difficult concussion or traumatic brain injury. I know I'm clearer because I now say no when people ask me to spend time and energy on things that don't fit my life priorities. In fact, I am the *queen* of saying no, whereas before my injury, I found it nearly impossible. I'm braver, because surviving my recovery gave me confidence in my resilience. It helped me find the courage to do life-changing things that seemed too scary or overwhelming before—like fighting my infertility to start a family with my husband and finally becoming a mom. And I know that I'm greater now because I have a new and more meaningful purpose in my work, which is to help others experience the same kind of transformative growth.

I f you are living by the seven gameful rules, *you too* are getting stronger, closer, clearer, braver, and greater.

You have improved your ability to control your attention and therefore your thoughts and feelings. You have developed the power to turn anyone into a potential ally and to strengthen your existing relationships. You have tapped into your natural capacity to motivate yourself and supercharge your heroic qualities, like willpower, compassion, and determination.

You know now how to play with purpose, so you can bring your gameful strengths to real-life obstacles. You have gotten better *at* challenge and adversity, so you can get better *through* challenge and adversity.

You have without a doubt proven that you are stronger than you knew. You are surrounded by allies. And you are definitely the hero of your own story.

Just remember:

*1. Challenge yourself.*

*2. Collect and activate power-ups.*

*3. Find and battle the bad guys.*

*4. Seek out and complete quests.*

*5. Recruit your allies.*

*6. Adopt a secret identity.*

*7. Go for an epic win.*

### *Skills Unlocked: How (and Why) to Keep Score*

- Keeping your own score is the best way to really internalize the seven gameful rules—and get a deeper understanding of your own play.
- Try to win the day. You win every time you get your daily dose of SuperBetter: three power-ups, one bad guy battle, and one quest.
- Go for personal records—for example, the most power-ups you can activate in a single hour.
- Keep a tally of behavior you're trying to increase, and set a target goal for how many times you'll do it.
- Level up your heroic strengths by inviting allies to award you points and achievements whenever you use your signature strengths.
- Take inventory of your growing strengths and other psychological changes, by completing the surveys at Areyougameful.com. Be sure to take the Gameful Strengths Inventory (GSI) once a month to track your increasing skills and abilities.
- Earn a multiplayer score with competitive or cooperative mini-games. Tap the motivational power of social play, and find new creative ways to get SuperBetter.
- Earn bonus time—up to three and a half hours a day—by practicing habits that increase your emotional, physical, social, and mental resilience. More important, *spend* your bonus time as soon as you earn it, on your top priorities and most urgent dreams.
- Track your post-ecstatic and post-traumatic growth by looking for five major benefits: you are becoming a stronger, closer, clearer, braver, and greater person because of the challenges you've tackled and the obstacles you've faced.

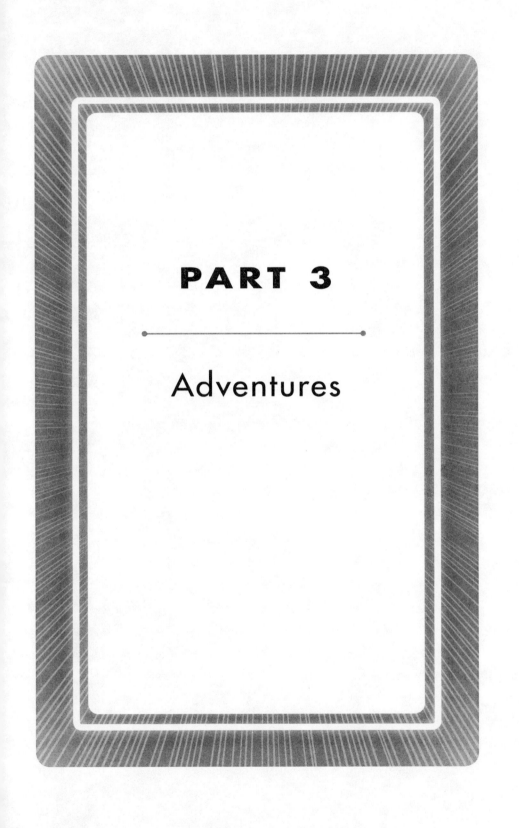

# PART 3

## Adventures

I t's time to put it all together—with three adventures that can help you practice all your new gameful strengths.

An *adventure* is a set of power-ups, bad guys, and quests designed to help you tackle a particular challenge. The adventures in this section will help you strengthen your most important relationships, energize your body, and discover a secret wealth of time each day to spend on the things that matter most.

I've created these adventures for you based on my own areas of expertise, developed through collaborations with the University of Pennsylvania's Positive Psychology Center, the American Heart Association, Nike, the Institute for the Future, the Ardmore Institute of Health, and UC Berkeley's Greater Good Science Center.

After you take an adventure or two, you'll be ready to create your own. It's easier than you think! Whatever you're an expert in—or *want* to become an expert in—can be the basis for an adventure.

SuperBetter players around the world have drawn on their personal experiences and life wisdom to design all kinds of adventures: how to survive the college admissions process, explore different religions, beat insomnia, become a part-time vegetarian, and write your first book, to name just a few.

All you have to do is collect the habits and skills that are important for success—those are your power-ups. Then list the obstacles that might get in someone's way—those are the bad guys. Finally, come up with one or two weeks' worth of tiny goals, or daily quests, that will help your players practice getting better at whatever your adventure is about.

It's especially fun to combine forces and design an adventure with a group. For example, you can collect power-ups, quests, and bad guys at your office, for a custom company adventure. That's what Zappos, the online apparel retailer, did when more than one hundred of its employees decided to get superbetter together. Teachers have created SuperBetter adventures with their students, navy officers with their direct reports, coaches with their athletes, resident assistants with their college dormitory residents, therapists with their patients, volunteer organizations with their members, ministers with their congregations, neighborhood associations with their neighbors, and even family members before a family reunion.

If you belong to a group, consider creating an adventure together. It can be a truly amazing way to collect the wisdom of your community and to empower and encourage each other.

To show you how it works, here are three adventures I've created:

## Adventure 1: Love Connection

*(Time to complete: 10 quests/10 days)*
Researchers can predict how much love you'll have in your life based on how you do five simple things. Learn what they are, and you'll master the secrets to happy relationships at work, at home, and in love.

On this adventure, you'll collect five new power-ups: celebrate like a true ally, deliver a super-powerful thank you, investigate something exciting, flip a lonely thought, and take a "hands over heart" moment. You'll also learn how to battle these five bad guys: passive congrats, the "it's too late to thank them now" monster, forgettable small talk, lonely thoughts, and the bully inside.

## Adventure 2: Ninja Body Transformation

*(Time to complete: 21 quests/21 days)*

Sneak up on change like a ninja! This adventure helps you energize, get fit, lose weight, increase your physical strength, and feel healthier—without dieting or stepping on a scale.

On this adventure, you'll collect ten new power-ups: eat a power food; listen to your power song; practice your power move; connect with the water element, *sui*; the earth element, *chi*; the wind element, *fū*; the fire element, *ka*; and the sky element, *kū*; practice *uzura-gakure*, the art of staying still as a stone; and practice *tanuki-gakure*, or "tree camoflauge." You'll also learn how to battle five sneaky bad guys: weighing yourself, counting calories, feeling guilty about what you eat, mentally checking out from your body, and ignoring your ninja powers.

## Adventure 3: Time Rich

*(Time to complete: 10 quests/10 days)*

Want to feel like you have all the time in the world to do the things you love most? That you have *more* than twenty-four hours in each day? This adventure is for you.

On this adventure, you'll collect six new power-ups: provoke awe, give someone ten minutes of your time, breathe, give yourself a power boost, and make a free and spontaneous choice. You'll also learn how to battle three tricky bad guys: time poverty, social jetlag, and mindless, stressful commuting.

I invite you to complete one, two, or all three, in any order. Taken together, these three adventures contain just enough quests for you to keep playing SuperBetter for six weeks. That's an important number, because six weeks is exactly how long participants followed the SuperBetter rules in our clinical trial and our randomized controlled study. In those studies, playing SuperBetter for six weeks resulted in significantly better mood, stronger social support, more optimism, less depression and anxiety, and higher self-confidence. If you complete all three of these adventures—by tackling just one quest a day—you'll have achieved a full, life-changing dose of the game.

# Love Connection

### Take this adventure if…

- You want more love in your life.
- You'd like to be more confident in social situations.
- You want to strengthen your closest relationships.
- You sometimes feel lonely, and you want to change that.
- You have a big heart, and you want to put it to good use!

### This adventure includes:

- 10 quests
- 5 power-ups
- 5 bad guys

### How to play:

- Complete one quest a day, until you finish all 10 quests.

▼

**LOVE CONNECTION QUEST 1:**
*Love the Good Stuff*

You're on an adventure to increase the love in your life. So let's start with what scientists have identified as the number-one secret to building strong relationships.

It's called *active constructive responding*, or ACR for short. It strengthens all kinds of relationships—not just romantic but also work and family relationships, as well as friendships. Although most people have never heard of this skill, the scientific research behind it is so strong, it's taught as the number-one most important relationship-building skill everywhere from the U.S. Army (as part of the Master Resilience course created by University of Pennsylvania psychologists) to the halls of the matchmaking site eHarmony .com (where senior research scientists contributed to peer-reviewed studies on the phenomenon).[1]

So what exactly *is* ACR? It involves celebrating someone else's success or good news with genuine enthusiasm and interest. Instead of offering a passive "congratulations" or "way to go" (or worse, actively sabotaging their celebration with a negative reaction!), you actively engage them in a positive conversation about the good news.

Here's how you do it:

1. **Show enthusiasm.** This is not the time to be distracted or seem disinterested. Stop what you're doing and give the person your full attention. Don't change the subject. Don't talk about yourself. Don't undermine their excitement. Try to match their enthusiasm with your own.

2. **Ask questions.** Draw them out about the news. "Tell me more!" "When will that happen?" "How long have you been waiting to find out?" "What will you do to celebrate?" It doesn't matter what you ask. What's important is giving them a chance to keep talking about it so they can relish the moment.

3. **Congratulate them and express your happiness for them.** It's a small thing, but be sure to tell them directly that you share their happiness. "I'm so pleased for you." "I'm so happy for you." "You deserve this." "I'm so proud of you." "This is truly the best news I've heard all week."

4. **Relive the experience with them.** Keep the conversation going. Success is something to be savored. Ask them to tell you about it in detail. If they've received good news, for example, you could ask them questions like "Where were you when you found out?" "What did you say when you heard the news?" "Who did you tell first?" "How did you feel when you found out?" Or if they're celebrating a success, simply ask them to tell you more about the most important moments. "What were you thinking when you crossed the finish line?" "How did your family react to the news?" Questions like these will put them right back in the happy moment and help them really savor it.

It sounds simple enough, but studies show that nothing contributes more to the long-term strength and success of relationships than whether its participants do ACR. Couples who do it stay married longer. (And new couples who do it fall in love faster.) Coworkers who do it are happier and more collaborative at work. Family members who do it report feeling closer to each other and experience less anxiety and depression. People who develop this skill and practice it regularly have more and stronger friendships.[2]

Now *you* know the secret. If you want more love in your life, celebrate others' good news with the enthusiasm and excitement of a true ally.

## LOVE CONNECTION QUEST 2:
### Savor a Moment

Your quest for today is to try out the new skill you learned yesterday: active constructive responding (ACR).

Ideally, the opportunity to try ACR will arise naturally today. But if no one comes to you, dying to share their good news, go ahead and create an ACR opportunity for yourself. Here's how:

**What to do:** Ask someone to tell you about one of their favorite memories. If you're eating together, ask them to tell you about the best meal they've ever had. If you're taking a walk together, ask them to tell you about the prettiest place they've ever been. If you're in a class together, ask them what they think the best class they've ever taken was. If there's no obvious natural topic for sharing memories, you can even say, "Just for fun, I've been asking people about their favorite memories. Do you mind if I ask you a question?" And then ask them about any kind of memory you want!

**Once they've started talking, actively celebrate their memory with them, like a true ally.** Remember to use all four ACR techniques: (1) show enthusiasm, (2) ask questions, (3) offer your congratulations and express your happiness for them, and (4) relive the experience with them.

*Tip:* When you're helping someone savor a favorite memory, steps 1, 2, and 4 should be very easy to do. But a memory may not necessarily be congratulations worthy, so for step 3, you can simply say something like: "That sounds like such an amazing experience." "You must be so thrilled that you had the chance to do that." "That memory must bring you a lot of happiness."

**Bonus mission:** Your conversation partner may return the favor and ask *you* about *your* favorite memory. If they do, pay attention to how *they* respond to your story. Do they actively and constructively respond to you? If so, notice how much fun you have savoring the memory, and how good it feels to have so much interest shown in your story. Or if they respond passively, take notice of the difference in the energy and warmth of the conversation. Whenever you don't quite get the same generous and active response you're looking for, it's a great reminder to be sure to give it to others every chance *you* get.

## LOVE CONNECTION QUEST 3:
### Love the Gratitude

Scientists have known for a long time that practicing gratitude makes people happier and healthier. It reduces stress, improves sleep, and even boosts immune function.[3] But they have only recently discovered that one form of gratitude is especially powerful—not just *feeling* grateful (or counting your blessings) but actively *expressing* gratitude to others.

Every time you express gratitude to others, it amplifies the positive emotion you feel. And it not only feels good in the moment: a powerful thank-you *changes the way you see the world for the next twenty-four hours*—making you more likely to see the good in anyone else you encounter, and increasing your optimism, hope, and compassion.[4]

A powerful thank-you also inspires and changes the person who receives your gratitude. Research shows that when you recognize the good in someone else, they become just a little more likely to do good again. That means that every time you thank someone, you make them just a little bit more of the best version of themselves.[5]

But not every thank-you delivers these powerful benefits! Sending someone a one-word "thanks!" by text message might boost your social connection a little bit, but if you really want to do good with your gratitude, you need to learn a special kind of thank-you.

The three-part "superpowerful thank-you" was created by Dr. Kelly McGonigal, a psychology professor at Stanford University, and an expert in the science of gratitude (as well as my twin sister and my first SuperBetter ally).[6] Here's how to do it:

1. **Find the benefit.** What good came to you because of this person? Be specific!
2. **Acknowledge the effort.** What might have been hard for them?
3. **Spot the strength.** What good do you see in the person you're thanking?

(And always start and end with "thank you.")

Here's what it looks like in action:

"Thank you for sending me those suggestions for new workout songs. They helped me get motivated today when I thought I was too exhausted to exercise." *(That's the benefit.)*

"You have so much to think about! It's really sweet of you to remember that I've been trying to work out more when you have so much else on your mind." *(That's the effort.)*

"You're so good at cheering everyone else on and helping us achieve our goals. You really make it seem as if you care as much about our success as you do your own." *(That's the strength.)*

"Thank you."

And another example:

"Thank you for keeping our secret (about being pregnant!). It meant so much to us to be able to tell the rest of the family in person. I'll never forget the looks on their faces." *(That's the benefit.)*

"I know it's not easy to keep such a big secret." *(That's the effort.)*

"I really respect how much honor and integrity you showed by keeping your promise." *(That's the strength.)*

"Thank you."

Do you think you have the hang of it? To lock it in, and complete this quest, repeat this out loud five times right now: **Find the benefit, acknowledge the effort, spot the strength.**

That's all it takes to give a life-changing thank-you.

---

## *LOVE CONNECTION QUEST 4: Unleash Your First Superpowerful Thank-You*

Now that you know *how* to deliver a superpowerful thank-you, it's time to put those skills to good use. **Pick someone—anyone—and thank them today.**

Make sure you follow the three steps: (1) find the benefit, (2) acknowledge the effort, and (3) spot the strength!

*Tip*: Most people find it easier to practice this skill *in writing* first—so you have time to really think about what you want to say. As an added bonus, if it's in writing, the recipient of your superpowerful thank-you will be able to reread it and really savor it!

## LOVE CONNECTION QUEST 5:
### Love What's Exciting

Dr. Robert Biswas-Diener is the world's leading practitioner of strengths coaching, a form of counseling that helps people recognize and utilize their own positive strengths. Although he often uses formal surveys, or inventories, with clients (like the ones you encountered in Chapter 12), he also recommends a more unusual method for spotting someone's signature strengths. It's called *conversational strengths-spotting*.[7] Here's how it works:

The next time you're catching up with someone, or when you're chatting with someone you don't know very well yet, **ask them about** *something exciting*. Like this:

- "So, what are you really excited about these days?"
- "What are you most looking forward to doing in the next few weeks?"
- "What's the most exciting thing you've done lately?"

Your goal, in listening to their response, is to *identify a positive strength* in their reply. For example, if the person mentions a new class they're taking, it shows off their curiosity. If they talk about seeing a grandchild, it shows the ability to love and be loved. If they're really excited about an upcoming sports game or a new movie, that's actually a sign of zest, enthusiasm, and energy. Whatever it is they're excited about or looking forward to, draw them out on the topic with follow-up questions until you can successfully identify at least one signature strength in their reply. ("Tell me more about that" or "What about it are you looking forward to?" do the trick just fine.)

Identifying a strength in someone else is always a win, because it means you're getting to know them better. But you'll make an even stronger connection if you reflect the strength back to them. It's easier than you might think. All it takes is a simple comment like "You really do have a lot of courage" or "I've always admired your love of learning" or "You have a greater appreciation of beauty than anyone else I know" or "Your enthusiasm is really contagious!" Don't worry if it doesn't come naturally at first. Like all new habits, it may take a few tries to feel comfortable.

The fastest way to see how this technique works is to try it on yourself. How would *you* answer any of these strengths-spotting questions? Try it now, and look for the strength in your own reply.

### LOVE CONNECTION QUEST 6: Practice Your Strengths-Spotting Questions

It's time to take your new strengths-spotting skill for a test drive.

**What to do:** Pick someone you'll see in the next twenty-four hours, and **plan to strike up a quick conversation around one of these topics:** "So, what are you really excited about these days?" or "What are you most looking forward to doing in the next few weeks?" or "What's the most exciting thing you've done lately?" Then carry out your plan.

This quest is complete when you've identified and reflected back at least one signature strength!

*Tip*: This skill works best face to face, so don't try to pull it off over text message!

## LOVE CONNECTION QUEST 7:
### Love Against Loneliness

Loneliness is one of the most common negative emotions in the world. Research shows that as many as 80 percent of people under eighteen, and 40 percent of adults over sixty-five, report being lonely at least sometimes. And for adults in their middle years, loneliness is as common as one in four.[8]

Loneliness is not the same as simply being alone. Many people can be relatively isolated from others and still be quite happy. Paradoxically, others can be surrounded by people constantly, yet still feel lonely. The *true* measure of loneliness is a sense of distress and dissatisfaction with the quality of your relationships. When you feel lonely, it means you are looking for a deeper, more satisfying connection with others.[9]

So what's the cure for loneliness? Recently, scientists analyzed the results from forty years' worth of loneliness research. They looked at more than fifty different studies of different methods to reduce the negative emotion, and the results were quite surprising.

The three techniques that psychologists most commonly suggested for reducing loneliness—increasing opportunities for social interaction, improving communication skills, and seeking counseling or joining support groups—were helpful, but not *that* helpful. The one truly helpful intervention was this: *Change your own negative expectations.*[10]

It turns out that when people feel lonely, they typically exhibit negative thought patterns. They're extrasensitive to potential negative feedback or criticism from others. They tend to focus on what went wrong instead of what went right. This leaves them feeling dissatisfied with, or hurt by, their social interactions. No matter what happened, they find a way to feel bad about it.

This kind of negative thinking creates a vicious cycle. It makes a lonely person less likely to participate or reach out to others. And when they do interact with others, they expect the worst—which becomes a self-fulfilling prophecy, fueled by their sensitivity to negative social information, like criticism or disagreement.

If you want to feel less lonely, the best thing you can do is *flip your lonely thoughts*. Instead of taking them at face value, challenge them. Ask yourself, *How do I know that's true? Can I find any evidence to the contrary? Is there any way to positively reframe this experience?* Remember those cognitive reappraisal techniques you learned in Chapter 5 (the challenge mindset) and Chapter 7 (battling the bad guys)—those are exactly the skills you're using when you flip a lonely thought!

According to research, changing your negative thoughts is *four times as effective* as any other method for curing loneliness. You'll have a chance to practice this skill in the next quest. For now, take a minute to consider whether *you* have a tendency to focus on the negative with others. See if you can identify a lonely thought that frequently pops into your mind—like "I don't fit in"; "I always embarrass myself when I try to be funny"; "I never have anything interesting to say"; or "They were probably looking down on me." Give it a moment's thought, and then congratulate yourself—this quest is a lot to wrap your mind around!

## LOVE CONNECTION QUEST 8: Flip Three Lonely Thoughts

Now that you know how important it is to flip your lonely thoughts, let's practice. Here are three negative thoughts that you might have after a social encounter. What could you think or say to yourself to counteract each one? (Remember your strategies for flipping a lonely thought: challenge your assumptions, look for disconfirming evidence, and reframe your perceptions!)

1. "I didn't have anything in common with the people I met tonight."
2. "No one was interested in what I had to say."
3. "Everyone was having such a good time except for me."

See what you can come up with on your own—then skip to the footnote on page 362 for a few more suggestions.*

*Tip:* Even if you've never had one of these thoughts, practice flipping them now—it's a skill that will serve you well if you ever suffer a lonely thought in the future.

---

* Here are some ways you might flip those lonely thoughts: 1. "That's not true. We must have something in common, even if it's just that we all know [X] or we're all interested in [Y] or we all live nearby." Or: "Well, I did meet that one guy who knew a lot about [Z], which I'd like to know more about." Or: "Maybe that just makes me a more interesting person to have around, since I'm so unique in this group." 2. "I can't really know that for sure. Nobody walked away when we were talking, so for all I know they were interested!" Or: "Maybe *I* didn't seem interested in what *they* had to say. I could ask more questions next time." Or: "Perhaps they didn't seem interested in what I had to say because it was really important to them to say what was on their minds tonight. I was a good listener, so that's something." 3. "It might have looked that way to me, but I'm probably not the only one who was having a bad day. I just didn't notice who else was feeling out of it." Or "Well, to be fair, even though it wasn't a great night overall, I *did* enjoy myself when . . ."

## *LOVE CONNECTION QUEST 9:*
## *Love Yourself*

"Self-compassion means treating yourself with the same type of kind, caring support and understanding that you would show to anyone you cared about." So says Dr. Kristin Neff, one of the world's leading experts on the subject. And according to her research, self-kindness is just as important as the love you show others. Not only does it lead to less depression, more optimism, greater happiness, and more life satisfaction, it also makes people kinder, more giving, and more supportive of their relationship partners. In other words, love yourself, and you will better love others.[11]

So what does it take to develop self-compassion? There are three steps.

1. Notice when you're suffering. Are you stressed? Are you in pain? Are you disappointed? Don't brush it off. Take a moment and acknowledge it.
2. Let yourself feel a desire to ease that suffering, just as you would try to ease the suffering of any friend or loved one. If this is hard for you—if your tendency is to be harsh with yourself or self-critical—imagine a beloved friend, family member, or even a cherished pet experiencing the same distress. How would you treat them?
3. Recognize that you're not alone in your suffering. It's part of the shared human experience that connects you to others.

It's not always easy to be kind to yourself when you're under extreme stress, or in pain, or failing to meet your own expectations. So what should you do?

**What to do:** Researchers have investigated many different ways people can tap into self-compassion, quickly, when they need it most. Here's the technique that experts recommend as one of the fastest and easiest ways to show yourself kindness:

"Place both hands on your heart as a reminder to be kind to yourself. Feel the warmth of your hands, and take three deep, relaxing breaths."[12]

It's called taking a *hands over heart* moment. To complete this quest, try it now for at least fifteen seconds. Do it again throughout the rest of today, whenever you need to give yourself a moment of kindness.

## LOVE CONNECTION QUEST 10: Say What You Need to Hear

You can double the power of the "hands over heart" moment if you add just one more thing.

When your hands are in position, ask yourself: *What do I need to hear right now to express kindness to myself?* See what phrase pops into your mind as the answer to this question. Let this be your self-kindness mantra for the day.

Here are some ideas:

- I accept myself as I am.
- I am strong today.
- I forgive myself.
- Whatever happens, I will be okay.
- I did everything I could today.
- Just for today, I don't need to change or fix anything.

*Congratulations!* You've completed all ten Love Connection quests.

So what's next? By taking this adventure, you've learned five powerful new skills (see the list below.) Activate these power-ups anytime you want to increase the love in your life. You've also identified five new bad guys (rounded up for you below). Keep battling them with the strategies you learned on this adventure!

## *Your Love Connection Power-ups*

### CELEBRATE LIKE A TRUE ALLY

Use your active constructive responding skills (Love Connection Quest 1) to celebrate someone else's good news, or to help them savor a great experience. Remember the four ways to do it: (1) show enthusiasm, (2) ask questions, (3) congratulate them, and (4) relive the experience with them.

### DELIVER A SUPERPOWERFUL THANK-YOU

Don't just *feel* grateful. Share your gratitude! Remember the three key steps (Love Connection Quest 3): (1) find the benefit, (2) acknowledge the effort, and (3) spot the strength.

### INVESTIGATE SOMETHING EXCITING

Ask someone one of your secret questions from Love Connection Quest 5: "What are you excited about these days?" or "What's something you're looking forward to in the next few weeks?" Try to spot the signature character strength they reveal in their answer—and let them know that you see it!

### FLIP A LONELY THOUGHT

If you've spotted a lonely thought, good job—now flip it! Think of at least one positive aspect to your social encounter (no matter how small or seemingly trivial). Whenever your mind starts obsessing over the lonely thought, bring your attention back to the positive one instead. The more you activate this power-up (learned in Love Connection Quest 7), the more you'll change how your brain reacts to social situations—helping you worry less, relate better, and create stronger connections with others.

## TAKE A "HANDS OVER HEART" MOMENT

Take a moment to be kind to yourself, and to feel your own strength. Place your hands over your heart, and breathe deeply for thirty seconds (learned in Love Connection Quest 9).

## *Your Love Connection Bad Guys*

●━━━━●

## PASSIVE CONGRATS

"Congrats." "That's cool." "Good for you." Is this the extent of your reaction to someone else's good news? If so, you're caught in the clutches of this relationship-killing bad guy. A passive congrats sucks the life out of someone else's positive emotion. Whatever you do, avoid this bad guy—and activate your Celebrate Like an Ally power-up instead.

## THE "IT'S TOO LATE TO THANK THEM NOW" MONSTER

This bad guy tries to talk you out of saying thanks to someone because "too much time has passed." It tells you a big fat lie: "It's too late to thank them now!" But that's not true. It's *never* too late to show gratitude. Not even if a month, a year, or a decade has passed. Combat this bad guy by delivering a three-part Superpowerful Thank-You.

## FORGETTABLE SMALL TALK

It's hard to make a memorable social connection when you're chatting about the weather, food, or celebrity gossip. If you find yourself talking to someone you'd like to know better, or someone you care about but haven't seen in a while, don't get trapped in forgettable small talk. Instead, make a memorable and meaningful connection by drawing out their strengths. Use your Investigate Something Exciting power-up!

## LONELY THOUGHTS

"She didn't seem to like me very much." "I can't believe I said something so stupid." "They seemed so bored by what I was talking about." "I made a terrible first impression." "Nobody even cared that I was there." If you're hearing any of these lonely thoughts after a social encounter, you may be caught up in a self-defeating cycle of negative perception. No matter how much time you spend with others, you'll still feel lonely—unless you defeat these bad guys! Try the Flip a Lonely Thought power-up to put them in their place.

## THE BULLY INSIDE

When you're under stress, this bad guy takes full advantage of it. It's the voice inside your head that says "You can't do this." "It's all your fault." "If only you'd done [X], this wouldn't be happening." "You're not strong enough." "You'll let them down." Don't let this bully get to you. Stand up to it by showing yourself the support and kindness you deserve. Your "Hands over Heart Moment" power-up will do just the trick.

## ADVENTURE 2

# Ninja Body Transformation

*Take this adventure if...*

- You want more energy.
- You're sick of diets.
- You're looking for a healthier way to lose or maintain your weight, or put on muscle.
- You want to develop more body confidence.
- You possibly have secret ninja superpowers just waiting to shine!*

*This adventure includes:*

- 21 quests
- 10 power-ups
- 5 bad guys

*How to play:*

- Complete one quest a day, until you finish all 21 quests.

▼

---

* *Ninja body transformation* refers to the art of adopting sneaky and unconventional weight-loss and fitness strategies, much as the Japanese ninjas of history and legend adopted sneaky and unconventional warfare strategies. Your adventure will *not* include throwing weapons, pyrotechnics, sword combat, stealth swimming, or other actual ninja-fighting techniques. (However, you *will* learn willpower methods and physical training techniques inspired by ninja culture.)

# QUESTS

## NINJA QUEST 1: Learn the Philosophy of Ninja Body Transformation

To master the art of ninja body transformation, you only have to follow four rules:

1. **Don't diet.**
2. **Ignore your scale.**
3. **Eat foods that make you feel stronger.**
4. **Do things that make you feel powerful.**

As you can see, ninja body transformation is very different from other weight loss methods you may have tried. In particular, *you aren't allowed to diet*. There are no foods you aren't "allowed" to eat. There is no calorie counting. Appetite suppressants are strongly discouraged.

Why? Because (as you probably already know if you've ever tried it) dieting rarely works. And worse, it's dangerous. Numerous scientific studies show that:

- Almost everyone who goes on a diet regains any weight they lost and then some.
- People who diet end up weighing *more* than people who start at the same weight but never diet.
- Even people who successfully lose weight and keep it off don't always end up healthier and happier.[1]

Meanwhile, repeated dieting:

- Raises cholesterol and blood pressure
- Suppresses the immune system
- Actually *increases* the risk of heart attack, stroke, diabetes, and all-cause mortality[2]

These harms are due to the extreme stress and strain that restricting food puts on your body.

So how are you going to change your body without dieting? This adventure will teach you unconventional, or "stealthy," weight loss and fitness strategies. It will focus your attention on foods that make you feel stronger and actions that make you feel powerful. It will develop your intuition for how to respect and nourish your body. And it will show you new, unexpected techniques for cultivating your physical strength. By completing these quests, you will sneak up on weight loss and energy gain—achieving your physical transformation goals without aiming at them directly.

Over the next twenty quests, you'll learn all about how and why these rules work. For now, simply make a commitment to follow them for at least three weeks.

To complete this first quest, **write the four rules of ninja body transformation somewhere where you can see them daily.** (But maybe, because you're in ninja training, put them somewhere where *no one else* can see them. Remember, ninjas are sneaky!)

## NINJA QUEST 2: Banish the Scale

To transform like a ninja, you have to learn to *ignore* your weight.

Check the scale today or tomorrow if you want. Then you must banish the scale for the rest of this adventure. **For the next three weeks, you will not weigh yourself.**

Why not? Because your goal is to feel healthier, happier, stronger. And that goal is not a *number*. That goal is a *feeling*.

To get to your true goal, you have to learn to pay attention to how your mind and body feel—not to what a machine says.

**On this adventure, you will learn to pay closer attention to other signs of health and vitality:** how much energy you have, what mood you're in, how well you sleep, how often you get sick, and the increasingly powerful actions you can take with your body.

Banishing your scale will also help you avoid one of the biggest mistakes people make when they diet: adopting short-term habits that they'll never be able to sustain. By focusing on how you feel instead of how much you weigh, you'll develop more sustainable habits, a powerful intuition, and true self-control.

**What to do:** Weigh yourself one last time—and then physically remove the scale from where you normally use it. Put it in the back of a closet, in the garage, or on a very high shelf.

*Tip:* If you think it will be really hard for you to go three weeks without weighing yourself, recruit a friend or family member to hide the scale for you!

## NINJA QUEST 3: Eat Like a Ninja

The third rule of ninja body transformation is: *Eat foods that make you feel stronger.*

You're not counting calories on this adventure. And you're not restricting or avoiding food. Instead, your primary mission is to *pay attention to how you feel after you eat*—and figure out which foods make you feel happier, healthier, and stronger.

Look for foods that make you feel more energized, alert, or in a better mood. Foods that make you feel calm and confident. Or perfectly fueled for a workout. Or more beautiful. Or better connected to nature. Check in with *your* mind and body to figure out exactly what feeling good means to you.

**What to do:** For the next twenty-four hours, investigate everything you eat. If a certain food makes you feel stronger, add it to your power-ups and plan to eat more of it over the next three weeks. A food that makes you feel sluggish, weighed down, or gross? That is *not* a power food. You don't have to eliminate it, but it won't count toward your daily power-ups. **Keep investigating until you've identified at least three power foods.**

**Keep in mind:** You're looking for foods that make you feel good for up to an hour or two *after* you eat them. Lots of foods taste amazing and make you happy *while* you're eating them, but make you feel slow, dull, bloated, heavy, or cranky afterward. Those are *not* power foods, even if you enjoy them. You want to enjoy how you feel *after* you eat, not just *while* you eat.

For the next three weeks, your mission is to **eat one food that makes you feel stronger with every meal.** Don't worry about eating *less* of anything. Instead, focus on eating *more* of the foods that make you feel good.

**Why it works:** Research shows that eating more power foods changes people's appetite and cravings over time, so eventually they eat fewer unhealthy foods without even trying.[3]

Everybody is different, so you should experiment with different foods to see what makes *you* feel more alert, full of energy, and in a better mood. Most likely, your power foods will be what food journalist Michael Pollan calls "real food, mostly plants." That means foods with a very short ingredient list, and as Pollan puts it, "ingredients your great-grandmother would recognize as food." (So no weird chemicals or additives.)[4]

**Examples:** Here are some potential power foods you can test for yourself:

- Roasted sunflower seeds
- Yogurt
- Sweet potatoes
- Scrambled eggs
- Popcorn
- Bananas
- Chickpeas (or hummus)
- Dark chocolate
- Blueberries
- Quinoa
- Spinach
- Almonds
- Vegetarian chili

**To be clear:** These aren't the *only* foods you should eat during this adventure. You just need to eat **at least one power food** with every meal and snack. Then you can eat whatever else you want.

## NINJA QUEST 4: Choose a Power Move

The fourth rule of ninja body transformation is: *Do things that make you feel powerful.* Here's one way to practice that habit.

**What to do:** Pick a tiny physical feat to accomplish. Choose something you don't think you can do now but would like to be able to do. A tiny physical feat should take only a few minutes (or even mere seconds!) to accomplish.

**Examples:** Here are some ideas:

- Do one fearless cartwheel
- Complete one perfect push-up (or 10, or 50, or 100 perfect push-ups!)
- Tread water for five minutes without stopping
- Learn the choreography to your favorite dance video
- Climb all the stairs at work in under three minutes
- Throw a Frisbee back and forth a hundred times with an ally, without dropping it once!
- Balance on one leg for thirty seconds with your eyes closed (harder than it sounds . . .)
- Complete one lap around the track in less than 90 seconds (or 120 seconds, or 240 seconds)
- Hold the yoga pose Downward Facing Dog, with your heels touching the floor, for ten breaths

As you can see from these examples, we're not talking about a major physical feat, like completing a triathlon. Instead, go for something small, something you can show off in a matter of minutes or seconds, and that you can reasonably master in a few weeks.

Just make sure it's something that you won't be able to complete on the first try! The idea is to pick something you can work toward, try a dozen times, improve upon, and accomplish by the end of your Ninja Body Transformation adventure.

Now choose your power move—**and make your first attempt at completing it today!**

## NINJA QUEST 5: Ninjas vs. Zombies!

Traditional diets often require calorie restriction and food deprivation—which have some rather unsettling effects on our brains. A 2011 study found that when we don't eat enough, we starve our brain cells—and over time the starved brain cells *start to eat themselves*.[5]

Scientists call this *autophagy*, or literally "self-eating." Neurons devour little bits of themselves, particularly in the hypothalamus, the part of the brain that controls your heart rate, blood pressure, appetite, and sleep cycles.

Your brain, understandably, wants to avoid eating its own neurons. So during self-eating, the hyopthalamus triggers hunger hormones that make you really, *really* want food. This is why you often feel so much hungrier when you're dieting—hungrier than you normally are. It's not just that you're eating less. It's that your brain is freaking out, cannibalizing itself, and telling you to eat *more* to stop the process!

This is one of the major reasons why traditional dieting doesn't work. It makes you weaker—not just physically but mentally.

To put it as plainly as possible: when you diet, you become a real-life zombie, eating your own brain.

To complete today's quest, simply **declare war on calorie restriction and food deprivation**. If your stomach grumbles, eat something. Make a promise to yourself today that you will never let yourself go hungry.

It's ninjas versus zombies—and you want to be a ninja, not a zombie!

### NINJA QUEST 6:
### Summon the Power of Water

Legend has it that ninjas were able to control all the elements of nature with only their minds—harnessing the power of water, earth, wind, fire, and sky for their own goals.[6]

This adventure will not help *you* develop any "supernatural" powers. However, over the next five quests, you *will* learn how to summon the very real mental, physical, and emotional powers that these five natural elements represent in Japanese culture.

Let's start with the first element: water, or *sui*.

In Japanese philosophy, water represents the fluid, flowing, and ever-changing life forces in nature. Water in nature is rarely still—think of the always changing tides of the ocean, the flowing river, or the falling rain. It adapts perfectly to whatever environment it fills or flows through.

You have these same abilities, to change and to adapt. You are changing and adapting *right now*, just by completing this quest. You're creating new memories, and wiring new neurons together. Like water, you are constantly adapting to new circumstances. You can take any form you want.

Keep this fundamental truth in mind as you think about your goals for your weight and your physical health. You are not stuck. Your life and your body are fluid, ever-changing.

Today's quest is simple: To connect with the element of water, **drink a glass of water.** While you drink the water, **remind yourself of your own ability to be like water—to adapt and change.**

## NINJA QUEST 7:
### Summon the Power of Earth

The second element is earth, or *chi*. In Japanese culture, it represents what is hard, solid, and unyielding in nature—from the ground you walk on to the mountains that stand strong through the centuries.

*You* have a hard, solid, and unyielding aspect, too: it is your determination and your steadfast commitment to your goals.

To connect with the element of *chi* in daily life, you need a small object from the earth to carry with you or put somewhere you'll see it often (on your desk at work, by your bed, on the kitchen counter). You need a *chi* stone—a small rock that can represent your own rock-hard willpower.

**What to do:** Choose a *chi* **stone.** When you have one, **hold it tightly in your hand for ten seconds and say to yourself,** *My commitment to my goals is as solid as this stone.*

Every time you mindfully hold this stone in the palm of your hand, you will remind yourself of your own solid, grounded, confident, and steadfast nature.

## *NINJA QUEST 8:*
## *Summon the Power of Wind*

The third element is wind, or *fū*. In Japanese culture, it represents things that expand and enjoy freedom of movement: the air all around us or smoke that rises from a fire.

There are two simple ways to summon the power of wind and connect with your own freedom of movement and expansiveness. Try them both today.

**What to do:** First, make yourself as big as possible for thirty seconds. Expand your body and take up as much room, physically, as you can. If you have a disability, illness, or injury that restricts your physical movement, focus on making *any* part of your body bigger—open your mouth as wide as you can or stretch your fingers as far apart as possible.

Then, move any part of your body through space in slow motion for thirty seconds. You can move your hands and arms, your whole body, or even just your head, slowly turning your neck in every possible direction. As you move in slow motion, put all your focus and attention on the air around you. Feel the air on your skin, and notice how you move through it. Pay attention to the powerful relationship between your body and the air around you, something we almost never notice.

Summoning the power of wind with these two quick actions will help you continue to develop respect and gratitude for the amazing capabilities of your body, exactly as it is, right now.

## NINJA QUEST 9:
### Summon the Power of Fire

The fourth element is fire, or *ka*. In Japanese culture, it represents the most forceful and powerful energies in the world, including not only physical heat (or literal fire) but also mental drive and emotional passion.

Japanese culture teaches that these powerful energies must be kept in balance. A physical fire can spiral quickly out of control and destroy everything in its path. But a life-sustaining fire can burn out too soon, leaving only coldness in its wake.

A candle lighting a safe path, a fire for cooking, a controlled burn in the forest that stimulates growth and clears the way for new life—these are all examples of just the right amount of fire.

Your mental drive and emotional passions must be kept in the same balance. Too much fire, and you feel anxiety or self-destructive anger. Too little fire, and you feel only boredom and apathy.

Boredom and anxiety are two of the most common causes of mindless, unhealthy eating. That's why finding a balance between them can help you achieve your weight loss goals.

Where to look for balance? Try the psychological state of *flow*, which you read about in Chapter 1. When you are in a flow state, you are motivated, interested, and fully engaged. You have a clear goal that fires you up—but you also have the needed skills and resources to achieve it without suffering undue anxiety or self-defeating thoughts.

**Your quest for today is to create at least five minutes of flow**. It can come from doing any goal-oriented activity: a physical workout, playing a video game, writing, dancing, making music, making art, cooking, cleaning, gardening . . . If you are motivated to do it and enjoy it, and if it fully absorbs your attention, you can get flow from it. (Just make sure you're not multitasking! Flow occurs only when you are *completely* absorbed.)

Once you are in flow, you have successfully balanced your most powerful source of energy—and are less likely to engage in mindless and unhealthy behavior. Remember, you can tap into your *ka* power whenever you want by taking just five minutes to find flow.

### NINJA QUEST 10:
### *Summon the Power of Sky*

The fifth element is sky, or *kū*. In Japanese culture, it represents the world beyond our everyday experience: the heavens above, the countless stars at night, and the boundless creative energy of the universe.

In your own life, sky represents spiritual strength and creativity. It's your ability to connect with something bigger than yourself, to feel awe and wonder, to create something out of a void. These elevating feelings can help you develop a better intuition about what you truly crave and want more of in life. This intuition will make it easier for you to break free of unhealthy habits.

To summon the power of sky, take a moment to connect with something greater than yourself. There are many ways to do this: through prayer, poetry, music, meditation, art, or even just literally by gazing up at the heavens. Today, **pick one of these rituals and devote at least one full minute to it, just before a snack or meal.**

If you enjoy this quest today, consider making it a daily habit.

### NINJA QUEST 11:
### *Take a Ninjitsu Break*

Sometime today schedule a *ninjitsu*, or ninja-training, break. Spend at least ten minutes practicing your power move. (If you've already mastered your power move, then it's time to pick a new one!)

## NINJA QUEST 12: Learn "Uzura-gakure"

*Uzura-gakure* is a ninja tactic that has been practiced since the fourteenth century as a way to develop willpower and go unseen by enemies.

The instructions are deceptively simple: **"Curl into a ball and remain motionless in order to appear like a stone."**

Why do ninjas practice this maneuver? According to martial arts historians, the *uzura-gakure* was an essential and effective technique for avoiding detection. By making themselves as small and still as possible, ninjas could hide in plain sight. But perhaps more important, it was also a way to teach ninjas to control their fear and to exercise total self-control.[7] As you will soon see for yourself, making yourself still, especially under extreme stress, takes tremendous mental *and* physical discipline.

*You* don't necessarily have to curl up into a ball every time you practice this traditional ninja tactic. Another option is to simply bow your head, cross your arms over your chest, and remain frozen.

**What to do:** Try *uzura-gakure* right now—and see how still you can be for one full minute.

## NINJA QUEST 13:
## Connect with Three Elements Today

You've already learned five different ways to summon the power of the natural elements (water, earth, wind, fire, and sky). Make today extra powerful by connecting with *three* of these five elements.

**What to do:** Before breakfast, lunch, and dinner today, make it a point to **spend one minute connecting with a different element**. Use the techniques you learned in the earlier quests, whether it's holding a stone in your hand or mindfully drinking a glass of water.

This simple ritual of connecting with an element before each meal will help you make better decisions, exercise greater willpower, and feel stronger throughout the day.

## NINJA QUEST 14: Pick a Power Song

On a low-energy day, it's all too easy to try to fuel up with sugar, caffeine, or junk food. But have you ever seen a ninja eat a doughnut? Probably not!

But there's an alternative source of energy: **power music**.

Scientists who study music have long known that it has powerful impacts on the mind and body: it improves your mood, distracts you from pain and fatigue, and increases your endurance. In fact, listening to music improves energy levels and athletic performance so much, Dr. Costas Karageorghis, a professor at Brunel University in

London and a leading sports psychologist, describes it as "a type of legal performance-enhancing drug."[8]

And there's more. Listening to music you love lowers your levels of the stress hormone cortisol more than taking antianxiety drugs. It also boosts levels of immunoglobin A, an important antibody linked to a strong immune system.[9]

So think of music as your new go-to source of energy and resilience.

**What to do:** Pick a power song now, and share it with at least one ally. Your power song should be any song that pumps you up and makes you want to move.

The next time you're feeling tired or in a bad mood, listen to your power song for energy!

## NINJA QUEST 15:
### Get Inspired by "Tanuki-gakure"

One of the ninja's favorite strategies to avoid detection was *tanuki-gakure*, or the practice of "climbing a tree and camouflaging oneself within the foliage."

You don't have to climb a tree or hide out for today's quest. But *tanuku-gakure* has a lot in common with the more modern Japanese practice known as forest bathing. It's a unique form of Japanese therapy, in which you stand around as many trees as you can in order to get a boost to your mood and your immune system.[10]

It sounds weird, but scientific research shows that it works. It turns out that trees emit airborne chemicals called phytoncides (which literally means "killed by a tree"). These chemicals protect trees by killing fungi, bacteria, and insects. These chemicals, strangely enough, *help* humans—boosting white blood cells that are essential to immune function and lowering cortisol (the stress hormone) levels.

**What to do:** To get inspired by the ancient ninja art of *tanuki-gakure,* or tree camouflage, **go spend five minutes next to or under a tree.** It will boost both your mental *and* your physical resilience.

## NINJA QUEST 16:
## Hunt for More Power Foods

You've been following Rule 3 from Ninja Quest 1, "Eat foods that make you feel stronger," for two weeks now, and eating the power foods you chose in Ninja Quest 3. It's time to increase your options!

Your next quest is to spend today hunting for more power foods.

**What to do:** Choose **at least three new power foods** to add to your power-up list. Remember, a power food is anything that makes you feel stronger after you eat it—more awake, full of energy, in a better mood.

**Examples:** To help you in your hunt, here are some more foods that research has shown improve mood, alertness, resilience, and energy levels:

- *Strawberries*. They're rich in vitamin C, which you need to produce the "happy hormone," endorphins.
- *Mashed potatoes*. They not only feel comforting, they're also packed with energy-boosting and cell-repairing potassium.
- *Peanut butter*. It's high in protein, which helps you avoid sugar crashes and maintain steady willpower.
- *Grilled chicken*. It has lots of B vitamins, which help control your mood.
- *Oatmeal*. It's high in fiber, which slows digestion and gives you longer-lasting energy.
- *Green tea*. It has enough caffeine to increase your alertness without causing a dramatic energy drop later.
- *Walnuts*. They offer plenty of omega-3 fatty acids, which boost mood and stimulate neuron repair.
- *Dark chocolate chips*. They provide tons of antioxidants, which help make every part of your body stronger and more resistant to injury or illness.

Whatever you choose, **make sure you actually *acquire* all three foods today**—whether you eat them today or just put them in the fridge for later.

## NINJA QUEST 17:
### Scale a Wall Together

Legend has it that in order to scale walls, ninjas carried each other on their backs. They called it "creating a human platform," and it allowed them to reach heights that no single ninja could reach alone.[11]

Teamwork should be an essential part of *your* ninja maneuvers, too. But instead of asking for help today, you're going to help someone else.

**What to do:** Who could *you* help reach a greater height today? Make it your mission to be ready to spring into action, at a moment's notice, **to help someone else "scale a wall."** We're talking metaphorically here—you don't have to give someone a boost over a literal wall. Any way you can give someone an emotional, mental, *or* physical boost will work just fine.

Although doing a spontaneous favor for someone else might not seem like it's directly related to your health goals, remember Rule 4, "Do things that make you feel powerful." Helping someone else is one of the most powerful things you can do.

This quest is complete when you've successfully helped someone "scale a wall"!

## NINJA QUEST 18:
### Have a Five-Element Day

You're nearing the end of your ninja-inspired adventure—so today, demonstrate how far you've come.

**What to do:** Summon all your natural powers today by **connecting with all five elements** (water, earth, wind, fire, and sky). Try to spread them out across the day. Connect with an element before each meal, plus once more in the morning and evening.

Think of today as an opportunity to lock in these simple, life-changing habits before your ninja journey is finished!

## NINJA QUEST 19:
### Master "Uzura-gakure"

Today you have a chance to demonstrate one of the new skills you've developed during this adventure: *uzura-gakure*, or the art of staying as still as a stone.

As you know from Ninja Quest 12, *uzura-gakure* is a test of your mental strengths, including willpower and determination. With all the quests you've completed on this adventure, *your* mental strengths should be in absolute peak condition. See for yourself!

**What to do:** Today, you must attempt a more difficult *uzura-gakure* mission: **stay still as a stone for three entire minutes.** *That's six times as difficult* as the *uzura-gakure* mission in Ninja Quest 12.

Set a timer, and hold yourself to it. Yes, it will take tremendous mental discipline. But when you successfully complete this quest, you'll know that your ninja training has made you measurably and objectively that much mentally stronger.

## NINJA QUEST 20:
## The Legend of the Shape-Shifters

In Japanese legend, ninjas were said to have several fantastic powers—not the least of which was *shape-shifting*, or the ability to transform physically into another form, such as a fox, a wolf, or an old woman.

While you won't be transforming into another creature, you *have* been shifting your shape for the past three weeks. Today is the day you **celebrate your transformation**—no matter how small or subtle it may be. Here are some changes you may notice:

- You stand or sit up taller.
- You have more energy.
- Your clothes fit better.
- Muscles that usually tense up in your face, neck, or back are more relaxed.
- The muscles in your arms and legs feel more powerful.
- You feel more comfortable in your own skin.

**What to do:** Spend at least **two minutes looking for and appreciating the shifts *you've* made in your shape.** These changes are a reflection of the powerful shifts you've made in how you think about your health goals, and how you treat your body.

## NINJA QUEST 21: Share the Secret

For three weeks, you've practiced the art of adopting sneaky and unconventional weight-loss and fitness strategies. Now it's time to share your ninja wisdom with others.

**Take what you've learned, and pay it forward.** For your final quest, teach someone else the four rules of ninja body transformation:

1. Don't diet.
2. Ignore the scale.
3. Eat foods that make you feel stronger.
4. Do things that make you feel powerful.

**What to do:** Teach the rules to a friend, post them online, or share them on your favorite online forum. If you're feeling *really* superbetter, offer yourself as an ally or mentor to anyone who would like to give it a try.

## *Your Ninja Body Transformation Power-ups*

●━━━━━●

### PRACTICE YOUR POWER MOVE

See how close you are to perfecting your power move (from Ninja Quest 4)—whether it's doing one perfect and fearless cartwheel, climbing all the stairs at work in less than sixty seconds, completing one hundred push-ups, or holding the yoga pose Downward Facing Dog for ten slow breaths.

Whether you achieve your goal or not, every attempt makes you stronger.

### EAT A POWER FOOD

Energize yourself by eating a power food (Ninja Quests 3 and 16). That's anything you eat that makes you feel stronger—more awake, full of energy, in a better mood. Keep a list of your personal power foods, which could be anything from sunflower seeds, dark chocolate, or yogurt to a hard-boiled egg, a banana, or almonds. Try to activate this power-up at every single meal or snack for the next three weeks.

### LISTEN TO YOUR POWER SONG

Increase your endurance, fight fatigue, improve your mood, and boost your immune system with the proven power of music (Ninja Quest 14). Use this power-up whenever you want a healthier way to energize.

### PRACTICE *UZURA-GAKURE*

Take a minute to practice *uzura-gakure*, or becoming "as still as a stone" (Ninja Quests 12 and 19). Curl up into a ball like a real ninja, or simply bow your head and cross your arms over your chest. Use this technique to quiet your mind and increase your willpower.

## CONNECT WITH THE WATER ELEMENT

Water, or *sui*, represents the fluid, flowing, and ever-changing life forces in nature. Every time you drink a glass of water, remind yourself of your own ability to adapt and change (Ninja Quest 6).

## CONNECT WITH THE EARTH ELEMENT

Earth, or *chi*, represents what is hard and solid in nature. If you chose a *chi* stone in Ninja Quest 7, hold it tightly in your hand for ten seconds to remind yourself of your own power to be solid, grounded, determined, confident, and steadfast.

## CONNECT WITH THE WIND ELEMENT

Wind, or *fū*, represents things that expand and enjoy freedom of movement. To remind yourself of your own freedom and expansiveness, make yourself (or any part of your body) as big as possible for thirty seconds (Ninja Quest 8). Expand your body and take up as much room, physically, as you can. Or move any part of your body (such as your hands and arms) through space in slow motion for thirty seconds, putting all your focus and attention on the air as you move through it.

## CONNECT WITH THE FIRE ELEMENT

Fire, or *ka*, represents the most forceful and powerful energies in the world, including physical heat, mental drive, and emotional passion. You tap into your *ka* power whenever you take five minutes to find flow, or balance, between a lack of fire (boredom) and too much fire (anxiety). As we saw in Ninja Quest 9, your flow can be any goal-oriented activity: playing a video game, writing, dancing, making music, making art, cooking, gardening . . .

## CONNECT WITH THE SKY ELEMENT

Sky, or *kū*, represents the world beyond our everyday experience. To remind yourself of your spiritual strength and creativity, take a minute for prayer, meditation, song, poetry, or art (Ninja Quest 10).

## PRACTICE *TANUKI-GAKURE*

Go outdoors and practice the art of *tanuki-gakure*, or "tree camouflage" (Ninja Quest 15). Get as close as you can to a tree and soak up its powerful phytoncides. Activating this power-up will help you reduce stress and boost your immune system.

## *Your Ninja Body Transformation Bad Guys*

## WEIGHING YOURSELF

For the duration of this adventure, you will not allow a number to define your health, power, or happiness.

For at least three weeks, avoid the scale!

## COUNTING CALORIES

Food is a source of energy and power, and one way to measure that potential energy is with calories. But it's not the best way. How you *feel* after you eat is a much better indicator of what will make you stronger and healthier than a simple calorie count.

During this adventure, ignore calories and focus on how you feel instead.

## FEELING GUILTY ABOUT WHAT YOU EAT

Your meals and snacks won't always go according to plan. But guilt will *not* help you make better decisions in the future. Instead, guilt will drain the emotional and physical energy that you need to strengthen your mind and body.

If you make an unwise food choice, skip the guilt—and use one of your ninja power-ups to reenergize instead.

## MENTALLY CHECKING OUT FROM YOUR BODY

During this adventure, your mission is keep the mind-body connection strong. Your body needs to move, it needs water, and it needs to eat. Don't allow mental distractions—like work, social media, books, movies, TV shows, or video games—to absorb you so fully that you ignore these physical needs.

Battle this bad guy until it becomes a natural habit to check in with your body at least once an hour. Try this strategy: Set a timer or calendar alert to remind you to check in with your body every hour. Every time it goes off, ask yourself: *Do I need to eat? Do I need some water? Do I need to move?* Or ask an ally to send you random texts or emails reminding you to check in with your body!

## IGNORING YOUR NINJA POWERS

You have the five elements at your disposal, always: water, earth, wind, fire, and sky. If you ignore these powers, they will diminish—so don't let a day go by without calling on at least one of these elements!

# Time Rich

***Take this adventure if...***

- You feel like the day isn't long enough to do everything you want.
- You could have more of any one thing, it would be more free time.
- You want to learn to *slow down time*, so you can use it more effectively.

***This adventure includes:***

- 10 quests
- 6 power-ups
- 3 bad guys

***How to play:***

- Complete one quest a day, until you finish all 10 quests.

▼

## TIME RICH QUEST 1:
### Learn What It Means to Be Time Rich

We all have the same twenty-four hours a day. By that measure, no one person should be "time richer" or "time poorer" than anyone else. But in fact, some people do experience what economists call *time affluence*. It's the feeling that you have abundant time to spend on all the things that matter most to you. When you're time affluent, no matter how busy you are, you feel like you always have enough time for your family, your health, and your passions.

But many more people experience *time poverty*, the feeling that you never have enough time to spend on your personal goals and priorities.[1] When you're time poor, it doesn't matter how motivated you are—you constantly feel deprived of the chance to put time and energy into your passions.

If you're like most people in the United States today, you're more likely to feel time poor than time rich. This adventure is designed to help you change that.

People who are time rich are happier, healthier, and more productive. They experience less chronic stress, and they dedicate more time each day to pursuing their personal goals and dreams. They have closer relationships. They volunteer and help others more. They make smarter choices about what to eat, how much to exercise, and how long to sleep.[2] All this makes perfect sense: **if you feel time rich, you'll spend time much more freely and generously with yourself.** In this way, time really is just like money.

Becoming time richer can make a huge and positive difference in your life. Economists have shown that time affluence is a better predictor of every kind of well-being (mental, physical, emotional, and social) than material affluence. People who feel time rich experience less stress, more happiness, closer relationships, and better physical health than people who feel time poor. These benefits accrue regardless of whether you have a lot of money. In fact, if you want to lead a better life, faster, economists recommend trying to increase your time wealth rather than your monetary wealth.[3]

But here's the strange thing about time affluence: *it doesn't actually correspond to how much "free time" you objectively have.* Except with individuals who work multiple jobs in order to stay above the poverty line, and those who have no control over unpredictable and frequently changing work schedules, perceived time affluence is almost completely unrelated to how many minutes or hours per day people have for personal pursuits or freely chosen activities.[4] Studies have found that most people who have a ton of free time don't feel time rich; they just feel bored or restless. On the other hand, many people with incredibly busy schedules and hardly a minute unaccounted for feel extremely time rich. Despite barely having a minute to themselves, they will tell you they have all the time in the world. So what makes the difference?

It turns out that, for the most part, time affluence is not related to a person's schedule but rather to a huge range of tiny mental, physical, emotional, and social habits. Little choices you make each day—how you sit, how you commute, even how fast or slowly you breathe—influence your perception of how much time is available to you. Meanwhile, the tiniest social interactions and seemingly trivial decisions (like "Which thirty-second video should I watch online today?") can make you feel dramatically time richer or time poorer.

This adventure will teach you the habits of the time rich. Over the next eight quests, you'll learn eight different techniques for increasing your time affluence *without changing how much free time you actually have.* These techniques have been developed and tested by researchers at Yale, Harvard, Stanford, Wharton, UC Berkeley, and other leading business schools and psychology departments.

**What to do:** Simply **accept this challenge:** "Over the next ten days, I will accumulate a small fortune of time to spend on the things that matter most to me!"

### TIME RICH QUEST 2:
### Get Rich with Power

"Time is money"—so goes the common saying. But according to a team of psychology researchers at the University of California at Berkeley, a more apt saying would be "Time is *power.*"

People in positions of power, such as CEOs, often feel time rich. The UC Berkeley researchers wanted to find out *why.* Is it because powerful people actually have more free and abundant time? Or does having power change our perception of time, helping us use it more effectively, regardless of how much free time we actually have?

To investigate this question, the researchers conducted a series of five experiments in which they cleverly increased and decreased participants' feelings of power while asking them to evaluate how much time they had to do the things that were most important to them in daily life.

Here are some of the power-increasing techniques they tested:

- **High-power seating:** Adjust your seat higher than you normally sit.
- **Power memory:** Remember a time when you had the power to make an important decision or impact someone else's life.
- **Power stance:** Raise your arms over your head as high as you can, plant your feet firmly and widely on the ground, and stick your chest up and out. (You may be familiar with this technique from Harvard Business School professor Amy Cuddy's widely cited "power posing" research.)[5]

As it turned out, all three of these psychological techniques successfully increased both feelings of power *and* time affluence. And there was a direct relationship between the two. The bigger the increase in perceived power, the more time participants said they had to pursue their own goals.[6]

Why did it work? The researchers theorized that feeling powerful increases our sense of control over *all* aspects of our lives—and control over time is just one aspect.

"Of course, in reality, the powerful don't control time," the Berkeley researchers wrote in a study published in the *Journal of Experimental Social Psychology*. "Unlike other resources, such as food or money, time is constantly being spent and can never be replaced." However, believing you control your own time *does* increase the likelihood that you will spend time on your own personal goals. "In this way," the researchers wrote, "the powerful really do have a monopoly on time."

Making yourself feel more powerful, even just for a moment, can help you discover time for yourself that you didn't realize you had. This is the first step to becoming time richer.

**What to do:** To gain some of the time you deserve, **choose one of the three high-power techniques used in the Berkeley study, and practice it right now.**

## TIME RICH QUEST 3:
### Discover the Time Gift Paradox

It sounds counterintuitive, but it's true: **giving time away to someone else will make you feel time richer.**

A team of Yale, Harvard, and Wharton researchers conducted a series of four experiments to test this theory. They found that spending as little as ten minutes helping someone else—for example, proofreading someone's essay or writing a supportive letter to a child in a hospital—increased time affluence significantly. In fact, giving time away made the study participants feel *more* time rich than participants who actually, objectively, got time richer—that is, participants who received a "time windfall," or an hour of unexpected free time to do whatever they wanted.

The researchers argued that this surprising effect stems from the fact that helping others makes us feel powerful. And as you already know from Quest 2, people who feel powerful also feel time rich.[7]

**What to do:** Your quest for today is to **spend ten minutes helping someone else.** Any kind of help will do. Help a coworker do a task at work or clean up around the house, or write a thoughtful letter to someone who needs to hear encouraging words. If you think you don't have time to complete this quest, just remember: *giving away ten minutes of your free time will make you feel even more time rich than receiving sixty minutes of free time.* In other words, this is a trade well worth making.

## *TIME RICH QUEST 4: Get Rich with Awe*

Awe is the positive emotion we feel when we're humbled by something bigger or greater than ourselves. You might feel awe looking at a natural wonder, like a waterfall or the Grand Canyon. You might feel awe listening to a massive choir, with its hundreds of voices working together to make something beautiful. You might feel awe watching an athlete do something no one has ever done before, breaking a record and changing our entire perspective on what is humanly possible.

Awe is one of the most pleasurable and motivating positive emotions. It's also, researchers at Stanford University recently discovered, the single emotion most closely linked to time affluence.

In a series of three experiments, the Stanford psychologists tested the impact of awe on perceptions of time availability. They discovered that participants who felt awe for just a moment or two (triggered by watching a video of a natural wonder, for example) felt they had more time available later in the day for their own goals, were less impatient, and were also more willing to volunteer time to help others. All three changes are signs of increased time affluence.[8]

Why would awe change our feelings about time? The Stanford researchers explain that when we feel awe, we experience time differently. We experience it as *slow and expansive* rather than rushed and limited. "Awe focuses people's attention on what is currently unfolding before them," they wrote in the journal *Psychological Science*. "Focusing on the present moment elongates time perception."

In other words, awe makes seconds and minutes literally feel longer. And this expansive, elongated experience of time makes us feel like there is simply more of it.

So how can you take practical advantage of this scientific finding? It's easy: just try to stimulate a little bit of awe each and every day. The researchers tested two main techniques for provoking awe, both of which you can easily replicate at home.

**What to do:** The first way to provoke awe is to **watch a video of something awesome**. That might mean watching a video of one of the world's best surfers charging a giant wave, or a panda giving birth to triplets, or a scene of a massive social protest, or a volcano erupting, or images of a distant galaxy collected by powerful telescopes. Whatever gives you goose bumps or makes you feel humbled by its greatness, *that* will do the trick.

The second way to provoke awe is to write for one or two minutes about something awesome you experienced or witnessed in the past. Here are the exact instructions that the Stanford researchers used in their studies, so you can replicate the effect: "Awe is a response to things perceived as vast and overwhelming that alters the way you understand the world. **Write about a personal experience that made you feel this way.**" You don't have to write a long essay! A few sentences will work just fine.

To complete this quest, pick either of these two awe-provoking techniques and do it today.

## TIME RICH QUEST 5:
## Avoid Social Jet Lag

Do you know your chronotype? If not, you may inadvertently be throwing away some of the best hours of your day.

A *chronotype* is a biological preference for when to sleep and when to be active. Types range from "extreme early" to "extreme late," and everything in between. Extreme early types are the so-called early birds, able to wake up at sunrise and be mentally and physically active right away. Extreme late types, on the other hand, are night owls. They aren't ready to perform at their best until ten a.m. or so. But they are mentally sharp and physically energized well into late evening, much more so than early types.

*Your* chronotype changes over the course of your life. Most people are extreme late types when they're teenagers and extreme early types when they're seniors. During the years in between, chronotypes are harder to predict. They vary based on what scientists call our *clock genes*: the bits of DNA that help determine our most comfortable waking and sleeping rhythms.

Why do chronotypes matter? If your biological clock doesn't match your social clock—the traditional start times for school and work—then you will be unable to think or perform at your best. Physiologically and mentally, being off your biological clock is a state very much like jet lag. You feel sluggish and sleep-deprived and have difficulty concentrating. Hence scientists call it *social jet lag*. Researchers estimate that currently more than half of the U.S. working population and a whopping 80 percent of high school students suffer from social jet lag—resulting in huge costs to workplace productivity and making it harder for most students to succeed.[9]

Social jet lag has physical consequences. People who suffer from it are more likely to be obese, more likely to smoke, and more likely to become dependent on high-caffeine products and other stimulants. That's because they're in a constant state of sleep deprivation and body clock misalignment—and so they use sugar, nicotine, and caffeine as a crutch to get through the day or night.[10]

Social jet lag has emotional consequences as well: it is thought to contribute to depression and flare-ups of mental illness, due to the stress it puts on the brain and body.[11]

So what is the solution? As science writer Stefan Klein, author of *The Secret Pulse of Time*, advises: "We should stop seeing calendar times as a corset we have to squeeze into. We need to move away from the one-size-fits-all model of time, and recognize and respect the fact that each person has—and needs—an individual rhythm and inner time."[12]

In practical terms, this means adjusting school and work schedules. For example, many schools have experimented with starting an hour or two later. Results from such experiments prove that such adjustments can indeed dramatically improve performance and quality of life. One school in Minneapolis, for example, found that starting school at 9:40 a.m. instead of 8:40 a.m. improved the average grade for all students by a full letter, and absenteeism fell by half. Workplaces have also experimented to positive effect, allowing employees to flexibly choose start times and scheduling important group meetings no earlier than ten a.m. to accommodate later chronotypes.

Let's be realistic: you aren't going to be able to implement sweeping social change in the next twenty-four hours. But you *can* take stock of your own chronotype and start scheduling your life as close to your biological rhythms as possible.

**What to do: Identify your chronotype.** Are you an early type, a late type, or somewhere in between?

If you naturally fall asleep by ten p.m., you're extreme early. If you can't sleep until after midnight, you're extreme late. In between, and you're . . . in between. Once you know your chronotype, make it a point to schedule your most important activities at the right time for you. Whenever you have a choice, schedule exams, meetings, presentations, first dates, workouts, study sessions, and any physically or mentally demanding activity in your chronotype sweet spot—typically *no earlier* than nine to ten hours after you naturally want to fall asleep, and *no later* than three hours before you naturally want to go to bed.

Paying attention to your chronotype will help make sure that you have the mental focus and physical energy when you need them most—giving you more "good hours" every day.

### TIME RICH QUEST 6:
### Make Your Day Longer

To make the day seem longer, do something for the first time.

Eat a new food. Meet a new person. Visit a new place. Learn a new fact. Try a new exercise. Play a new game. Go to a shop you've never been to before. Listen to a song you've never heard before.

According to Dr. David Eagleman, a neuroscientist at Baylor College of Medicine and an expert on the subjective experience of time, doing *anything* for the first time changes how your brain processes the passing minutes and hours. Specifically, it slows time down. [13]

Here's why: the more predictable and familiar an experience is to you, the less work your brain has to do to understand it. If you've seen it before or done it before, your brain can take a shortcut, drawing on its previous learning to process what's happening. This is good for saving mental energy but terrible for accumulating time riches. That's because the less work your brain has to do, the faster time flies. If your brain processes an event quickly, it thinks the event *happened* quickly. Time seems shorter, more compressed— the opposite of what you want and need to feel time rich.

Fortunately, you can take advantage of this phenomenon by forcing your brain to slow down and take in new information. Doing something for the first time requires it to process everything more slowly— and therefore you will experience time as moving more slowly. And the more slowly time moves for you, the more abundant it will feel.

**What to do:** Do one thing you normally do every day **differently**. Brush your teeth with your nondominant hand. (That is, if you're right-handed, brush your teeth with your left hand.) Or walk backward from your bedroom to the kitchen, instead of forward. Or eat your breakfast with your eyes closed. Making a small change in your routine will make time slow down ever so slightly—which means you'll be more likely to take time for your most important priorities and goals later in the day.[14]

### TIME RICH QUEST 7:
### Get Rich with Oxygen

Perhaps the easiest way to start feeling more time rich, especially when you're under pressure, is to *take long, slow breaths for five minutes*.

Researchers at the Stanford University Graduate School of Business conducted a series of laboratory experiments—and found that this simple action changed time perception dramatically. According to a study published in the *Journal of Consumer Psychology*, "Subjects who were instructed to take long and slow breaths for five minutes," they wrote, "not only felt there was more time available to get things done, but also perceived their day to be longer."[15] People who took shorter, quicker breaths, on the other hand, were much more likely to feel time poor.

Why does this technique work? The body influences the mind: quick breathing tells your brain that you're rushing, hurried, and stressed. Slow breathing, however, tells your brain that you have all the time in the world.

**What to do:** Set a timer for five minutes. Focus on taking **long, slow breaths** the entire time. Return to this technique as a power-up whenever you need it.

## TIME RICH QUEST 8: Get Rich on the Go

How you get from A to B each day is a major factor in how time rich or time poor you'll feel.

According to research from the University of North Carolina at Chapel Hill, people who drive are significantly time poorer than people who walk, bicycle, or take public transportation. Crucially, this is true even when drivers spend *less time* commuting each day than someone who walks, bikes, or takes public transportation. Driving itself, and not the time spent doing it, seems to create feelings of time poverty.[16]

Why is this the case? UNC's study of nearly one thousand commuters showed that driving was the most stressful mode of travel. Driving, particularly during heavy rush-hour traffic, also provokes negative emotions such as frustration, anxiety, and anger. Increased stress and negative emotions are both associated with increased feelings of time poverty. (Remember from Time Rich Quest 2 that when you feel powerless, you feel time poor.)

On the other hand, other forms of travel—especially walking and bicycling—promote reduced stress and feelings of self-efficacy. They increase mindfulness, or active and compassionate attention paid to our thoughts, feelings, and surroundings. Increased self-efficacy and mindfulness are associated with increased time affluence.

So what can you do, in the next twenty-four hours, to take advantage of this research? *Any* change you can make to your commute to decrease the time you spend driving and increase the time you spend walking, bicycling, or taking public transportation will help make you feel time richer. This is true *even if your new commute takes longer than driving.*

Every small change helps. For example, park farther away and spend ten minutes walking to work at the end of your commute. Or see if you can change your commute time to avoid the most stressful driving periods. Or carpool, so you can reduce the number of days you feel the strain of driving yourself. (As an added bonus, driving others can help you feel powerful—which may balance out the impact of driving on your time affluence!)

Another option—one that may be easier for you—is to *adopt mindful driving habits.* The mindfulness experts at Wildmind Buddhist Meditation recommend the following simple changes:

- Turn off the radio.
- Slow down, and try driving at or just below the speed limit. This will free up the energy (and eliminate the tension) you otherwise spend constantly trying to push the speed limit and pass other vehicles.
- Take one or two deep breaths at every stop sign or red light.[17]

These habits will decrease stress and increase mindfulness, helping you reap some of the benefits of getting time richer on the go.

**What to do:** Try making **a small change in how you get from A to B** over the next twenty-four hours. If you're not going anywhere today, complete this quest by making a plan to make a small change!

## TIME RICH QUEST 9:
### Choose Your Own Quest!

Today's quest is . . . do whatever you want!

That's right. This quest has no instructions, other than **take five minutes today to do something, anything, of your own choosing.**

Take a nap. Call your mom. Lift some weights. Window-shop online. Play a game. Go enjoy a view. Whatever it is, it should be something you weren't already planning to do today.

**Why it works:** Research shows that freely and spontaneously chosen activities increase time affluence, while routine or obligatory activities decrease it.[18] This makes sense: whenever you exercise control over how to spend your time, it reminds you of how much power you have to *make time* for what's important.

Of course, you can't (and shouldn't) avoid routines and obligations. But if you do *only* what is routine and obligatory, you'll eventually feel less and less in control of your time. Making a free and spontaneous choice about what to do reminds you of the power you have over your own time—even if it's only for a few minutes!

So make a free choice about how to spend five minutes today. By doing so, you'll actively shift your attention from what you *have* to do to what you *want* to do—and that's a huge component of feeling time rich.

You have total control over your quest for the day. **Do whatever you want for five minutes!**

## TIME RICH QUEST 10:
### *Measure Your Time Wealth*

Congratulations! You've learned eight powerful techniques for increasing your time affluence. But how will you know that these techniques are working? Time affluence is a lot harder to measure than monetary riches. You still only have twenty-four hours a day, after all, no matter how time rich you feel.

To measure *your* time wealth, you'll need to do what psychologists do. They use several different specially designed surveys to measure time affluence and its opposite, time poverty, such as the Perceived Time Availability Index, the Material Affluence and Time Affluence Survey, the Time Constriction Index, and the Future Time Perspective Scale.

You don't have to take the full surveys to get a sense of your growing time wealth.

Here are ten of the most important questions from these measurement tools. You can use these questions as a way to check in, periodically, with yourself. Are you feeling time rich or time poor this week?

## TIME POVERTY

**How many of these statements do you agree with?**
- My life has been too rushed.
- There have not been enough minutes in the day.
- I'm pressed for time.
- I'm not in control of my time.
- Time is slipping away.

## TIME AFFLUENCE

**How many of these statements do you agree with?**
- I have had enough time to do the things that are important to me.
- I have lots of time in which I can get things done.
- I have plenty of time in my future.
- I am in control of how I spend my time.
- Time is boundless.

If you agree with more of the *time poverty* than *time affluence* statements, make an extra effort to activate your Time Rich power-ups (listed below). If you agree with more of the *time affluence* than *time poverty* statements, then congratulations—you're building up real time wealth.

## *Your Time Rich Power-ups*

## GIVE YOURSELF A POWER BOOST

To increase feelings of power and time affluence, use one of the three proven techniques from Time Rich Quest 2.
- **High-power seating:** Adjust your seat higher than you normally sit.
- **Power memory:** Think of a time in the past when you had the power to make an important decision or impact someone's life.
- **Power stance:** Plant your feet, raise your hands, and lift your chest.

## GIVE SOMEONE TEN MINUTES OF YOUR TIME

Help someone else for ten minutes today (Time Rich Quest 3). It gives you a greater feeling of time affluence than a windfall of one hour of unexpected free time!

## PROVOKE AWE

Make time feel long and expansive by watching an awe-inspiring video, or spend two minutes writing about a time when you felt humbled and awed by something bigger than yourself (Time Rich Quest 4).

## DO SOMETHING FOR THE FIRST TIME

Slow down your experience of time by making your brain work a little bit harder: do something for the first time or do something you normally do just a little bit differently (Time Rich Quest 6).

## BREATHE

Take long and slow breaths for five minutes (Time Rich Quest 7). It will slow down your entire day, helping you find more time to do the things that are most important to you.

## MAKE A FREE AND SPONTANEOUS CHOICE

Carve out a block of five minutes to do something spontaneous (Time Rich Quest 9). Show yourself that you really are in control of how you spend your own time.

## *Your Time Rich Bad Guys*

### TIME POVERTY

Time poverty is the feeling that there aren't enough hours in the day to do what you want. It fogs your mind and makes you time-stingy, preventing you from spending the free minutes and hours you do have on the things that matter most: your health, your dreams, your closest relationships. Battle this bad guy with any of your time rich power-ups!

### SOCIAL JET LAG

This bad guy puts your mind and body's natural rhythms out of sync with your daily responsibilities. Even if you can't change your overall schedule, you can still fight this bad guy (as in Time Rich Quest 5). Whenever possible, schedule the activities that are most important to you *at the right time for you*. If you are comfortable with speaking up, advocate for flexible start times, or fairer meeting times, at your school or workplace. And in the future, when you have the choice, actively seek out a schedule that better matches your chronotype.

### MINDLESS, STRESSFUL COMMUTING

The more stress and distraction you experience during your daily commute, the more time poor you're likely to feel. Fight this bad guy by changing how you commute (as in Time Rich Quest 8). If you drive, switch to walking, bicycling, carpooling, or public transportation. Even if your commute takes longer, you will feel time richer. If this is not feasible, practice mindful driving—turn off the radio, slow down slightly and drive at the speed limit, and take deep breaths at stop signs or red lights. And if you already have a more mindful method of commuting, or don't have a commute, even better—no need to fight this bad guy!

# About the Science

This book is based on five years of research, including a randomized, controlled study of the SuperBetter method with the University of Pennsylvania; a clinical trial of the SuperBetter method with Ohio State University Wexner Medical Center and Cincinnati Children's Hospital, which was funded by the National Institutes of Health; and a literature review of more than one thousand peer-reviewed, scientific papers on the topics of game-related psychology and neuroscience, post-traumatic and post-ecstatic growth, and resilience, particularly as it is related to positive emotion, physical activity, and social support. The most relevant papers— roughly five hundred—are cited in the endnotes of this book.

To make it easier for you to explore the science yourself, I have created a directory of these studies online at Showmethescience.com. Wherever possible, I have linked to the free, public version of the full scientific paper. Academic publishing, unfortunately, often requires a subscription or university affiliation to access the research; where this is the case, I have linked to descriptions of the research as well as to the original study. I will continue to update these resources as additional research into the psychology and neuroscience of games become available.

For scientifically curious readers, I want to provide a more detailed description of the University of Pennsylvania and Ohio State University

Wexner Medical Center studies. How did these collaborations come about? What were the goals of the studies? What were the methods? Who were the participants, and what were the results? While the University of Pennsylvania study was completed in 2013, and its findings recently published, the OSU trial is ongoing. Updates to the trial, as well as any further studies conducted and scientific papers published, will be available at Showmethe science.com.

*Please note: None of the researchers or doctors who conducted the Super-Better studies at the University of Pennsylvania, Ohio State University Wexner Medical Center, or Cincinnati Children's Hospital have any financial interest in video games in general or SuperBetter in particular; nor were they compensated in any way for conducting this research.*

## THE UNIVERSITY OF PENNSYLVANIA SUPERBETTER STUDY

"We need something new and creative to help people with depression, because there are still many people who don't benefit from existing therapies and medications," said Ann Marie Roepke, a clinical psychologist and doctoral candidate at the University of Pennsylvania's Positive Psychology Center, when I asked what inspired her to conduct a randomized, controlled study of SuperBetter. "I was struck by SuperBetter's playful, lighthearted approach. It's not often that you see something so fresh and new come along."

I first met Roepke at a scientific conference in Philadelphia in 2011, where she was presenting her work on post-ecstatic growth, a concept she pioneered. (Her talk was how I first discovered the idea!) Meanwhile, I was presenting my games research at a panel about technology and psychological health. We spent several hours talking about our work, and I told her my personal SuperBetter story. We immediately realized that we had a great many overlapping research interests. In particular, we both shared a passion for developing and testing novel interventions to help encourage post-traumatic—and I now know, post-ecstatic—growth.

We stayed in touch for more than a year, sharing our latest research and looking for the right way to team up. Eventually, the perfect opportunity arose: Roepke found two colleagues at Penn who were interested in helping her conduct a formal study of SuperBetter's effectiveness for treating depression.

To help Penn prepare for this study, I teamed up with two collaborators at SuperBetter Labs, science writer Bez Maxwell and data scientist Rose Broome, to create a special set of depression-related power-ups, bad guys, and quests. The three of us also helped the Penn researchers design the study—how long it would last, how often we would encourage participants to play, and what questions we would ask. But the actual trial, including all recruitment, data collection, and data analysis, was conducted independently by the research team at the University of Pennsylvania. This was to ensure maximum scientific validity. I found out the results of the trial only when the Penn researchers prepared their independent report for presentation at the annual Association for Psychological Science conference.

The study was set up as a thirty-day randomized, controlled trial. Two-thirds of the participants were given access to the SuperBetter method, while the other third were put on a wait list. This allowed the researchers to compare the effects of playing SuperBetter against other possible factors in getting better, such as time passing or receiving treatment in the form of therapy or medication.

The playing group was instructed to spend ten minutes a day with Super-Better. They were also encouraged to continue any other treatment they were already engaged with, including therapy or prescription medication. Roughly one half of the participants reported that they were currently in therapy or taking antidepressants.

We enrolled 236 participants in total. All the participants were eighteen or older, and all met the criteria for clinical depression. They were recruited online at a popular self-help website, Authentic Happiness. They were not compensated in any way. This was very important for us—we wanted to learn how SuperBetter works for typical players, so we avoided giving them any kind of special motivation or reward that ordinary SuperBetter players don't have.

We also wanted to find out how different approaches to getting Super-

Better might work differently, so we divided the SuperBetter group into two subgroups. One was given a set of power-ups, bad guys, and quests specific to depression and anxiety. The other was simply set loose in the SuperBetter world and given a set of the game's most popular power-ups, bad guys, and quests (as judged by number of activations by other SuperBetter users). This included content related to self-compassion, physical activity, and social resilience. Our hypothesis was that both groups with access to SuperBetter would do better than the wait-list group, but that the players receiving depression-specific content would do even better.

Both groups took four psychological surveys—one at the beginning, and the others every two weeks until the conclusion of the study. This included a follow-up survey two weeks after the official thirty-day period of play or waiting. The study has recently completed the scientific peer-review process and has been published in the journal *Games for Health*.[1] Here's what we learned.

SuperBetter players experienced significantly greater relief from symptoms of depression than the wait-list participants. By the end of the study, on average, the players had *six fewer symptoms of depression*, while the wait-list group had two fewer. The players also had significantly less anxiety, developed more self-efficacy, experienced stronger social support, and reported higher overall life satisfaction. In short the SuperBetter players felt better, faster, in every way we measured. Moreover, they kept getting better even after the thirty-day period; two weeks after they stopped playing, they were still experiencing the same rate of improvement. They continued to get less depressed and anxious, to develop greater self-efficacy, and to feel more supported, at a rate that was faster and more significant than participants on the wait list. This suggests a possible "upward spiral" effect: once you start getting superbetter, it's easier to keep getting superbetter. (For those of you interested in statistics, the Cohen's effect size for SuperBetter at the end of six weeks was $d = 0.67$, which is a very strong result. An effect size higher than 0.2 means something had a small effect on an outcome, while 0.5 or higher means it had a moderate effect on an outcome, and 0.8 is considered a large effect. So SuperBetter had a moderate to large impact on players' well-being.)

What else did we find out? Lots! One of the factors we investigated was whether SuperBetter worked differently for individuals who were also in therapy or taking prescription psychiatric medication, such as antidepressants. We found that they experienced similar results *regardless of whether* they were engaging in another form of treatment. We take this as an indication that SuperBetter works well in conjunction with traditional treatment and therefore does not need to be considered an alternative to therapy or medication. At the same time, strong evidence suggests that it can offer significant benefits to individuals who, for whatever reason, have chosen not to or are unable to pursue therapy or medication.

We also observed that the playing group logged into the online version of SuperBetter an average of twenty times over the course of thirty days. This was an interesting result, because although we recommended a daily check-in with the game, a daily check-in did not ultimately prove necessary to have significant benefit. Something closer to *every other day* was enough to make a positive difference.

Finally, we noticed that the players who were simply set loose in the SuperBetter environment and given a popular set of power-ups, bad guys, and quests improved even better and faster than players who were given a depression-specific set! Both groups improved significantly, more so and faster than the wait-list group. But the group that was not asked to focus specifically on their depression did the best of all. This was a fascinating and unexpected finding. There are several possible explanations for it. The one that the Penn researchers consider most likely is that the most popular SuperBetter content might be popular for a reason—namely, that it works really well. The players who received the most popular power-ups, bad guys, and quests as suggestions, therefore, were particularly well set up for success. (This, by the way, is the reason why I have included so many of them in this book!) Another possibility is that it's more empowering to have lots of creative options for how to get better than to be prescribed one particular approach. This is actually more typical of how most people use the Super-Better method. They decide for themselves which power-ups, bad guys, and quests are right for them.

Despite these promising findings, the Penn study should be looked at as a starting point for evaluating the SuperBetter method and not as a final or definitive answer to the question "Who can SuperBetter help?" The results were both positive and, statistically speaking, significant. However, as we note in the scientific paper, several factors about the study limit the conclusions we can draw from it. For example, the study size—236 participants—is fairly large for a first-time study of a novel psychological intervention, but even larger studies would provide more compelling evidence. We also know that because we recruited participants who were already seeking self-help solutions for depression, they may have been more motivated to get better than the general population of people who suffer from depression and therefore better able to benefit from SuperBetter. A future study that enrolls participants using other methods—for example, by offering screenings for depression to a wider population not already seeking solutions—might provide a better understanding of how much self-motivation is needed to benefit from the method.

Another limiting factor is that we followed participants for only six weeks; therefore, while the results show that most players experienced significant benefits, this particular study provides no evidence either way as to whether or for how long the benefits last, beyond the initial two-week follow-up. Finally, as is common in studies seeking to study "natural usage"—that is, studies in which participants are not paid or otherwise compensated—the study lost quite a few users by the end of the six weeks to attrition, particularly in the wait-list group. (That is, some participants never came back to answer later surveys.) Complete data sets were collected from 63 participants; partial data sets were collected from another 102 participants. For this reason, it's worth considering again the possibility that the SuperBetter method may only appeal to or work for individuals who are actively seeking solutions and who are particularly motivated to get better. This would confirm what we've observed among the more than 400,000 users of the online version: the method seems to be the most effective for people who are actively struggling with a very difficult personal challenge and therefore may be more motivated and open to trying something new.

After the study was completed and presented at two scientific conferences, I asked Roepke what she thought accounted for SuperBetter's demonstrated effectiveness. She offered several theories. First, she zoomed in on its "playful, lighthearted approach." She said: "We all sometimes take ourselves and our thoughts too seriously. By reframing things in gameful ways, SuperBetter can help us gain some perspective and separate ourselves from unhelpful thoughts."

She also cited the underlying science as a crucial element to the game. "Research psychologists have made really wonderful and useful discoveries," she said, "but the field needs people to help translate hard-to-access, hard-to-read journal articles into something more approachable. SuperBetter does this by taking important research and translating it into power-ups, bad guys, and quests."

She also thinks the secret identity and epic wins are a key part of its power to create positive change. "The idea of a heroic journey is really important and compelling," she said. "Stories are central to our lives. We understand others by the stories they tell, and we come to understand ourselves by the stories *we* tell. SuperBetter offers us a powerful and fun way to change the story. Instead of telling ourselves a story about victimhood or tragedy, we can tell a story about adventure and redemption." That, to her, was potentially the most important piece of SuperBetter. "It reminds us that we can be the hero of our own story."

# THE OHIO STATE UNIVERSITY STUDY

"Can we turn doctors' advice and medical guidelines into a game, so patients have an easier time following it?" That's the idea that Lise Worthen-Chaudhari, a research scientist and faculty member at the College of Medicine at Ohio State University, wanted to explore when she reached out to me in the summer of 2010.

Worthen-Chaudhari has been in the field of rehabilitation research for twenty years, and she knew that most patients typically have a difficult time keeping up with all their doctors' recommendations at home. She wanted to find something that could help patients remember their doctors' advice, and improve their ability to follow it consistently.

She also knew that when family members are aware of the recommendations, a patient is more likely to follow them successfully. But too often caretakers feel overwhelmed and anxious and forget the advice they've heard. So Worthen-Chaudhari wondered what could help family members feel more empowered to help their loved ones get better, faster.

She conducted a review of innovations in patient care, specifically looking for a tool that would engage patients over a long rehabilitation period and create a stronger support system. "After looking at everything," she explained to me. "SuperBetter is the only thing I've found that seems to be doing both effectively."

Her timing was incredibly fortuitous—I had just begun to develop a digital version of the SuperBetter method with my collaborators at the social gaming startup Social Chocolate. With Worthen-Chaudhari's help, we were able to start interviewing medical practitioners at OSU immediately for their input on how to improve the SuperBetter method and how to make it more useful for both patients and doctors. We embarked on a collaboration that, over a three-year period, helped us strengthen the design and incorporate specific medical guidance for players using the game for concussions and traumatic brain injury recovery.

As a result of our ongoing collaboration, we were awarded a research grant from the National Institutes of Health. We were tasked with conducting a pilot study of SuperBetter in a clinical setting—in official terms, a phase-one clinical trial. Patients would use the SuperBetter method for six weeks; their doctor would play as their ally.

You'll notice that both the Penn and the OSU studies tested a relatively short play period (thirty days and six weeks in duration, respectively). That decision was based on our observations of and interviews with other Super-Better players at large; most of them, we were finding, experienced the majority of emotional and social gains, and the biggest shift in their thinking, within the first thirty days of play.

For the pilot study, OSU enrolled twenty patients from Cincinnati Children's Hospital. Aged thirteen to twenty, they were all dealing with difficult recoveries from a mild traumatic brain injury or concussion. They were introduced to SuperBetter by their doctor and given a quick tutorial on how to use the digital version. They were then encouraged to get their "daily SuperBetter dose"—three power-ups, one bad guy battle, and at least one quest—every day for the next six weeks of their treatment. They were also given a starter list of ten power-ups they might find useful (such as wearing sunglasses inside to protect against bright lights), twenty bad guys they might encounter (such as difficulty concentrating or dizziness), and daily quests (such as "Find one fun activity you can do for at least twenty minutes that doesn't hurt your brain—such as drawing or listening to a favorite movie with your eyes closed"). Based on their symptoms and recovery progress, they were sent new, personalized suggestions from their doctor for additional power-ups, bad guys, and quests several times throughout the study. The patients were not compensated for their participation; expenses of up to $40 were reimbursed to cover their transportation to two follow-up interviews.

The primary purpose of this clinical trial was to assess the feasibility of the SuperBetter method for use in hospitals—in other words, to find out if doctors and patients would be able to use it effectively, and if both groups would report a positive experience with it. By all measures, it was a success.

The qualitative data collected over a four-month period showed that all twenty patients were able to learn the method quickly and implement it effectively at home. Roughly 75 percent were able to achieve the recommended dose of play throughout their six-week trial.

The most common sentiment among patients was that "SuperBetter helped me do more of the important things I need to do to take care of myself." Indeed, simply introducing the idea of a game into a clinical conversation was observed to increase patient interest and attention to their doctors' medical advice. "When you bring up the game, they react with surprise," according to Worthen-Chaudhari. "It's consistently delightful. It piques their interest. A teenager's not even listening to you and all of a sudden they register what you're saying. It's an extremely positive result."

The data also showed that the game helped the patients' primary caretakers, mostly parents. They were able to learn the language of power-ups and bad guys quickly and reported playing the role of allies in the game consistently through the duration of the study. The most frequent response from caretakers in follow-up interviews was that SuperBetter provided them with a feeling of "relief"—that they worried less about their loved ones' ability to successfully recover, and that they had more positive interactions with them as a result.

The OSU research team reported that medical practitioners were able to learn the method quickly and were effective in translating their advice and treatment plans into power-ups, bad guys, and quests.

In addition to this qualitative observation, we used the clinical trial as an opportunity to collect quantitative data on how the SuperBetter method impacted players' mood, quality of life, and postconcussion symptoms. Not only did participants have significantly fewer symptoms of postconcussion syndrome by the end of the study, they also were significantly less depressed and more optimistic. Their rates of improvement for depression and optimism were similar to those in the Penn study, helping to show that an even wider range of people can benefit from the SuperBetter method. One particularly interesting finding was that the participants who had the most severe depression before playing benefited the most from the game. Four out of five participants with severe depression at the start of the trial had improved to "nondepressed" by the end.

Crucially, despite the possibility that game play can trigger postconcussion symptoms such as headache, nausea, and exhaustion, none of the participants reported that playing SuperBetter triggered such symptoms. Worthen-Chaudhari summarizes the findings: "The data clearly suggest that SuperBetter works as a powerful complement to traditional medical care."

The next step will be to conduct a controlled version of the clinical trial, similar to the Penn study. This will allow us to compare the experiences of patients who do not have access to SuperBetter with patients who do. In the meantime, the results of the pilot study are providing guidance to medical practitioners for the best practices to adopt while engaging patients with the SuperBetter method. This is an important step for this line of research, because as Worthen-Chaudhari reports, "Many of the doctors and fellows at OSU have expressed a desire to explore using the SuperBetter method for a wider range of illness and injury rehabilitation."

*For updates on studies of SuperBetter, visit Showmethescience.com.*

# Acknowledgments

To all of the SuperBetter heroes, thank you. Your secret identities amaze me, your power-ups encourage me, and your epic wins inspire me. I am especially grateful to the players who shared their stories for this book. You are extraordinary examples of what it means to possess gameful strength and resilience. You have my utmost admiration and respect.

SuperBetter has had many important allies over the past six years, particularly in the area of scientific research. I am very grateful to Dr. Ann Marie Roepke, who brilliantly led the randomized controlled trial of SuperBetter at the University of Pennsylvania, and to Rose Broome and Bez Maxwell, our coauthors on the Penn study. I am also greatly indebted to Professor Lise Worthen-Chaudhari at the Ohio State University Wexner Medical Center for her endless optimism and her tireless work on our clinical trial. Thank you also to the National Institutes of Health for funding our research, and to John Yost for your unshakable dedication to making Super-Better available to as many people as possible.

Over the past four years, I've had the great honor to work with an amazing creative and production team on the SuperBetter apps and online game. To everyone who contributed and collaborated at Social Chocolate, Super-

Better Labs, Natron Baxter, and the Ardmore Institute of Health, I want to celebrate your talent, dedication, and hard work. I hope you are as proud as I am of what we built together. I especially want to recognize Chelsea Howe, Nathan Verrill, and Finlay Cowan for their huge creative contributions, and Keith Wakeman for his commitment to taking SuperBetter to the next level.

I am so grateful to Scott Moyers and Ann Godoff for giving SuperBetter a home at Penguin Press. It is a dream come true for any writer to work with such a brilliant editor and such a visionary publisher. Your support for this book means the world to me.

Thank you to the entire production team at Penguin Press, whose superpowers in book design and copyediting have been essential to creating this book!

Thank you to the incredible Chris Parris-Lamb for encouraging me to write this book. Something important to know about Chris: He is not only a book genius, he is also an incredibly talented and accomplished marathon runner. Thank you, Chris, for coaching me and Kiyash to run a full marathon this year. That was a huge epic win! (And as many runner-writers know, running every day is the key to staying sane while writing a book.)

Many thanks also to Andy Kifer, Rebecca Gardner, and Will Roberts at the Gernert Agency for their invaluable advice, and for creating audiences for this book worldwide. And to everyone at the Leigh Bureau, thank you for helping me share the ideas in this book with as many people as possible.

And to a few more extraordinary allies...

Kelly, my better half, thank goodness we're identical twins so that whenever you do something amazing, a small part of me thinks, "We have the same DNA! Maybe someday I can do that too!"

To my parents, Judy and Kevin, and my parents-in-law, Paula and Mike, thank you for all of your support, encouragement, love, and excitement over the past extremely adventurous year.

A huge and special thank-you to my hero Jennifer Sibilla for being the best ally anyone could ever hope to have. While I was writing this book, you were doing something much greater, and you have changed our lives forever.

And finally, Kiyash—I would have dedicated this book to *you* if we hadn't had such wonderful luck this year. So this is a second dedication. You are the person I always want to be superbetter for—which is easy, because every day you make me stronger, braver, and happier. Let's always do three great things.

# Notes

*Introduction*

1. Jessica L. Mackelprang et al., "Rates and Predictors of Suicidal Ideation During the First Year After Traumatic Brain Injury," *American Journal of Public Health* 104, no. 7 (2014): e100–e107; Nazanin H. Bahraini et al., "Suicidal Ideation and Behaviours After Traumatic Brain Injury: A Systematic Review," *Brain Impairment* 14.01 (2013): 92–112.
2. Richard G. Tedeschi and Lawrence G. Calhoun, "Posttraumatic Growth: Conceptual Foundations and Empirical Evidence," *Psychological Inquiry* 15, no. 1 (2004): 1–18.
3. I arrived at this list of the five most common signs of post-traumatic growth after an extensive review of the scientific literature on PTG, including the following important sources: Birgit Wagner, Christine Knaevelsrud, and Andreas Maercker, "Post-Traumatic Growth and Optimism as Outcomes of an Internet-Based Intervention for Complicated Grief," *Cognitive Behaviour Therapy* 36, no. 3 (2007): 156–61; Lawrence G. Calhoun and Richard G. Tedeschi, "Beyond Recovery from Trauma: Implications for Clinical Practice and Research," *Journal of Social Issues* 54, no. 2 (1998): 357–71; Laura Quiros, "Trauma, Recovery, and Growth: Positive Psychological Perspectives on Posttraumatic Stress," (2010): 118–21; Stephen Joseph and P. Alex Linley, "Growth Following Adversity: Theoretical Perspectives and Implications for Clinical Practice," *Clinical Psychology Review* 26, no. 8 (2006): 1041–53; Richard G. Tedeschi and Lawrence G. Calhoun, "The Posttraumatic Growth Inventory: Measuring the Positive Legacy of Trauma," *Journal of Traumatic Stress* 9, no. 3 (1996): 455–71; Matthew J. Cordova et al., "Posttraumatic Growth Following Breast Cancer: A Controlled Comparison Study," *Health Psychology* 20, no. 3 (2001): 176; Susan Cadell, Cheryl Regehr, and David Hemsworth, "Factors Contributing to Posttraumatic Growth: A Proposed Structural Equation Model," *American Journal of Orthopsychiatry* 73, no. 3 (2003): 279–28; Mary Beth Werdel and Robert J. Wicks, *Primer on Posttraumatic Growth: An Introduction and Guide* (Hoboken, NJ: John Wiley and Sons, 2012); Kenneth W. Phelps et al., "Enrichment, Stress, and Growth from Parenting an Individual with an Autism Spectrum Disorder," *Journal of Intellectual and Developmental Disability* 34, no. 2 (2009): 133–41; Katie A. Devine et al., "Posttraumatic Growth in Young Adults Who Experienced Serious Childhood Illness: A Mixed-Methods Approach," *Journal of Clinical Psychology in Medical Settings* 17, no. 4 (2010): 340–48; Stephen Joseph, *What Doesn't Kill Us Makes Us Stronger: The New Psychology of Posttraumatic Growth* (New York: Basic Books, 2011); and Janelle M. Jones et al., "That Which Doesn't Kill Us Can Make Us Stronger (and More Satisfied with Life): The Contribution of

Personal and Social Changes to Well-Being After Acquired Brain Injury," *Psychology and Health* 26, no. 3 (2011): 353–69.

4. Bronnie Ware, "Regrets of the Dying," November 19, 2009, http://bronnieware.com/regrets-of -the-dying. The article was subsequently expanded to a full-length book, *The Top Five Regrets of the Dying* (Bloomington, IN: Hay House, 2012).

5. Ann Marie Roepke, "Psychosocial Interventions and Post-traumatic Growth: A Meta-Analysis," *Journal of Consulting and Clinical Psychology* (May 19, 2014): n.p.

6. Ann Marie Roepke, "Gains Without Pains? Growth After Positive Events," *Journal of Positive Psychology* 8, no. 4 (2013): 280–91.

7. Mark Stephen Tremblay et al., "Physiological and Health Implications of a Sedentary Lifestyle," *Applied Physiology, Nutrition, and Metabolism* 35, no. 6 (2010): 725–40.

8. Ruth M. Barrientos et al., "Little Exercise, Big Effects: Reversing Aging and Infection-Induced Memory Deficits, and Underlying Processes," *Journal of Neuroscience* 31, no. 32 (2011): 11578–86; Genevieve N. Healy et al., "Breaks in Sedentary Time Beneficial Associations with Metabolic Risk," *Diabetes Care* 31, no. 4 (2008): 661–66; and Corby K. Martin et al., "Exercise Dose and Quality of Life: A Randomized Controlled Trial," *Archives of Internal Medicine* 169, no. 3 (2009): 269.

9. Martin S. Hagger et al., "Ego Depletion and the Strength Model of Self-Control: A Meta-Analysis," *Psychological Bulletin* 136, no. 4 (2010): 495.

10. Barbara L. Fredrickson "The Role of Positive Emotions in Positive Psychology: The Broaden-and-Build Theory of Positive Emotions," *American Psychologist* 56, no. 3 (2001): 218; Barbara L. Fredrickson, "What Good Are Positive Emotions?," *Review of General Psychology* 2, no. 3 (1998): 300; and Sarah D. Pressman and Sheldon Cohen, "Does Positive Affect Influence Health?," *Psychological Bulletin* 131, no. 6 (2005): 925.

11. Todd B. Kashdan, Paul Rose, and Frank D. Fincham, "Curiosity and Exploration: Facilitating Positive Subjective Experiences and Personal Growth Opportunities," *Journal of Personality Assessment* 82, no. 3 (2004): 291–305; and Todd Kashdan, *Curious?: Discover the Missing Ingredient to a Fulfilling Life* (New York: Harper, 2010), 352.

12. Hiroshi Nittono et al., "The Power of Kawaii: Viewing Cute Images Promotes a Careful Behavior and Narrows Attentional Focus," *PLOS ONE* 7, no. 9 (2012): e46362. There's a bonus benefit, too: viewing baby animals also makes you more productive!

13. Julianne Holt-Lunstad, Wendy A. Birmingham, and Kathleen C. Light, "Influence of a 'Warm Touch' Support Enhancement Intervention Among Married Couples on Ambulatory Blood Pressure, Oxytocin, Alpha Amylase, and Cortisol," *Psychosomatic Medicine* 70, no. 9 (2008): 976–85.

14. Robin I. M. Dunbar, "The Social Role of Touch in Humans and Primates: Behavioural Function and Neurobiological Mechanisms," *Neuroscience and Biobehavioral Reviews* 34, no. 2 (2010): 260–68; and Kerstin Uvnäs Moberg, *The Oxytocin Factor: Tapping the Hormone of Calm, Love, and Healing* (New York: Merloyd Lawrence Books, 2003).

15. As defined by leading gratitude researcher Dr. Robert Emmons. See Robert A. Emmons and Cheryl A. Crumpler, "Gratitude as a Human Strength: Appraising the Evidence," *Journal of Social and Clinical Psychology* 19, no. 1 (2000): 56–69; Sara B. Algoe, "Find, Remind, and Bind: The Functions of Gratitude in Everyday Relationships," *Social and Personality Psychology Compass* 6, no. 6 (2012): 455–69; and Sara B. Algoe, Jonathan Haidt, and Shelly L. Gable, "Beyond Reciprocity: Gratitude and Relationships in Everyday Life," *Emotion* 8, no. 3 (2008): 425.

## Part 1: Why Games Make Us Superbetter

1. The one billion number is a calculation based on my aggregation of more than twenty global game play demographic and marketplace reports, including the 2014 Entertainment Software Association's Demographic Report and Newzoo's 2013 Global Games Market Report, which estimates 1.23 billion active video game players worldwide. That estimate includes 192 million in North America, 446 million in Europe, the Middle East, and Africa, 477 million in Asia, and 116 million in Latin America.

2.   Amanda Lenhart et al., "Teens, Video Games and Civics," Pew Internet Life Report, September 16, 2008, http://www.pewinternet.org/2008/09/16/teens-video-games-and-civics.

3.   See Jane McGonigal, *Reality Is Broken: Why Games Make Us Better and How They Can Change the World* (New York: Penguin, 2011), chap. 4.

4.   John T. Cacioppo, Joseph R. Priester, and Gary G. Berntson, "Rudimentary Determinants of Attitudes: II. Arm Flexion and Extension Have Differential Effects on Attitudes," *Journal of Personality and Social Psychology* 65, no. 1 (1993): 5.

5.   Amy S. Pollick and Frans B.M. De Waal, "Ape Gestures and Language Evolution," *Proceedings of the National Academy of Sciences* 104, no. 19 (2007): 8184–89; and David McNeill et al., "Growth Points from the Very Beginning," *Interaction Studies* 9, no. 1 (2008): 117–32.

## Chapter 1: You Are Stronger Than You Know

1.   Hunter G. Hoffman et al., "Virtual Reality as an Adjunctive Non-Pharmacologic Analgesic for Acute Burn Pain During Medical Procedures," *Annals of Behavioral Medicine* 41, no. 2 (2011): 183–91.

2.   You can find up-to-date information about the availability of *Snow World* virtual reality for pain relief at www.hitl.washington.edu/projects/vrpain.

3.   Hunter G. Hoffman, "Virtual Reality Therapy," *Scientific American* (August 2004): 60–65.

4.   Hunter G. Hoffman et al., "Using fMRI to Study the Neural Correlates of Virtual Reality Analgesia," *CNS Spectrums* 11, no. 1 (2006): 45–51.

5.   Eleanor Jameson, Judy Trevena, and Nic Swain, "Electronic Gaming as Pain Distraction," *Pain Research and Management: Journal of the Canadian Pain Society* 16, no. 1 (2011): 27; Molly Greco, *Effectiveness of an iPad as a Distraction Tool for Children During a Medical Procedure*, Ph.D. diss., Ball State University, 2013; and Andrea Windich-Biermeier et al., "Effects of Distraction on Pain, Fear, and Distress During Venous Port Access and Venipuncture in Children and Adolescents with Cancer," *Journal of Pediatric Oncology Nursing* 24, no. 1 (2007): 8–19.

6.   Sharon A. Gutman and Victoria P. Schindler, "The Neurological Basis of Occupation," *Occupational Therapy International* 14, no. 2 (2007): 71–85; and Nancy Nainis et al., "Relieving Symptoms in Cancer: Innovative Use of Art Therapy," *Journal of Pain and Symptom Management* 31, no. 2 (2006): 162–69.

7.   Daniel M. Wegner et al., "Paradoxical Effects of Thought Suppression," *Journal of Personality and Social Psychology* 53, no. 1 (1987): 5; and George Lakoff, *Don't Think of an Elephant: Know Your Values and Frame the Debate* (White River Junction, Vt.: Chelsea Green, 2008).

8.   Emily A. Holmes et al., "Can Playing the Computer Game 'Tetris' Reduce the Build-up of Flashbacks for Trauma? A Proposal from Cognitive Science," *PLOS ONE* 4, no. 1 (2009): e4153.

9.   Emily A. Holmes et al., "Key Steps in Developing a Cognitive Vaccine Against Traumatic Flashbacks: Visuospatial Tetris Versus Verbal Pub Quiz," *PLOS ONE* 5, no. 11 (2010): e13706.

10.  Jessica Skorka-Brown, Jackie Andrade, and Jon May, "Playing 'Tetris' Reduces the Strength, Frequency and Vividness of Naturally Occurring Cravings," *Appetite* 76 (2014): 161–65.

11.  Jackie Andrade, Jon May, and D. K. Kavanagh, "Sensory Imagery in Craving: From Cognitive Psychology to New Treatments for Addiction," *Journal of Experimental Psychopathology* 3, no. 2 (2012): 127–45.

12.  Xiaomeng Xu et al., "An fMRI Study of Nicotine-Deprived Smokers' Reactivity to Smoking Cues During Novel/Exciting Activity," *PLOS ONE* 9, no. 4 (2014): e94598.

13.  Xiaomeng Xu et al., "Intense Passionate Love Attenuates Cigarette Cue-Reactivity in Nicotine-Deprived Smokers: An fMRI Study," *PLOS ONE* 7, no. 7 (2012): e42235.

14.  Anuradha Patel et al., "Distraction with a Hand-Held Video Game Reduces Pediatric Preoperative Anxiety," *Pediatric Anesthesia* 16, no. 10 (2006): 1019–27.

15.  Peggy Yip et al., "Cochrane Review: Non-Phamacological Interventions for Assisting the Induction of Anaesthesia in Children," *Evidence-Based Child Health: A Cochrane Review Journal* 6, no. 1 (2011): 71–134.

16.  Mihaly Csikszentmihalyi, *Beyond Boredom ad Anxiety: Experiencing Flow in Work and Play* (San Francisco: Jossey-Bass, 1975).

17. Mihaly Csikszentmihalyi, "The Flow Experience and Its Significance for Human Psychology," in Mihaly Csikszentmihalyi and Isabella Selega Csikszentmihalyi, eds., *Optimal Experience: Psychological Studies of Flow in Consciousness* (Cambridge, U.K.: Cambridge University Press, 1988).

18. Mihaly Csikszentmihalyi, "Activity and Happiness: Towards a Science of Occupation," *Journal of Occupational Science* 1, no. 1 (1993): 38–42.

19. Brenda E. Mansfield et al., "A Possible Physiological Correlate for Mental Flow," *Journal of Positive Psychology* 7, no. 4 (2012): 327–33.

20. Jenova Chen, "Flow in Games (And Everything Else)," *Communications of the ACM* 50, no. 4 (2007): 31–34.

21. Dennis Scimeca, "How Playing Casual Games Could Help Lead to Better Soldiers," *Ars Technica*, October 5, 2013.

22. Carmen V. Russoniello, Kevin O'Brien, and Jennifer M. Parks, "EEG, HRV and Psychological Correlates While Playing Bejeweled II: A Randomized Controlled Study," *Studies in Health Technology and Informatics* 144 (2009): 189–92.

23. C. V. Russoniello, Kevin O'Brien, and Jennifer M. Parks, "The Effectiveness of Casual Video Games in Improving Mood and Decreasing Stress," *Journal of Cyber Therapy and Rehabilitation* 2, no. 1 (2009): 53–66.

24. Brian A. Primack et al., "Role of Video Games in Improving Health-Related Outcomes: A Systematic Review," *American Journal of Preventive Medicine* 42, no. 6 (2012): 630–38.

25. Jayne Gackenbach and Johnathan Bown, "Mindfulness and Video Game Play: A Preliminary Inquiry," *Mindfulness* 2, no. 2 (2011): 114–22.

26. Paul Grossman et al., "Mindfulness-Based Stress Reduction and Health Benefits: A Meta-Analysis," *Journal of Psychosomatic Research* 57, no. 1 (2004): 35–43; Stefan G. Hofmann et al., "The Effect of Mindfulness-Based Therapy on Anxiety and Depression: A Meta-Analytic Review," *Journal of Consulting and Clinical Psychology* 78, no. 2 (2010): 169; and Alberto Chiesa and Alessandro Serretti, "Mindfulness-Based Stress Reduction for Stress Management in Healthy People: A Review and Meta-Analysis," *Journal of Alternative and Complementary Medicine* 15, no. 5 (2009): 593–600.

27. Jonathan R. Krygier et al., "Mindfulness Meditation, Well-Being, and Heart Rate Variability: A Preliminary Investigation into the Impact of Intensive Vipassana Meditation," *International Journal of Psychophysiology* 89, no. 3 (2013): 305–13.

28. Thomas William Rhys Davids, trans., *Dialogues of the Buddha* (1899; reprint Delhi: Motilal Banarsidass, 2000).

### Chapter 2: You Are Surrounded by Potential Allies

1. Michiel M. Spapé et al., "Keep Your Opponents Close: Social Context Affects EEG and fEMG Linkage in a Turn-Based Computer Game," *PLOS ONE* 8, no. 11 (2013): e78795.

2. Marco Iacoboni, "Imitation, Empathy, and Mirror Neurons," *Annual Review of Psychology* 60 (2009): 653–70; Kenneth R. Leslie, Scott H. Johnson-Frey, and Scott T. Grafton, "Functional Imaging of Face and Hand Imitation: Towards a Motor Theory of Empathy," *Neuroimage* 21, no. 2 (2004): 601–7; Ruth Feldman et al., "Mother and Infant Coordinate Heart Rhythms Through Episodes of Interaction Synchrony," *Infant Behavior and Development* 34, no. 4 (2011): 569–77; Piercarlo Valdesolo, Jennifer Ouyang, and David Desteno, "The Rhythm of Joint Action: Synchrony Promotes Cooperative Ability," *Journal of Experimental Social Psychology* 46, no. 4 (2010): 693–95; and Piercarlo Valdesolo and David Desteno, "Synchrony and the Social Tuning of Compassion," *Emotion* 11, no. 2 (2011): 262.

3. Guillaume Chanel, J. Matias Kivikangas, and Niklas Ravaja, "Physiological Compliance for Social Gaming Analysis: Cooperative Versus Competitive Play," *Interacting with Computers* 24, no. 4 (2012): 306–16; and Inger Ekman et al., "Social Interaction in Games Measuring Physiological Linkage and Social Presence," *Simulation and Gaming* 43, no. 3 (2012): 321–38.

4. Barbara Fredrickson, *Love 2.0: How Our Supreme Emotion Affects Everything We Think, Do, Feel, and Become* (New York: Hudson Street Press, 2013).

5. Tiffany Field, Brian Healy, and William G. Leblanc, "Sharing and Synchrony of Behavior States

and Heart Rate in Nondepressed Versus Depressed Mother-Infant Interactions," *Infant Behavior and Development* 12, no. 3 (1989): 357–76.

6.  Greg J. Stephens, Lauren J. Silbert, and Uri Hasson, "Speaker–Listener Neural Coupling Underlies Successful Communication," *Proceedings of the National Academy of Sciences* 107, no. 32 (2010): 14425–30.

7.  Bethany E. Kok and Barbara L. Fredrickson, "Upward Spirals of the Heart: Autonomic Flexibility, as Indexed by Vagal Tone, Reciprocally and Prospectively Predicts Positive Emotions and Social Connectedness," *Biological Psychology* 85, no. 3 (2010): 432–36.

8.  Robert W. Levenson and John M. Gottman, "Marital Interaction: Physiological Linkage and Affective Exchange," *Journal of Personality and Social Psychology* 45, no. 3 (1983): 587.

9.  Fredrickson, *Love 2.0.*

10. Charles J. Walker, "Experiencing Flow: Is Doing It Together Better Than Doing It Alone?," *Journal of Positive Psychology* 5, no. 1 (2010): 3–11.

11. Simo Järvelä et al., "Physiological Linkage of Dyadic Gaming Experience," *Simulation and Gaming* 45, no. 1 (2014): 24–40.

12. Sarah M. Coyne et al., "Game on . . . Girls: Associations Between Co-Playing Video Games and Adolescent Behavioral and Family Outcomes," *Journal of Adolescent Health* 49, no. 2 (2011): 160–65; Laura M. Padilla-Walker, Sarah M. Coyne, and Ashley M. Fraser, "Getting a High-Speed Family Connection: Associations Between Family Media Use and Family Connection," *Family Relations* 61, no. 3 (2012): 426–40; and Lydia Buswell et al., "The Relationship Between Father Involvement in Family Leisure and Family Functioning: The Importance of Daily Family Leisure," *Leisure Sciences* 34, no. 2 (2012): 172–90.

13. Daphne Bavelier et al., "Brains on Video Games," *Nature Reviews Neuroscience* 12, no. 12 (2011): 763–68; J. Wainer, K. Dautenhahn, B. Robins, and F. Amirabdollahian, "A Pilot Study with a Novel Setup for Collaborative Play of the Humanoid Robot KASPAR with Children with Autism," *International Journal of Social Robotics* 6, no. 1 (2014): 45–65; and Bill Ferguson et al., "Game Interventions for Autism Spectrum Disorder," *Games for Health Journal* 1, no. 4 (August 2012): 248–53.

14. "Video Games Can Benefit Autistic Children: Study," Agence France-Presse, March 7, 2014.

15. Valdesolo, Ouyang, and Desteno, "The Rhythm of Joint Action: Synchrony Promotes Cooperative Ability"; Natalie Sebanz, Harold Bekkering, and Günther Knoblich, "Joint Action: Bodies and Minds Moving Together," *Trends in Cognitive Sciences* 10, no. 2 (2006): 70–76; and Lynden K. Miles, Louise K. Nind, and C. Neil Macrae, "The Rhythm of Rapport: Interpersonal Synchrony and Social Perception," *Journal of Experimental Social Psychology* 45, no. 3 (2009): 585–89.

16. C. Daniel Batson et al., "Empathy, Attitudes, and Action: Can Feeling for a Member of a Stigmatized Group Motivate One to Help the Group?," *Personality and Social Psychology Bulletin* 28, no. 12 (2002): 1656–66; and C. Daniel Batson et al., "Empathy and Attitudes: Can Feeling for a Member of a Stigmatized Group Improve Feelings Toward the Group?," *Journal of Personality and Social Psychology* 72, no. 1 (1997): 105.

17. Jennifer N. Gutsell and Michael Inzlicht, "Empathy Constrained: Prejudice Predicts Reduced Mental Simulation of Actions During Observation of Outgroups," *Journal of Experimental Social Psychology* 46, no. 5 (2010): 841–45.

18. "Games for Peace: Bridging Conflict Through Online Games," http://gamesforpeace.org, acessed April 20, 2014.

19. Donghee Yvette Wohn et al., "The 'S' in Social Network Games: Initiating, Maintaining, and Enhancing Relationships," *Proceedings of the 44th Hawaii International Conference on System Sciences* (IEEE, 2011): 1–10.

20. Donghee Yvette Wohn et al., "Building Common Ground and Reciprocity Through Social Network Games," *CHI EA'10 Extended Abstracts on Human Factors in Computing Systems* (ACM, 2010): 4423–28.

21. Sabine Trepte, Leonard Reinecke, and Keno Juechems, "The Social Side of Gaming: How Playing Online Computer Games Creates Online and Offline Social Support," *Computers in Human Behavior* 28, no. 3 (2012): 832–39.

22. Jonathan Oxford, Davidé Ponzi, and David C. Geary, "Hormonal Responses Differ When Playing Violent Video Games Against an Ingroup and Outgroup," *Evolution and Human Behavior* 31, no. 3 (2010): 201–9; and Samuele Zilioli and Neil V. Watson, "The Hidden Dimensions of the Competition Effect: Basal Cortisol and Basal Testosterone Jointly Predict Changes in Salivary Testosterone After Social Victory in Men," *Psychoneuroendocrinology* 37, no. 11 (2012): 1855–65.

23. Erno Jan Hermans, Peter Putman, and Jack Van Honk, "Testosterone Administration Reduces Empathetic Behavior: A Facial Mimicry Study," *Psychoneuroendocrinology* 31, no. 7 (2006): 859–66; and Paul J. Zak et al., "Testosterone Administration Decreases Generosity in the Ultimatum Game," *PLOS ONE* 4, no. 12 (2009): e8330.

24. Allan Mazur, Elizabeth J. Susman, and Sandy Edelbrock, "Sex Difference in Testosterone Response to a Video Game Contest," *Evolution and Human Behavior* 18, no. 5 (1997): 317–26.

25. Justin M. Carré, Susan K. Putnam, and Cheryl M. McCormick, "Testosterone Responses to Competition Predict Future Aggressive Behaviour at a Cost to Reward in Men," *Psychoneuroendocrinology* 34, no. 4 (2009): 561–70; Justin M. Carré, Cheryl M. McCormick, and Ahmad R. Hariri, "The Social Neuroendocrinology of Human Aggression," *Psychoneuroendocrinology* 36, no. 7 (2011): 935–44; and Pranjal H. Mehta, Amanda C. Jones, and Robert A. Josephs, "The Social Endocrinology of Dominance: Basal Testosterone Predicts Cortisol Changes and Behavior Following Victory and Defeat," *Journal of Personality and Social Psychology* 94, no. 6 (2008): 1078.

26. Andrew K. Przybylski et al., "Competence-Impeding Electronic Games and Players' Aggressive Feelings, Thoughts, and Behaviors," *Journal of Personality and Social Psychology* 106, no. 3 (2014): 441–57.

27. Robert Mihan, Yvonne Anisimowicz, and Richard Nicki, "Safer with a Partner: Exploring the Emotional Consequences of Multiplayer Video Gaming," *Computers in Human Behavior* 44 (2015): 299–304.

## Chapter 3: You Are the Hero of Your Own Story

1. Pamela M. Kato et al., "A Video Game Improves Behavioral Outcomes in Adolescents and Young Adults with Cancer: A Randomized Trial," *Pediatrics* 122, no. 2 (2008): e305–e317.

2. Richard Tate, Jana Haritatos, and Steve Cole, "HopeLab's Approach to *Re-Mission*," *International Journal of Learning and Media* 1, no. 1 (2009): 29–35.

3. Hye-Sue Song and Paul M. Lehrer, "The Effects of Specific Respiratory Rates on Heart Rate and Heart Rate Variability," *Applied Psychophysiology and Biofeedback* 28, no. 1 (2003): 13–23; and Paul M. Lehrer, "Biofeedback Training to Increase Heart Rate Variability," *Principles and Practice of Stress Management* 3 (2007): 227–48.

4. Jeffrey J. Goldberger et al., "Relationship of Heart Rate Variability to Parasympathetic Effect," *Circulation* 103, no. 15 (2001): 1977–83; and Harald M. Stauss, "Heart Rate Variability," *American Journal of Physiology-Regulatory, Integrative and Comparative Physiology* 285, no. 5 (2003): R927-R931.

5. Matthias J. Koepp et al., "Evidence for Striatal Dopamine Release During a Video Game," *Nature* 393, no. 6682 (1998): 266–68.

6. Matilda Hellman et al., "Is There Such a Thing as Online Video Game Addiction? A Cross-Disciplinary Review," *Addiction Research and Theory* 21, no. 2 (2013): 102–12; Florian Rehbein et al., "Prevalence and Risk Factors of Video Game Dependency in Adolescence: Results of a German Nationwide Survey," *Cyberpsychology, Behavior, and Social Networking* 13, no. 3 (2010): 269–77; Antonius J. Van Rooij et al., "Online Video Game Addiction: Identification of Addicted Adolescent Gamers," *Addiction* 106, no. 1 (2011): 205–12; and Douglas Gentile, "Pathological Video-Game Use Among Youth Ages 8 to 18 a National Study," *Psychological Science* 20, no. 5 (2009): 594–602.

7. Irma Triasih Kurniawan, Marc Guitart-Masip, and Ray J. Dolan, "Dopamine and Effort-Based Decision Making," *Frontiers in Neuroscience* 5 (2011).

8. M. E. Walton et al., "Weighing Up the Benefits of Work: Behavioral and Neural Analyses of Effort-Related Decision Making," *Neural Networks* 19, no. 8 (2006): 1302–14; and Michael T.

Treadway et al., "Worth the 'EEfRT'? The Effort Expenditure for Rewards Task as an Objective Measure of Motivation and Anhedonia," *PLOS ONE* 4, no. 8 (2009): e6598.

9. Michael T. Treadway et al., "Dopaminergic Mechanisms of Individual Differences in Human Effort-Based Decision-Making," *Journal of Neuroscience* 32, no. 18 (2012): 6170–76.

10. Marie-Laure Cléry-Melin et al., "Why Don't You Try Harder? An Investigation of Effort Production in Major Depression," *PLOS ONE* 6, no. 8 (2011): e23178.

11. Loan T.K. Vo et al., "Predicting Individuals' Learning Success from Patterns of Pre-Learning MRI Activity," *PLOS ONE* 6, no. 1 (2011): e16093; Caterina Breitenstein et al., "Hippocampus Activity Differentiates Good from Poor Learners of a Novel Lexicon," *NeuroImage* 25, no. 3 (2005): 958–68; and Roy A. Wise "Dopamine, Learning and Motivation," *Nature Reviews Neuroscience* 5, no. 6 (2004): 483–94.

12. Jane McGonigal, *Reality Is Broken: Why Games Make Us Better and How They Can Change the World* (New York: Penguin, 2011).

13. Matthew Ventura, Valerie Shute, and Weinan Zhao, "The Relationship Between Video Game Use and a Performance-Based Measure of Persistence," *Computers and Education* 60, no. 1 (2013): 52–58.

14. Treadway et al., "Dopaminergic Mechanisms of Individual Differences."

15. Simone Kühn et al., "The Neural Basis of Video Gaming," *Translational Psychiatry* 1, no. 11 (2011): e53.

16. Simone Kühn et al., "Playing Super Mario Induces Structural Brain Plasticity: Gray Matter Changes Resulting from Training with a Commercial Video Game," *Molecular Psychiatry* 19 (2013): 265–71.

17. C. Shawn Green and Daphne Bavelier, "The Cognitive Neuroscience of Video Games," in P. Messaris and L. Humphreys, eds., *Digital Media: Transformations in Human Communication* (New York: Peter Lang, 2006): 211–23; Matthew W.G. Dye, C. Shawn Green, and Daphne Bavelier, "Increasing Speed of Processing with Action Video Games," *Current Directions in Psychological Science* 18, no. 6 (2009): 321–26; and C. Shawn Green, Alexandre Pouget, and Daphne Bavelier, "Improved Probabilistic Inference as a General Learning Mechanism with Action Video Games," *Current Biology* 20, no. 17 (2010): 1573–79.

18. Daphne Bavelier et al., "Removing Brakes on Adult Brain Plasticity: From Molecular to Behavioral Interventions," *Journal of Neuroscience* 30, no. 45 (2010): 14964–71.

19. Daniela Oltea JOJA, "Learning Experience and Neuroplasticity—A Shifting Paradigm," *Nature Reviews Neuroscience* 3, no. 1 (2002): 65–71.

20. Steven W. Cole, Daniel J. Yoo, and Brian Knutson, "Interactivity and Reward-Related Neural Activation During a Serious Videogame," *PLOS ONE* 7, no. 3 (2012): e33909; Jari Kätsyri et al., "The Opponent Matters: Elevated fMRI Reward Responses to Winning Against a Human Versus a Computer Opponent During Interactive Video Game Playing," *Cerebral Cortex* 23, no. 12 (2013): 2829–39; Klaus Mathiak and René Weber, "Toward Brain Correlates of Natural Behavior: fMRI During Violent Video Games," *Human Brain Mapping* 27, no. 12 (2006): 948–56; Keiichi Saito, Naoki Mukawa, and Masao Saito, "Brain Activity Comparison of Different-Genre Video Game Players," *Second International Conference on Innovative Computing, Information and Control, ICICIC '07* (IEEE, 2007); Martin Klasen et al., "Neural Contributions to Flow Experience During Video Game Playing," *Social Cognitive and Affective Neuroscience* 7, no. 4 (2012): 485–95; and Jari Kätsyri et al., "When Just Looking Ain't Enough: Phasic fMRI Reward Responses During Playing Versus Watching a Video Game," *Frontiers in Psychology* (2013).

21. Jesse Fox and Jeremy N. Bailenson, "Virtual Self-Modeling: The Effects of Vicarious Reinforcement and Identification on Exercise Behaviors," *Media Psychology* 12, no. 1 (2009): 1–25.

22. Jeremy N. Bailenson, "Doppelgangers—A New Form of Self?," *Psychologist* 25, no. 1 (2012): 36–38.

23. Jesse Fox and Jeremy N. Bailenson, "The Use of Doppelgängers to Promote Health Behavior Change," *Cybertherapy and Rehabilitation* 3, no. 2 (2010): 16–17.

24. Robin S. Rosenberg, Shawnee L. Baughman, and Jeremy N. Bailenson, "Virtual Superheroes: Using Superpowers in Virtual Reality to Encourage Prosocial Behavior," *PLOS ONE* 8, no. 1 (2013): e55003.

25. Leif D. Nelson and Michael I. Norton, "From Student to Superhero: Situational Primes Shape Future Helping," *Journal of Experimental Social Psychology* 41, no. 4 (2005): 423–30.

## Chapter 4: You Can Make the Leap from Games to Gameful

1. Rune Aune Mentzoni et al., "Problematic Video Game Use: Estimated Prevalence and Associations with Mental and Physical Health," *Cyberpsychology, Behavior, and Social Networking* 14, no. 10 (2011): 591–96; Douglas A. Gentile et al., "Pathological Video Game Use Among Youths: A Two-Year Longitudinal Study," *Pediatrics* 127, no. 2 (2011): e319–e329; and Douglas Gentile, "Pathological Video Game Use Among Youth Ages 8 to 18: A National Study," *Psychological Science* 20, no. 5 (2009): 594–602.

2. Lily Shui-Lien Chen, Hill Hung-Jen Tu, and Edward Shih-Tse Wang, "Personality Traits and Life Satisfaction Among Online Game Players," *Cyberpsychology and Behavior* 11, no. 2 (2008): 145–49; Patricia E. Kahlbaugh et al., "Effects of Playing Wii on Well-Being in the Elderly: Physical Activity, Loneliness, and Mood," *Activities, Adaptation and Aging* 35, no. 4 (2011): 331–44; Younbo Jung et al., "Games for a Better Life: Effects of Playing Wii Games on the Well-Being of Seniors in a Long-Term Care Facility," *Proceedings of the Sixth Australasian Conference on Interactive Entertainment* (ACM, 2009); Mark Griffiths, "Video Games and Health: Video Gaming Is Safe for Most Players and Can Be Useful in Health Care," *BMJ: British Medical Journal* 331, no. 7509 (2005): 122; and Jason C. Allaire et al., "Successful Aging Through Digital Games: Socioemotional Differences Between Older Adult Gamers and Non-Gamers," *Computers in Human Behavior* 29, no. 4 (2013): 1302–06.

3. Laura M. Padilla-Walker et al., "More Than a Just a Game: Video Game and Internet Use During Emerging Adulthood," *Journal of Youth and Adolescence* 39, no. 2 (2010): 103–13; and Vivek Anand, "A Study of Time Management: The Correlation Between Video Game Usage and Academic Performance Markers," *Cyberpsychology and Behavior* 10, no. 4 (2007): 552–59.

4. Rani A. Desai et al., "Video-Gaming Among High School Students: Health Correlates, Gender Differences, and Problematic Gaming," *Pediatrics* 126, no. 6 (2010): e1414–e1424; and Paul J.C. Adachi and Teena Willoughby, "More Than Just Fun and Games: The Longitudinal Relationships Between Strategic Video Games, Self-Reported Problem Solving Skills, and Academic Grades," *Journal of Youth and Adolescence* 42, no. 7 (2013): 1041–52.

5. Rosalina Richards et al., "Adolescent Screen Time and Attachment to Parents and Peers," *Archives of Pediatrics and Adolescent Medicine* 164, no. 3 (2010): 258–62; and Shao-Kang Lo, Chih-Chien Wang, and Wenchang Fang, "Physical Interpersonal Relationships and Social Anxiety Among Online Game Players," *CyberPsychology and Behavior* 8, no. 1 (2005): 15–20.

6. Sarah M. Coyne et al., "Game on . . . Girls: Associations Between Co-Playing Video Games and Adolescent Behavioral and Family Outcomes," *Journal of Adolescent Health* 49, no. 2 (2011): 160–65.

7. Julia Kneer and Sabine Glock, "Escaping in Digital Games: The Relationship Between Playing Motives and Addictive Tendencies in Males," *Computers in Human Behavior* 29, no. 4 (2013): 1415–20.

8. Joseph Benjamin Hilgard, Christopher R. Engelhardt, and Bruce D. Bartholow, "Individual Differences in Motives, Preferences, and Pathology in Video Games," *Frontiers in Psychology* 4 (2013): 608.

9. Andrew K. Przybylski, C. Scott Rigby, and Richard M. Ryan, "A Motivational Model of Video Game Engagement," *Review of General Psychology* 14, no. 2 (2010): 154.

10. Andrew K. Przybylski et al., "Having to Versus Wanting to Play: Background and Consequences of Harmonious Versus Obsessive Engagement in Video Games," *CyberPsychology and Behavior* 12, no. 5 (2009): 485–92.

11. Frode Stenseng, Jostein Rise, and Pål Kraft, "Activity Engagement as Escape from Self: The Role of Self-Suppression and Self-Expansion," *Leisure Sciences* 34, no. 1 (2012): 19–38.

12. Frode Stenseng, Jostein Rise, and Pål Kraft, "The Dark Side of Leisure: Obsessive Passion and Its Covariates and Outcomes," *Leisure Studies* 30, no. 1 (2011): 49–62; and Frode Stenseng, "The Two Faces of Leisure Activity Engagement: Harmonious and Obsessive Passion in Rela-

tion to Intrapersonal Conflict and Life Domain Outcomes," *Leisure Sciences* 30, no. 5 (2008): 465–81.

13. Isabela Granic, Adam Lobel, and Rutger C.M.E. Engels, "The Benefits of Playing Video Games," *American Psychologist* 69, no. 1 (2014): 66–78.

14. Matthew W.G. Dye, C. Shawn Green, and Daphne Bavelier, "Increasing Speed of Processing with Action Video Games," *Current Directions in Psychological Science* 18, no. 6 (2009): 321–26; C. Shawn Green, Alexandre Pouget, and Daphne Bavelier, "Improved Probabilistic Inference as a General Learning Mechanism with Action Video Games," *Current Biology* 20, no. 17 (2010): 1573–79; Bjorn Hubert Wallander, C. Shawn Green, and Daphne Bavelier, "Stretching the Limits of Visual Attention: The Case of Action Video Games," *Wiley Interdisciplinary Reviews: Cognitive Science* 2, no. 2 (2011): 222–30; Daphne Bavelier et al., "Brain Plasticity Through the Life Span: Learning to Learn and Action Video Games," *Annual Review of Neuroscience* 35 (2012): 391–416; C. Shawn Green et al., "The Effect of Action Video Game Experience on Task-Switching," *Computers in Human Behavior* 28, no. 3 (2012): 984–94; and Jyoti Mishra et al., "Neural Basis of Superior Performance of Action Videogame Players in an Attention-Demanding Task," *Journal of Neuroscience* 31, no. 3 (2011): 992–98.

15. Constance Steinkuehler and Sean Duncan, "Scientific Habits of Mind in Virtual Worlds," *Journal of Science Education and Technology* 17, no. 6 (2008): 530–43; Tsung-Yen Chuang and Wei-Fan Chen, "Effect of Computer-Based Video Games on Children: An Experimental Study," *First IEEE International Workshop on Digital Game and Intelligent Toy Enhanced Learning, DIGITEL'07* (IEEE, 2007); and Paul J.C. Adachi and Teena Willoughby, "More Than Just Fun and Games: The Longitudinal Relationships Between Strategic Video Games, Self-Reported Problem Solving Skills, and Academic Grades," *Journal of Youth and Adolescence* 42, no. 7 (2013): 1041–52.

16. Linda A. Jackson, Edward A. Witt, and Ivan Alexander Games, "Videogame Playing and Creativity: Findings from the Children and Technology Project," *National Social Science Proceedings* vol. 47, Seattle Summer Seminar, 2011; Linda A. Jackson, "The Upside of Videogame Playing," *Games for Health: Research, Development, and Clinical Applications* 1, no. 6 (2012): 452–55.

17. "A Consensus on the Brain Training Industry from the Scientific Community," Max Planck Institute for Human Development and Stanford Center on Longevity, October 20, 2014, http://longevity3.stanford.edu/blog/2014/10/15/the-consensus-on-the-brain-training-industry-from-the-scientific-community.

18. Valerie Shute, Matthew Ventura, and Fengfeng Ke, "The Power of Play: The Effects of Portal 2 and Lumosity on Cognitive and Noncognitive Skills," *Computers and Education* 80 (2014): 58–67; and Laura A. Whitlock, Anne Collins Mclaughlin, and Jason C. Allaire, "Individual Differences in Response to Cognitive Training: Using a Multi-Modal, Attentionally Demanding Game-Based Intervention for Older Adults," *Computers in Human Behavior* 28, no. 4 (2012): 1091–96.

19. Andrew K. Przybylski, C. Scott Rigby, and Richard M. Ryan, "A Motivational Model of Video Game Engagement," *Review of General Psychology* 14, no. 2 (2010): 154; Christopher Bateman, "Top Ten Emotions of Videogames—Results of the DGD2 Global Survey," *Only a Game* (2008); and Niklas Ravaja et al., "The Psychophysiology of Video Gaming: Phasic Emotional Responses to Game Events," in Authors Digital Games and Nicolas Esposito, eds., *Proceedings of DIGRA 2005 Conference: Changing Views—Worlds in Play* (2005).

20. Cheryl K. Olson, "Children's Motivations for Video Game Play in the Context of Normal Development," *Review of General Psychology* 14, no. 2 (2010): 180; Christopher J. Ferguson and Cheryl K. Olson, "Friends, Fun, Frustration and Fantasy: Child Motivations for Video Game Play," *Motivation and Emotion* 37, no. 1 (2013): 154–64; and Jeroen Jansz, "The Emotional Appeal of Violent Video Games for Adolescent Males," *Communication Theory* 15, no. 3 (2005): 219–41.

21. Jayne Gackenbach, Beena Kuruvilla, and Raelyne Dopko, "Video Game Play and Dream Bizarreness," *Dreaming* 19, no. 4 (2009): 218; Jayne Gackenbach, "Electronic Media and Lucid-Control Dreams: Morning After Reports," *Dreaming* 19, no. 1 (2009): 1; Jayne Gackenbach and Beena Kuruvilla, "The Relationship Between Video Game Play and Threat Simulation Dreams,"

*Dreaming* 18, no. 4 (2008): 236; and Jayne Gackenbach, "Video Game Play and Lucid Dreams: Implications for the Development of Consciousness," *Dreaming* 16, no. 2 (2006): 96.

22. David R. Ewoldsen et al., "Effect of Playing Violent Video Games Cooperatively or Competitively on Subsequent Cooperative Behavior," *Cyberpsychology, Behavior, and Social Networking* 15, no. 5 (2012): 277–80; John A. Velez et al., "Ingroup Versus Outgroup Conflict in the Context of Violent Video Game Play: The Effect of Cooperation on Increased Helping and Decreased Aggression," *Communication Research* (2012); Tobias Greitemeyer and Christopher Cox, "There's No 'I' in Team: Effects of Cooperative Video Games on Cooperative Behavior," *European Journal of Social Psychology* 43, no. 3 (2013): 224–28; Tobias Greitemeyer, "Playing Video Games Cooperatively Increases Empathic Concern," *Social Psychology* 44, no. 6 (2013): 408; and Jessica M. Jerabeck and Christopher J. Ferguson, "The Influence of Solitary and Cooperative Violent Video Game Play on Aggressive and Prosocial Behavior," *Computers in Human Behavior* 29, no. 6 (2013): 2573–78.

23. Christopher J. Ferguson and Adolfo Garza, "Call of (Civic) Duty: Action Games and Civic Behavior in a Large Sample of Youth," *Computers in Human Behavior* 27, no. 2 (2011): 770–75; Nicolas Ducheneaut and Robert J. Moore, "More Than Just 'XP': Learning Social Skills in Massively Multiplayer Online Games," *Interactive Technology and Smart Education* 2, no. 2 (2005): 89–100; and Timothy C. Lisk, Ugur T. Kaplancali, and Ronald E. Riggio, "Leadership in Multiplayer Online Gaming Environments," *Simulation and Gaming* 43, no. 1 (2012): 133–49.

24. Steven C. Hayes et al., "Measuring Experiential Avoidance: A Preliminary Test of a Working Model," *Psychological Record* 54, no. 4 (2004); Todd B. Kashdan et al., "Experiential Avoidance as a Generalized Psychological Vulnerability: Comparisons with Coping and Emotion Regulation Strategies," *Behaviour Research and Therapy* 44, no. 9 (2006): 1301–20; and Jonathan W. Kanter, David E. Baruch, and Scott T. Gaynor, "Acceptance and Commitment Therapy and Behavioral Activation for the Treatment of Depression: Description and Comparison," *Behavior Analyst* 29, no. 2 (2006): 161.

25. Most recently, Andrew K. Przybylski, "Electronic Gaming and Psychosocial Adjustment," *Pediatrics*, August 4, 2014, doi: 10.1542/peds.2013-4021.

26. Zaheer Hussain and Mark D. Griffiths, "Excessive Use of Massively Multi-Player Online Role-Playing Games: A Pilot Study," *International Journal of Mental Health and Addiction* 7, no. 4 (2009): 563–71.

27. Daniel King and Paul Delfabbro, "Motivational Differences in Problem Video Game Play," *Journal of Cybertherapy and Rehabilitation (JCR)* 2, no. 2 (2009).

28. Amelia McDonell-Parry, "Seven Incredibly Deep Life Lessons from Candy Crush Saga," July 8, 2013, *Frisky*, http://www.thefrisky.com/2013-07-08/7-incredibly-deep-life-lessons-from-candy-crush-saga.

## Part 2: How to Be Gameful

1. Ann Marie Roepke et al., "Randomized Controlled Trial of SuperBetter, a Smartphone-Based/Internet-Based Self-Help Tool to Reduce Depressive Symptoms," *Games for Health* (in progress); and Ann Marie Roepke, "Results of a Randomized Controlled Trial: The Effects of SuperBetter on Depression," University of Pennsylvania, July 15, 2013, http://annmarieroepke.files .wordpress.com/2013/08/superbetter-study-results-bulletin-8-15-13.pdf.

2. "Clinical Trial of a Rehabiliation Game—SuperBetter," NIH-funded trial in collaboration with Ohio State University Medical Research Center, http://clinicaltrials.gov/show/NCT01398566.

## Chapter 5: Challenge Yourself

1. Although players do report sometimes feeling frustration, anger, and sadness during game play, they also report that the "pretend" context of game play creates a safe environment to practice controlling or changing these negative emotions. A good summary of this phenomenon is found in Isabela Granic, Adam Lobel, and Rutger C.M.E. Engels, "The Benefits of Playing Video Games," *American Psychologist* 69, no. 1 (2014): 66–78.

2. Robert J. Harmison, "Peak Performance in Sport: Identifying Ideal Performance States and Developing Athletes' Psychological Skills," *Professional Psychology: Research and Practice* 37, no. 3 (2011): 233–43.

3. Alison Wood Brooks, "Get Excited: Reappraising Pre-Performance Anxiety as Excitement," *Journal of Experimental Psychology: General* 143, no. 3 (2014): 1144–58.

4. The seminal work on the subject of threat versus challenge mindset is Susan Folkman et al., "Dynamics of a Stressful Encounter: Cognitive Appraisal, Coping, and Encounter Outcomes," *Journal of Personality and Social Psychology* 50, no. 5 (1986): 992.

5. Richard M. Ryan, C. Scott Rigby, and Andrew Przybylski, "The Motivational Pull of Video Games: A Self-Determination Theory Approach," *Motivation and Emotion* 30, no. 4 (2006): 344–60; and Jesper Juul, "Fear of Failing?: The Many Meanings of Difficulty in Video Games," in Mark J. P. Wolf and Bernard Perron, eds., *Video Game Theory Reader 2* (New York: Routledge, 2009): 237–52.

6. This has been a particularly consistent finding in digital game research over the past thirty years, starting with Robert F. McClure and F. Gary Mears, "Video Game Players: Personality Characteristics and Demographic Variables," *Psychological Reports* 55, no. 1 (1984): 271–76; continuing through John L. Sherry et al., "Video Game Uses and Gratifications as Predictors of Use and Game Preference," in Peter Vorderer and Jennings Bryant, eds., *Playing Video Games: Motives, Responses, and Consequences* (n.p.: Lawrence Erlbaum Associates, 2006): 213–24; Kristen Lucas and John L. Sherry, "Sex Differences in Video Game Play: A Communication-Based Explanation," *Communication Research* 31, no. 5 (2004): 499–523; and Cheryl K. Olson, "Children's Motivations for Video Game Play in the Context of Normal Development," *Review of General Psychology* 14, no. 2 (2010): 180.

7. For an excellent overview of this research, see Anat Drach-Zahavy and Miriam Erez, "Challenge Versus Threat Effects on the Goal-Performance Relationship," *Organizational Behavior and Human Decision Processes* 88, no. 2 (2002): 667–82.

8. Allison S. Troy et al., "Seeing the Silver Lining: Cognitive Reappraisal Ability Moderates the Relationship Between Stress and Depressive Symptoms," *Emotion* 10, no. 6 (2010): 783.

9. Jim Blascovich et al., "Predicting Athletic Performance from Cardiovascular Indexes of Challenge and Threat," *Journal of Experimental Social Psychology* 40, no. 5 (2004): 683–88.

10. Drach-Zahavy and Erez, "Challenge Versus Threat Effects on the Goal–Performance Relationship."

11. Kenneth I. Pakenham and Machelle Rinaldis, "The Role of Illness, Resources, Appraisal, and Coping Strategies in Adjustment to HIV/AIDS: The Direct and Buffering Effects," *Journal of Behavioral Medicine* 24, no. 3 (2001): 259–79; Heather M. Franks and Scott C. Roesch, "Appraisals and Coping in People Living with Cancer: A Meta Analysis," *Psycho Oncology* 15, no. 12 (2006): 1027–37.

12. Annette L. Stanton et al., "Cognitive Appraisal and Adjustment to Infertility," *Women and Health* 17, no. 3 (1991): 1–15.

13. Michele M. Tugade and Barbara L. Fredrickson, "Resilient Individuals Use Positive Emotions to Bounce Back from Negative Emotional Experiences," *Journal of Personality and Social Psychology* 86, no. 2 (2004): 320.

14. Ulrike Sirsch, "The Impending Transition from Primary to Secondary School: Challenge or Threat?," *International Journal of Behavioral Development* 27, no. 5 (2003): 385–95.

15. Kathleen A. Gass and Audrey S. Chang, "Appraisals of Bereavement, Coping, Resources, and Psychosocial Health Dysfunction in Widows and Widowers," *Nursing Research* 38, no. 1 (1989): 31–36.

16. John M. Schaubroeck et al., "Resilience to Traumatic Exposure among Soldiers Deployed in Combat," *Journal of Occupational Health Psychology* 16, no. 1 (2011): 18; Alan Fontana and Robert Rosenheck, "Psychological Benefits and Liabilities of Traumatic Exposure in the War Zone," *Journal of Traumatic Stress* 11, no. 3 (1998): 485–503.

17. Bernard Suits, *The Grasshopper: Games, Life and Utopia* (Peterborough, ON: Broadview Press, 2014).

18. Gerard H. Seijts and Gary P. Latham, "Learning Versus Performance Goals: When Should Each Be Used?," *Academy of Management Executive* 19, no. 1 (2005): 124–31; and Kieran M. Kingston

and Lew Hardy, "Effects of Different Types of Goals on Processes That Support Performance," *Sport Psychologist* 11 (1997): 277–93.

19. Drach-Zahavy and Erez, "Challenge Versus Threat Effects on the Goal–Performance Relationship."


## *Chapter 6: Power-ups*

1. Duncan A. Groves and Verity J. Brown, "Vagal Nerve Stimulation: A Review of Its Applications and Potential Mechanisms That Mediate Its Clinical Effects," *Neuroscience and Biobehavioral Reviews* 29, no. 3 (2005): 493–500.

2. Beginning with Stephen W. Porges, "Vagal Tone: A Physiologic Marker of Stress Vulnerability," *Pediatrics* 90, no. 3 (1992): 498–504; and continuing through Luca Carnevali and Andrea Sgoifo, "Vagal Modulation of Resting Heart Rate in Rats: The Role of Stress, Psychosocial Factors, and Physical Exercise," *Frontiers in Physiology* 5 (2014): 118.

3. For a basic overview of respiratory sinus arrhythmia research, see Paul Grossman and Edwin W. Taylor, "Toward Understanding Respiratory Sinus Arrhythmia: Relations to Cardiac Vagal Tone, Evolution and Biobehavioral Functions," *Biological Psychology* 74, no. 2 (2007): 263–85.

4. Julian F. Thayer and Richard D. Lane, "The Role of Vagal Function in the Risk for Cardiovascular Disease and Mortality," *Biological Psychology* 74, no. 2 (2007): 224–42; Georg Schmidt et al., "Respiratory Sinus Arrhythmia Predicts Mortality After Myocardial Infarction," *Journal of the American College of Cardiology* 63, no. 12_S (2014); Al Hazzouri, Adina Zeki et al., "Reduced Heart Rate Variability Is Associated with Worse Cognitive Performance in Elderly Mexican Americans," *Hypertension* 63, no. 1 (2014): 181–87; Carmilla M.M. Licht, Eco J.C. De Geus, and Brenda W.J.H. Penninx, "Dysregulation of the Autonomic Nervous System Predicts the Development of the Metabolic Syndrome," *Journal of Clinical Endocrinology and Metabolism* 98, no. 6 (2013): 2484–93; Steve Bibevski and Mark E. Dunlap, "Evidence for Impaired Vagus Nerve Activity in Heart Failure," *Heart Failure Reviews* 16, no. 2 (2011): 129–35; and Julian F. Thayer, "Vagal Tone and the Inflammatory Reflex," *Cleveland Clinic Journal of Medicine* 76, supp. 2 (2009): S23–S26.

5. Zhenhong Wang, Wei Lü, and Rongcai Qin, "Respiratory Sinus Arrhythmia Is Associated with Trait Positive Affect and Positive Emotional Expressivity," *Biological Psychology* 93, no. 1 (2013): 190–96; Michelle A. Patriquin et al., "Respiratory Sinus Arrhythmia: A Marker for Positive Social Functioning and Receptive Language Skills in Children with Autism Spectrum Disorders," *Developmental Psychobiology* 55, no. 2 (2013): 101–12; Christopher P. Fagundes et al., "Attachment Style and Respiratory Sinus Arrhythmia Predict Post-Treatment Quality of Life in Breast Cancer Survivors," *Psycho-Oncology* 23, no. 7 (2014): 820–26; Lauren M. Bylsma et al., "Respiratory Sinus Arrhythmia Reactivity in Current and Remitted Major Depressive Disorder," *Psychosomatic Medicine* 76, no. 1 (2014): 66–73; John A. Sturgeon, Ellen Wanheung Yeung, and Alex J. Zautra, "Respiratory Sinus Arrhythmia: A Marker of Resilience to Pain Induction," *International Journal of Behavioral Medicine* (2014): 1–5; and Bruce H. Friedman, "An Autonomic Flexibility–Neurovisceral Integration Model of Anxiety and Cardiac Vagal Tone," *Biological Psychology* 74, no. 2 (2007): 185–99.

6. Barbara L. Fredrickson, "Updated Thinking on Positivity Ratios," *American Psychologist* 68, no. 9 (2013): 814–22.

7. Yoichi Chida and Andrew Steptoe, "Positive Psychological Well-Being and Mortality: A Quantitative Review of Prospective Observational Studies," *Psychosomatic Medicine* 70, no. 7 (2008): 741–56; and Ryan T. Howell, Margaret L. Kern, and Sonja Lyubomirsky, "Health Benefits: Meta-Analytically Determining the Impact of Well-Being on Objective Health Outcomes," *Health Psychology Review* 1, no. 1 (2007): 83–136.

8. Ed Diener and Micaela Y. Chan, "Happy People Live Longer: Subjective Well-Being Contributes to Health and Longevity," *Applied Psychology: Health and Well-Being* 3, no. 1 (2011): 1–43; Julia K. Boehm and Laura D. Kubzansky, "The Heart's Content: The Association Between Positive Psychological Well-Being and Cardiovascular Health," *Psychological Bulletin* 138, no. 4 (2012): 655; and Sheldon Cohen et al., "Positive Emotional Style Predicts Resistance to Illness

After Experimental Exposure to Rhinovirus or Influenza A Virus," *Psychosomatic Medicine* 68, no. 6 (2006): 809–15.

9.  Bethany E. Kok et al., "How Positive Emotions Build Physical Health: Perceived Positive Social Connections Account for the Upward Spiral Between Positive Emotions and Vagal Tone," *Psychological Science* 24, no. 7 (2013): 1123–32; and Bethany E. Kok and Barbara L. Fredrickson, "Upward Spirals of the Heart: Autonomic Flexibility, as Indexed by Vagal Tone, Reciprocally and Prospectively Predicts Positive Emotions and Social Connectedness," *Biological Psychology* 85, no. 3 (2010): 432–36.

10. Barbara L. Fredrickson, "The Role of Positive Emotions in Positive Psychology: The Broaden-and-Build Theory of Positive Emotions," *American Psychologist* 56, no. 3 (2001): 218.

11. Barbara Fredrickson, *Positivity: Top-Notch Research Reveals the 3 to 1 Ratio That Will Change Your Life* (New York: Random House, 2009).

12. John Mordechai Gottman, *What Predicts Divorce?: The Relationship Between Marital Processes and Marital Outcomes* (London: Psychology Press, 2014).

13. Robert M. Schwartz et al., "Optimal and Normal Affect Balance in Psychotherapy of Major Depression: Evaluation of the Balanced States of Mind Model," *Behavioural and Cognitive Psychotherapy* 30, no. 4 (2002): 439–50.

14. Arménio Rego et al., "Optimism Predicting Employees' Creativity: The Mediating Role of Positive Affect and the Positivity Ratio," *European Journal of Work and Organizational Psychology* 21, no. 2 (2012): 244–70.

15. Amit Shrira et al., "The Positivity Ratio and Functioning Under Stress," *Stress and Health* 27, no. 4 (2011): 265–71.

16. Ibid.

17. Mara Mather and Laura L. Carstensen, "Aging and Motivated Cognition: The Positivity Effect in Attention and Memory," *Trends in Cognitive Sciences* 9, no. 10 (2005): 496–502; and Suzanne Meeks et al., "Positivity and Well-Being Among Community-Residing Elders and Nursing Home Residents: What Is the Optimal Affect Balance?," *Journals of Gerontology Series B: Psychological Sciences and Social Sciences* 67, no. 4 (2012): 460–67.

18. Ed Diener, Ed Sandvik, and William Pavot, "Happiness Is the Frequency, Not the Intensity, of Positive Versus Negative Affect," *Subjective Well-Being: An Interdisciplinary Perspective* 21 (1991): 119–39.

19. John F. Cryan and Timothy G. Dinan, "Mind-Altering Microorganisms: The Impact of the Gut Microbiota on Brain and Behaviour," *Nature Reviews Neuroscience* 13, no. 10 (2012): 701–12.

20. See Kok and Fredrickson, "Upward Spirals of the Heart."

21. Brian M. Curtis and James H. O'Keefe, Jr., "Autonomic Tone as a Cardiovascular Risk Factor: The Dangers of Chronic Fight or Flight," *Mayo Clinic Proceedings* 77, no. 1 (2002).

22. June Gruber et al., "Risk for Mania and Positive Emotional Responding: Too Much of a Good Thing?," *Emotion* 8, no. 1 (2008): 23.

23. Adam M. Grant and Barry Schwartz, "Too Much of a Good Thing: The Challenge and Opportunity of the Inverted U," *Perspectives on Psychological Science* 6, no. 1 (2011): 61–76.

24. Patricia E. Suess, Stephen W. Porges, and Dana J. Plude, "Cardiac Vagal Tone and Sustained Attention in School-Age Children," *Psychophysiology* 31, no. 1 (1994): 17–22; Lynn Fainsilber Katz and John M. Gottman, "Vagal Tone Protects Children from Marital Conflict," *Development and Psychopathology* 7, no. 1 (1995): 83–92; and Bonny Donzella et al., "Cortisol and Vagal Tone Responses to Competitive Challenge in Preschoolers: Associations with Temperament," *Developmental Psychobiology* 37, no. 4 (2000): 209–20.

25. See Kok and Fredrickson, "Upward Spirals of the Heart."

## Chapter 7: Bad Guys

1.  Stacey Kennelly, "When Guilt Stops Gratitude," *Greater Good: The Science of a Meaingful Life*, January 14, 2014, http://greatergood.berkeley.edu/article/item/when_guilt_stops_gratitude.

2.  The SuperBetter science advisers included James Doty at the Stanford School of Medicine; Dacher Keltner at UC Berkeley's Greater Good Science Center; Kelly McGonigal at Stanford Uni-

versity's Center for Compassion and Altruism Research and Education; Ann Marie Roepke, a Ph.D. candidate in clinical psychology at the University of Pennsylvania; and Lise Worthen-Chaudhari, a research scientist at Ohio State University's School of Medicine. Science writer Bez Maxwell contributed as well.

3.  Todd B. Kashdan and Jonathan Rottenberg, "Psychological Flexibility as a Fundamental Aspect of Health," *Clinical Psychology Review* 30, no. 7 (2010): 865–78.

4.  Todd B. Kashdan and Jennifer Q. Kane, "Post-Traumatic Distress and the Presence of Post-traumatic Growth and Meaning in Life: Experiential Avoidance as a Moderator," *Personality and Individual Differences* 50, no. 1 (2011): 84–89; and Holly K. Orcutt, Scott M. Pickett, and E. Brooke Pope, "Experiential Avoidance and Forgiveness as Mediators in the Relation Between Traumatic Interpersonal Events and Post-traumatic Stress Disorder Symptoms," *Journal of Social and Clinical Psychology* 24, no. 7 (2005): 1003–29.

5.  Steven C. Hayes et al., "Acceptance and Commitment Therapy: Model, Processes and Outcomes," *Behaviour Research and Therapy* 44, no. 1 (2006): 1–25; Neharika Chawla and Brian Ostafin, "Experiential Avoidance as a Functional Dimensional Approach to Psychopathology: An Empirical Review," *Journal of Clinical Psychology* 63, no. 9 (2007): 871–90; Frank W. Bond and David Bunce, "The Role of Acceptance and Job Control in Mental Health, Job Satisfaction, and Work Performance," *Journal of Applied Psychology* 88, no. 6 (2003): 1057; and Jodie Butler and Joseph Ciarrochi, "Psychological Acceptance and Quality of Life in the Elderly," *Quality of Life Research* 16, no. 4 (2007): 607–15.

6.  Martine Fledderus, Ernst T. Bohlmeijer, and Marcel E. Pieterse, "Does Experiential Avoidance Mediate the Effects of Maladaptive Coping Styles on Psychopathology and Mental Health?," *Behavior Modification* (2010); and Todd B. Kashdan et al., "Experiential Avoidance as a Generalized Psychological Vulnerability: Comparisons with Coping and Emotion Regulation Strategies," *Behaviour Research and Therapy* 44, no. 9 (2006): 1301–20.

7.  Alexander L. Chapman, Matthew W. Specht, and Tony Cellucci, "Borderline Personality Disorder and Deliberate Self-Harm: Does Experiential Avoidance Play a Role?," *Suicide and Life-Threatening Behavior* 35, no. 4 (2005): 388–99; Orcutt, Pickett, and Pope, "Experiential Avoidance and Forgiveness as Mediators in the Relation Between Traumatic Interpersonal Events and Post-traumatic Stress Disorder Symptoms"; Neharika Chawla and Brian Ostafin, "Experiential Avoidance as a Functional Dimensional Approach to Psychopathology: An Empirical Review," *Journal of Clinical Psychology* 63, no. 9 (2007): 871–90; Todd B. Kashdan, Nexhmedin Morina, and ˙ efan Priebe, "Post-Traumatic Stress Disorder, Social Anxiety Disorder, and Depression in Survivors of the Kosovo War: Experiential Avoidance as a Contributor ʈ Distress and Quality of Life," *Journal of Anxiety Disorders* 23, no. 2 (2009): 185–96; Laura E. Boeschen et al., "Experiential Avoidance and Post-Traumatic Stress Disorder: A Cognitive Mediational Model of Rape Recovery," *Journal of Aggression, Maltreatment and Trauma* 4, no. 2 (2001): 211–45; and Matthew T. Tull and Kim L. Gratz, "Further Examination of the Relationship Between Anxiety Sensitivity and Depression: The Mediating Role of Experiential Avoidance and Difficulties Engaging in Goal-Directed Behavior When Distressed," *Journal of Anxiety Disorders* 22, no. 2 (2008): 199–10.

8.  Brian L. Thompson and Jennifer Waltz, "Mindfulness and Experiential Avoidance as Predictors of Post-traumatic Stress Disorder Avoidance Symptom Severity," *Journal of Anxiety Disorders* 24, no. 4 (2010): 409–15.

9.  Julie M. Fritz, Steven Z. George, and Anthony Delitto, "The Role of Fear-Avoidance Beliefs in Acute Low Back Pain: Relationships with Current and Future Disability and Work Status," *Pain* 94, no. 1 (2001): 7–15; Gordon Waddell et al., "A Fear-Avoidance Beliefs Questionnaire (FABQ) and the Role of Fear-Avoidance Beliefs in Chronic Low Back Pain and Disability," *Pain* 52, no. 2 (1993): 157–68; Maaike Leeuw et al., "The Fear-Avoidance Model of Musculoskeletal Pain: Current State of Scientific Evidence," *Journal of Behavioral Medicine* 30, no. 1 (2007): 77–94; and Steve R. Woby et al., "Are Changes in Fear-Avoidance Beliefs, Catastrophizing, and Appraisals of Control Predictive of Changes in Chronic Low Back Pain and Disability?," *European Journal of Pain* 8, no. 3 (2004): 201–10.

10. G. Lorimer Moseley, "A New Direction for the Fear Avoidance Model?," *Pain* 152, no. 11 (2011): 2447–48.

11. Baltasar Rodero et al., "Relationship Between Behavioural Coping Strategies and Acceptance in Patients with Fibromyalgia Syndrome: Elucidating Targets of Interventions," *BMC Musculoskeletal Disorders* 12, no. 1 (2011): 143; Lance M. McCracken and Edmund Keogh, "Acceptance, Mindfulness, and Values-Based Action May Counteract Fear and Avoidance of Emotions in Chronic Pain: An Analysis of Anxiety Sensitivity," *Journal of Pain* 10, no. 4 (2009): 408–15; Rikard K. Wicksell et al., "Avoidance and Cognitive Fusion—Central Components in Pain Related Disability? Development and Preliminary Validation of the Psychological Inflexibility in Pain Scale (PIPS)," *European Journal of Pain* 12, no. 4 (2008): 491–500; Brjánn Ljótsson et al., "Exposure and Mindfulness Based Therapy for Irritable Bowel Syndrome—An Open Pilot Study," *Journal of Behavior Therapy and Experimental Psychiatry* 41, no. 3 (2010): 185–90; Paul R. Martin and Colin MacLeod, "Behavioral Management of Headache Triggers: Avoidance of Triggers Is an Inadequate Strategy," *Clinical Psychology Review* 29, no. 6 (2009): 483–95; and Christine Chiros and William H. O'Brien, "Acceptance, Appraisals, and Coping in Relation to Migraine Headache: An Evaluation of Interrelationships Using Daily Diary Methods," *Journal of Behavioral Medicine* 34, no. 4 (2011): 307–20.

12. *Measuring Experiential Avoidance.* Steven C. Hayes, Richard T. Bissett, Jacqueline Pistorello, and Dosheen T. Cook, University of Nevada, Reno; Kirk Strosahl, Mountainview Consulting Group; Kelly G. Wilson, University of Mississippi; Melissa A. Polusny, Minneapolis VA Medical Center; Thane A. Dykstra, Trinity Services; Sonja V. Batten, Yale University School of Medicine; Sherry H. Stewart, Dalhousie University; Michael J. Zvolensky, University of Vermont; George H. Eifert, Chapman University; Frank W. Bond, Goldsmiths College, University of London; John P. Forsyth and Maria Karekla, State University of New York at Albany; and Susan M. McCurry, University of Washington. See also Steven C. Hayes et al., "Measuring Experiential Avoidance: A Preliminary Test of a Working Model," *Psychological Record* 54 (2004): 553–78.

13. The Chicago-based mindfulness training center Integrative Health Partners has several different psychology flexibility measures. You can review the forty-nine-question inventory at http://integrativehealthpartners.org/downloads/ACTmeasures.pdf.

### Chapter 8: Quests

1. Iris W. Hung and Aparna A. Labroo, "From Firm Muscles to Firm Willpower: Understanding the Role of Embodied Cognition in Self-Regulation," *Journal of Consumer Research* 37, no. 6 (2011): 1046–64.

2. Barbara Vann and Neil Alperstein, "Dream Sharing as Social Interaction," *Dreaming* 10, no. 2 (2000): 111; Murray L. Wax, "Dream Sharing as Social Practice," *Dreaming* 14, nos. 2–3 (2004): 83; Antonietta Curci and Bernard Rimé, "Dreams, Emotions, and Social Sharing of Dreams," *Cognition and Emotion* 22, no. 1 (2008): 155–67; and Michael Schredl and Joelle Alexandra Schawinski, "Frequency of Dream Sharing: The Effects of Gender and Personality," *American Journal of Psychology* 123, no. 1 (2010): 93–101.

3. Eddie Weitzberg and Jon O.N. Lundberg, "Humming Greatly Increases Nasal Nitric Oxide," *American Journal of Respiratory and Critical Care Medicine* 166, no. 2 (2002): 144–45; M. Maniscalco et al., "Assessment of Nasal and Sinus Nitric Oxide Output Using Single-Breath Humming Exhalations," *European Respiratory Journal* 22, no. 2 (2003): 323–29.

4. Lysann Damisch, Barbara Stoberock, and Thomas Mussweiler, "Keep Your Fingers Crossed! How Superstition Improves Performance," *Psychological Science* 21, no. 7 (2010): 1014–20.

5. Mark Muraven and Roy F. Baumeister, "Self-Regulation and Depletion of Limited Resources: Does Self-Control Resemble a Muscle?," *Psychological Bulletin* 126, no. 2 (2000): 247.

6. Steven C. Hayes and Kirk D. Strosahl, eds., A *Practical Guide to Acceptance and Commitment Therapy* (n.p.: Springer, 2004).

7. Steven C. Hayes et al., "Acceptance and Commitment Therapy: Model, Processes and Outcomes," *Behaviour Research and Therapy* 44, no. 1 (2006): 1–25; and Lance M. McCracken, "Committed Action: An Application of the Psychological Flexibility Model to Activity Patterns in Chronic Pain," *Journal of Pain* 14, no. 8 (2013): 828–35.

8. Barry J. Zimmerman and Dale H. Schunk, "Competence and Control Beliefs: Distinguishing the

Means and Ends," in Patricia A. Alexander and Philip H. Winne, eds., *Handbook of Educational Psychology* (New York: Routledge, 2006): 349–67; Philip R. Magaletta and J. M. Oliver, "The Hope Construct, Will, and Ways: Their Relations with Self-Efficacy, Optimism, and General Well-Being," *Journal of Clinical Psychology* 55, no. 5 (1999): 539–51; James Carifio and Lauren Rhodes, "Construct Validities and the Empirical Relationships Between Optimism, Hope, Self-Efficacy, and Locus of Control," *Work: A Journal of Prevention, Assessment and Rehabilitation* 19, no. 2 (2002): 125–36; and Cecil Robinson and Karla Snipes, "Hope, Optimism and Self-Efficacy: A System of Competence and Control," *Multiple Linear Regression Viewpoints* 35, no. 2 (2009): 16–26.

9.  C. Richard Snyder, ed., *Handbook of Hope: Theory, Measures, and Applications* (New York: Academic Press, 2000).

10. Sonja Lyubomirsky, Laura King, and Ed Diener, "The Benefits of Frequent Positive Affect: Does Happiness Lead to Success?" *Psychological Bulletin* 131, no. 6 (2005): 803.

11. Albert Bandura, "Self-Efficacy: Toward a Unifying Theory of Behavioral Change," *Psychological Review* 84, no. 2 (1977): 191.

12. The idea of values-driven or "committed" action was first described in Steven C. Hayes, Kirk D. Strosahl, and Kelly G. Wilson, *Acceptance and Commitment Therapy: An Experiential Approach to Behavior Change* (New York: Guilford, 1999). For a summary of studies of its effectiveness, see Francisco J. Ruiz, "A Review of Acceptance and Commitment Therapy (ACT) Empirical Evidence: Correlational, Experimental Psychopathology, Component and Outcome Studies," *International Journal of Psychology and Psychological Therapy* 10, no. 1 (2010): 125–62.

13. Kelly G. Wilson et al., "The Valued Living Questionnaire: Defining and Measuring Valued Action Within a Behavioral Framework," *Psychological Record* 60, no. 2 (2011): 4.

14. Russ Harris, *ACT Made Simple: An Easy-to-Read Primer on Acceptance and Commitment Therapy* (Oakland, CA: New Harbinger Publications, 2009). If you're interested in trying more exercises to explore your values, you can also check out Dr. Harris's website, www.thehappinesstrap.com.

15. Ibid.

16. Ibid. See also Russ Harris, *The Happiness Trap: Stop Struggling, Start Living* (Auckland, NZ: Exisle Publishing, 2007).

17. Edward L. Deci, Richard Koestner, and Richard M. Ryan, "A Meta-Analytic Review of Experiments Examining the Effects of Extrinsic Rewards on Intrinsic Motivation," *Psychological Bulletin* 125, no. 6 (1999): 627.

18. Carolina O.C. Werle, Brian Wansink, and Collin R. Payne, "Is It Fun or Exercise? The Framing of Physical Activity Biases Subsequent Snacking," *Marketing Letters* (2014): 1–12.

## Chapter 9: Allies

1.  "2014 Global Games Market Report," *NewZoo Games Market Research*, May 2014.

2.  Although there are no global stats on general leisure time (whereas there are global stats for video game play; see the previous endnote), we can make an educated guess that nondigital play consumes at least as many social hours, from national time use surveys that track card games, board games, and sports, such as the 2014 American Time Use Survey by the Bureau of Labor Statistics. Other national time use surveys are collected by the United Nations here: http://unstats.un.org/unsd/demographic/sconcerns/tuse.

3.  Wendy Birmingham et al., "Social Ties and Cardiovascular Function: An Examination of Relationship Positivity and Negativity During Stress," *International Journal of Psychophysiology* 74, no. 2 (2009): 114–19; Sheldon Cohen and Thomas A. Wills, "Stress, Social Support, and the Buffering Hypothesis," *Psychological Bulletin* 98, no. 2 (1985): 310; Debra Umberson and Jennifer Karas Montez, "Social Relationships and Health: A Flashpoint for Health Policy," *Journal of Health and Social Behavior* 51, no. 1 supp. (2010): S54–S66; and Ralf Schwarzer and Anja Leppin, "Social Support and Health: A Theoretical and Empirical Overview," *Journal of Social and Personal Relationships* 8, no. 1 (1991): 99–127.

4.  Julianne Holt-Lunstad, Timothy B. Smith, and J. Bradley Layton, "Social Relationships and Mortality Risk: A Meta-Analytic Review," *PLOS Medicine* 7, no. 7 (2010): e1000316.

5. These are the two most common items on scientific measures of perceived social support, such as the Multidimensional Scale of Perceived Social Support (MSPSS), the Social Support Network Inventory (SSNI), the Brief Measure of Social Support (BMSS), and the Social Support Questionnaire (SSQ). See Gregory D. Zimet et al., "The Multidimensional Scale of Perceived Social Support," *Journal of Personality Assessment* 52, no. 1 (1988): 30–41; Joseph A. Flaherty, F. Moises Gaviria, and Dev S. Pathak, "The Measurement of Social Support: The Social Support Network Inventory," *Comprehensive Psychiatry* 24, no. 6 (1983): 521–29; Irwin G. Sarason et al., "A Brief Measure of Social Support: Practical and Theoretical Implications," *Journal of Social and Personal Relationships* 4, no. 4 (1987): 497–510; and Irwin G. Sarason et al., "Assessing Social Support: The Social Support Questionnaire," *Journal of Personality and Social Psychology* 44, no. 1 (1983): 127.

6. "Six Weeks of Superbetter," November 18, 2011, *On the Media*, archived at http://www.onthemedia.org/story/171259-six-weeks-superbetter.

7. Alex Goldman "The Superbetter Diaries," *On the Media* blog, http://www.onthemedia.org/blogs/on-the-media/2011/oct/04/superbetter-diaries-entry-1.

8. Julianne Holt-Lunstad, Wendy A. Birmingham, and Kathleen C. Light, "Influence of a 'Warm Touch' Support Enhancement Intervention Among Married Couples on Ambulatory Blood Pressure, Oxytocin, Alpha Amylase, and Cortisol," *Psychosomatic Medicine* 70, no. 9 (2008): 976–85; Diana Lynn Woods and Margaret Dimond, "The Effect of Therapeutic Touch on Agitated Behavior and Cortisol in Persons with Alzheimer's Disease," *Biological Research for Nursing* 4, no. 2 (2002): 104–14; Ruth Feldman, Magi Singer, and Orna Zagoory, "Touch Attenuates Infants' Physiological Reactivity to Stress," *Developmental Science* 13, no. 2 (2010): 271–78; Yu-Shen Lin and Ann Gill Taylor, "Effects of Therapeutic Touch in Reducing Pain and Anxiety in an Elderly Population," *Integrative Medicine* 1, no. 4 (1998): 155–62; Tiffany Field et al., "Cortisol Decreases and Serotonin and Dopamine Increase Following Massage Therapy," *International Journal of Neuroscience* 115, no. 10 (2005): 1397–413; Tiffany Field et al., "Brief Report: Autistic Children's Attentiveness and Responsivity Improve After Touch Therapy," *Journal of Autism and Developmental Disorders* 27, no. 3 (1997): 333–38; Maria Henricson et al., "The Outcome of Tactile Touch on Oxytocin in Intensive Care Patients: A Randomised Controlled Trial," *Journal of Clinical Nursing* 17, no. 19 (2008): 2624–33; Matthew J. Hertenstein et al., "Touch Communicates Distinct Emotions," *Emotion* 6, no. 3 (2006): 528; and Michael W. Kraus, Cassey Huang, and Dacher Keltner, "Tactile Communication, Cooperation, and Performance: An Ethological Study of the NBA," *Emotion* 10, no. 5 (2010): 745.

9. Manuel Barrera, Jr., "Distinctions Between Social Support Concepts, Measures, and Models," *American Journal of Community Psychology* 14, no. 4 (1986): 413–45; and Sheldon Cohen, "Social Relationships and Health," *American Psychologist* 59, no. 8 (2004): 676.

10. Lynn M. Martire et al., "Is It Beneficial to Involve a Family Member? A Meta-Analysis of Psychosocial Interventions for Chronic Illness," *Health Psychology* 23, no. 6 (2004): 599.

11. Miller McPherson, Lynn Smith-Lovin, and Matthew E. Brashears, "Social Isolation in America: Changes in Core Discussion Networks over Two Decades," *American Sociological Review* 71, no. 3 (2006): 353–75.

### Chapter 10: Secret Identity

1. I recommend the following online name generators: www.seventhsanctum.com/index-name.php and http://fantasynamegenerators.com, as well as the helpful article "Tricks and Tips for Naming Superheroes and Supervillians" at www.springhole.net/writing/naming-superheroes-and-supervillains.htm.

2. P. Alex Linley et al., "Using Signature Strengths in Pursuit of Goals: Effects on Goal Progress, Need Satisfaction, and Well-Being, and Implications for Coaching Psychologists," *International Coaching Psychology Review* 5, no. 1 (2010): 6–15.

3. Martin E. P. Seligman et al., "Positive Psychology Progress: Empirical Validation of Interventions," *American Psychologist* 60, no. 5 (2005): 410.

4. Carmel Proctor, John Maltby, and P. Alex Linley, "Strengths Use as a Predictor of Well-Being and Health-Related Quality of Life," *Journal of Happiness Studies* 12, no. 1 (2011): 153–69.

5. Christopher Peterson, Nansook Park, and Martin E. P. Seligman, "Greater Strengths of Character and Recovery from Illness," *Journal of Positive Psychology* 1, no. 1 (2006): 17–26.
6. For a list of 340 ways to use signature character strengths, see http://tayyabrashid.com/pdf/via_strengths.pdf.
7. Ethan Kross and Özlem Ayduk, "Making Meaning Out of Negative Experiences by Self-Distancing," *Current Directions in Psychological Science* 20, no. 3 (2011): 187–91.
8. Ethan Kross et al., "Self-Talk as a Regulatory Mechanism: How You Do It Matters," *Journal of Personality and Social Psychology* 106, no. 2 (2014): 304.
9. Kentaro Fujita et al., "Construal Levels and Self-Control," *Journal of Personality and Social Psychology* 90, no. 3 (2006): 351; Hedy Kober et al., "Prefrontal-Striatal Pathway Underlies Cognitive Regulation of Craving," *Proceedings of the National Academy of Sciences* 107, no. 33 (2010): 14811–16; and Walter Mischel and Monica L. Rodriguez, "Psychological Distance in Self-Imposed Delay of Gratification," in Rodney R. Cocking and K. Ann Renninger, eds., *The Development and Meaning of Psychological Distance* (Hillsdale, NJ: Lawrence Erlbaum Associates, 1993).
10. Kross and Ayduk, "Making Meaning."
11. Kross et al., "Self-Talk as a Regulatory Mechanism."
12. Özlem Ayduk and Ethan Kross, "From a Distance: Implications of Spontaneous Self-Distancing for Adaptive Self-Reflection," *Journal of Personality and Social Psychology* 98, no. 5 (2010): 809.
13. Steven C. Hayes et al., "Acceptance and Commitment Therapy: Model, Processes and Outcomes," *Behaviour Research and Therapy* 44, no. 1 (2006): 1–25; and John D. Teasdale et al., "Metacognitive Awareness and Prevention of Relapse in Depression: Empirical Evidence," *Journal of Consulting and Clinical Psychology* 70, no. 2 (2002): 275.
14. Kross et al., "Self-Talk as a Regulatory Mechanism."
15. Barbara E. Abernathy, "Who Am I Now?: Helping Trauma Clients Find Meaning, Wisdom, and a Renewed Sense of Self," in Garry R. Walz, Jeanne C. Bleuer, and Richard K. Yep, eds., *Compelling Counseling Interventions: Celebrating VISTAS' Fifth Anniversary* (Ann Arbor, MI: Counseling Outfitters, 2008).
16. Jennifer L. Pals and Dan P. McAdams, "The Transformed Self: A Narrative Understanding of Post-Traumatic Growth," *Psychological Inquiry* (2004): 65–69; Laura A. King et al., "Stories of Life Transition: Subjective Well-Being and Ego Development in Parents of Children with Down Syndrome," *Journal of Research in Personality* 34, no. 4 (2000): 509–36; and Jack J. Bauer, Dan P. McAdams, and Jennifer L. Pals, "Narrative Identity and Eudaimonic Well-Being," *Journal of Happiness Studies* 9, no. 1 (2008): 81–104.

### Chapter 11: Epic Wins

1. Vicki S. Helgeson, Kerry A. Reynolds, and Patricia L. Tomich, "A Meta-Analytic Review of Benefit Finding and Growth," *Journal of Consulting and Clinical Psychology* 74, no. 5 (2006): 797.
2. Julienne E. Bower et al., "Benefit Finding and Physical Health: Positive Psychological Changes and Enhanced Allostasis," *Social and Personality Psychology Compass* 2, no. 1 (2008): 223–44; Dean G. Cruess et al., "Cognitive-Behavioral Stress Management Reduces Serum Cortisol by Enhancing Benefit Finding Among Women Being Treated for Early Stage Breast Cancer," *Psychosomatic Medicine* 62, no. 3 (2000): 304–8; Michael H. Antoni et al., "Cognitive-Behavioral Stress Management Intervention Decreases the Prevalence of Depression and Enhances Benefit Finding Among Women Under Treatment for Early-Stage Breast Cancer," *Health Psychology* 20, no. 1 (2001): 20; Roger C. Katz et al., "The Psychosocial Impact of Cancer and Lupus: A Cross Validation Study That Extends the Generality of 'Benefit-Finding' in Patients with Chronic Disease," *Journal of Behavioral Medicine* 24, no. 6 (2001): 561–71; Charles S. Carver and Michael H. Antoni, "Finding Benefit in Breast Cancer During the Year After Diagnosis Predicts Better Adjustment 5 to 8 Years After Diagnosis," *Health Psychology* 23, no. 6 (2004): 595; Sharon Danoff-Burg and Tracey A. Revenson, "Benefit-Finding Among Patients with Rheumatoid Arthritis: Positive Effects on Interpersonal Relationships," *Journal of Behavioral Medicine* 28, no. 1 (2005): 91–103; and Eric L. Garland, Susan A. Gaylord, and Barbara L. Fredrickson, "Positive Reappraisal Mediates the Stress-Reductive Effects of Mindfulness: An Upward Spiral Process," *Mindfulness* 2, no. 1 (2011): 59–67.

3.  Kennon M. Sheldon and Linda Houser-Marko, "Self-Concordance, Goal Attainment, and the Pursuit of Happiness: Can There Be an Upward Spiral?," *Journal of Personality and Social Psychology* 80, no. 1 (2001): 152.

4.  Kate C. McLean and Michael W. Pratt, "Life's Little (and Big) Lessons: Identity Statuses and Meaning-Making in the Turning Point Narratives of Emerging Adults," *Developmental Psychology* 42, no. 4 (2006): 714; Jack J. Bauer, Dan P. McAdams, and April R. Sakaeda, "Interpreting the Good Life: Growth Memories in the Lives of Mature, Happy People," *Journal of Personality and Social Psychology* 88, no. 1 (2005): 203; Colette Hillebrand Duggan and Marcel Dijkers, "Quality of Life—Peaks and Valleys: A Qualitative Analysis of the Narratives of Persons with Spinal Cord Injuries," *Canadian Journal of Rehabilitation* 12, no. 3 (1999): 179–89; James Mcintosh and Neil McKeganey, "Addicts' Narratives of Recovery from Drug Use: Constructing a Non-Addict Identity," *Social Science and Medicine* 50, no. 10 (2000): 1501–10; M.R.E.G.K.P.A. Harney, "In the Aftermath of Sexual Abuse: Making and Remaking Meaning in Narratives of Trauma and Recovery," *Narrative Inquiry* 10, no. 2 (2001): 291–311; Clare Woodward and Stephen Joseph, "Positive Change Processes and Post Traumatic Growth in People Who Have Experienced Childhood Abuse: Understanding Vehicles of Change," *Psychology and Psychotherapy: Theory, Research and Practice* 76, no. 3 (2003): 267–83; Jack J. Bauer, Dan P. McAdams, and Jennifer L. Pals, "Narrative Identity and Eudaimonic Well-Being," *Journal of Happiness Studies* 9, no. 1 (2008): 81–104; and Sally Maitlis, "Who Am I Now? Sensemaking and Identity in Post-traumatic Growth," in Laura Morgan Roberts and Jane E. Dutton, eds., *Exploring Positive Identities and Organizations: Building a Theoretical and Research Foundation* (New York: Taylor and Francis, 2009).

5.  Eric J. Nestler and William A. Carlezon, Jr., "The Mesolimbic Dopamine Reward Circuit in Depression," *Biological Psychiatry* 59, no. 12 (2006): 1151–59; Moria J. Smoski et al., "fMRI of Alterations in Reward Selection, Anticipation, and Feedback in Major Depressive Disorder," *Journal of Affective Disorders* 118, no. 1 (2009): 69–78; and Jane H. Powell et al., "Motivational Deficits After Brain Injury: Effects of Bromocriptine in 11 Patients," *Journal of Neurology, Neurosurgery and Psychiatry* 60, no. 4 (1996): 416–21.

6.  Kennon M. Sheldon and Andrew J. Elliot, "Goal Striving, Need Satisfaction, and Longitudinal Well-Being: The Self-Concordance Model," *Journal of Personality and Social Psychology* 76, no. 3 (1999): 482.

7.  Alisha L. Brosse et al., "Exercise and the Treatment of Clinical Depression in Adults," *Sports Medicine* 32, no. 12 (2002): 741–60; Andrea L. Dunn et al., "Exercise Treatment for Depression: Efficacy and Dose Response," *American Journal of Preventive Medicine* 28, no. 1 (2005): 1–8; A. Byrne and D. G. Byrne, "The Effect of Exercise on Depression, Anxiety and Other Mood States: A Review," *Journal of Psychosomatic Research* 37, no. 6 (1993): 565–74.

8.  Kelli F. Koltyn et al., "Perception of Pain Following Aerobic Exercise," *Medicine and Science in Sports and Exercise* 28, no. 11 (1996): 1418–21; Deborah S. Nichols and Terri M. Glenn, "Effects of Aerobic Exercise on Pain Perception, Affect, and Level of Disability in Individuals with Fibromyalgia," *Physical Therapy* 74, no. 4 (1994): 327–32; Kelli F. Koltyn and R. W. Arbogast, "Perception of Pain After Resistance Exercise," *British Journal of Sports Medicine* 32, no. 1 (1998): 20–24; Martin D. Hoffman et al., "Experimentally Induced Pain Perception Is Acutely Reduced by Aerobic Exercise in People with Chronic Low Back Pain," *Journal of Rehabilitation Research and Development* 42, no. 2 (2005): 183–90; Karen E. Kuphal, Eugene E. Fibuch, and Bradley K. Taylor, "Extended Swimming Exercise Reduces Inflammatory and Peripheral Neuropathic Pain in Rodents," *Journal of Pain* 8, no. 12 (2007): 989–97.

9.  Edwin A. Locke and Gary P. Latham, "Building a Practically Useful Theory of Goal Setting and Task Motivation: A 35-Year Odyssey," *American Psychologist* 57, no. 9 (2002): 705.

10. Edwin A. Locke and Gary P. Latham, "New Directions in Goal-Setting Theory," *Current Directions in Psychological Science* 15, no. 5 (2006): 265–68.

11. Edward L. Deci and Richard M. Ryan, "Self-Determination Theory: A Macrotheory of Human Motivation, Development, and Health," *Canadian Psychology/Psychologie Canadienne* 49, no. 3 (2008): 182.

## Chapter 12: Keeping Score

1.   C. P. Stack, "The Pleasure and Profit of Keeping Score," *Baseball Magazine,* 1914, quoted in Paul Dickson, *The Joy of Keeping Score* (1966; reprint New York: Walker, 2007).

2.   J. Lethem et al., "Outline of a Fear-Avoidance Model of Exaggerated Pain Perception—I," *Behaviour Research and Therapy* 21, no. 4 (1983): 401–8; Geert Crombez et al., "Pain-Related Fear Is More Disabling Than Pain Itself: Evidence on the Role of Pain-Related Fear in Chronic Back Pain Disability," *Pain* 80, no. 1 (1999): 329–39; Predrag Petrovic et al., "Pain-Related Cerebral Activation Is Altered by a Distracting Cognitive Task," *Pain* 85, no. 1 (2000): 19–30.

3.   James Carse, *Finite and Infinite Games: A Vision of Life as Play and Possibility* (1986; reprint New York: Simon and Schuster, 2011).

4.   Steven C. Moore et al., "Leisure Time Physical Activity of Moderate to Vigorous Intensity and Mortality: A Large Pooled Cohort Analysis," *PLOS Medicine* 9, no. 11 (2012): e1001335.

5.   Matthew Pantell et al., "Social Isolation: A Predictor of Mortality Comparable to Traditional Clinical Risk Factors," *American Journal of Public Health* 103, no. 11 (2013): 2056–62.

6.   Deborah D. Danner, David A. Snowdon, and Wallace V. Friesen, "Positive Emotions in Early Life and Longevity: Findings from the Nun Study," *Journal of Personality and Social Psychology* 80, no. 5 (2001): 804.

7.   Jingping Xu and Robert E. Roberts, "The Power of Positive Emotions: It's a Matter of Life or Death—Subjective Well-Being and Longevity Over 28 Years in a General Population," *Health Psychology* 29, no. 1 (2010): 9; Ed Diener and Micaela Y. Chan, "Happy People Live Longer: Subjective Well-Being Contributes to Health and Longevity," *Applied Psychology: Health and Well-Being* 3, no. 1 (2011): 1–43; Yoichi Chida and Andrew Steptoe, "Positive Psychological Well-Being and Mortality: A Quantitative Review of Prospective Observational Studies," *Psychosomatic Medicine* 70, no. 7 (2008): 741–56; Teije A. Koopmans et al., "Effects of Happiness on All-Cause Mortality During 15 Years of Follow-Up: The Arnhem Elderly Study," *Journal of Happiness Studies* 11, no. 1 (2010): 113–24; and Kokoro Shirai et al., "Perceived Level of Life Enjoyment and Risks of Cardiovascular Disease Incidence and Mortality; The Japan Public Health Center–Based Study," *Circulation* 120, no. 11 (2009): 956–63.


## Adventure 1: Love Connection

1.   Karen J. Reivich, Martin E. P. Seligman, and Sharon McBride, "Master Resilience Training in the US Army," *American Psychologist* 66, no. 1 (2011): 25; and Shelly L. Gable, Gian C. Gonzaga, and Amy Strachman, "Will You Be There for Me When Things Go Right?: Supportive Responses to Positive Event Disclosures," *Journal of Personality and Social Psychology* 91, no. 5 (2006): 904.

2.   Shelly L. Gable et al., "What Do You Do When Things Go Right?: The Intrapersonal and Interpersonal Benefits of Sharing Positive Events," *Journal of Personality and Social Psychology* 87, no. 2 (2004): 228; Harry T. Reis et al., "Are You Happy for Me?: How Sharing Positive Events with Others Provides Personal and Interpersonal Benefits," *Journal of Personality and Social Psychology* 99, no. 2 (2010): 311; Gable, Gonzaga, and Strachman, "Will You Be There for Me When Things Go Right?"; Natalya C. Maisel, Shelly L. Gable, and Amy Strachman, "Responsive Behaviors in Good Times and in Bad," *Personal Relationships* 15, no. 3 (2008): 317–38; Shelly L. Gable and Harry T. Reis, "Good News!: Capitalizing on Positive Events in an Interpersonal Context," *Advances in Experimental Social Psychology* 42 (2010): 195–257; Remus Ilies, Jessica Keeney, and Brent A. Scott, "Work-Family Interpersonal Capitalization: Sharing Positive Work Events at Home," *Organizational Behavior and Human Decision Processes* 114, no. 2 (2011): 115–26; and Shannon M. Smith *"Wow! That's Great!": Correlates of and Variability in Responding Enthusiastically,* Ph.D. diss., University of Rochester, 2012.

3.   Alex M. Wood, Jeffrey J. Froh, and Adam W. A. Geraghty, "Gratitude and Well-Being: A Review and Theoretical Integration," *Clinical Psychology Review* 30, no. 7 (2010): 890–905; Alex M. Wood et al., "The Role of Gratitude in the Development of Social Support, Stress, and Depression:

Two Longitudinal Studies," *Journal of Research in Personality* 42, no. 4 (2008): 854–71; and Robert A. Emmons and Anjali Mishra, "Why Gratitude Enhances Well-Being: What We Know, What We Need to Know," in Kennon M. Sheldon and Todd B. Kashdan, eds., *Designing Positive Psychology: Taking Stock and Moving Forward* (New York: Oxford University Press, 2011).

4. Nathaniel M. Lambert et al., "Benefits of Expressing Gratitude: Expressing Gratitude to a Partner Changes One's View of the Relationship," *Psychological Science* 21, no. 4 (2010): 574–80; also Kennon M. Sheldon and Sonja Lyubomirsky, "How to Increase and Sustain Positive Emotion: The Effects of Expressing Gratitude and Visualizing Best Possible Selves," *Journal of Positive Psychology* 1, no. 2 (2006): 73–82.

5. Robert A. Emmons, "Gratitude, Subjective Well-Being, and the Brain," in Michael Eid and Randy J. Larsen, eds., *The Science of Subjective Well-Being* (New York: Guilford, 2008): 469–89; Sara B. Algoe and Jonathan Haidt, "Witnessing Excellence in Action: The 'Other-Praising' Emotions of Elevation, Gratitude, and Admiration," *Journal of Positive Psychology* 4, no. 2 (2009): 105–27; and Sara B. Algoe, Jonathan Haidt, and Shelly L. Gable, "Beyond Reciprocity: Gratitude and Relationships in Everyday Life," *Emotion* 8, no. 3 (2008): 425.

6. Dr. Kelly McGonigal and I created the three-part thank-you as part of a special SuperBetter collaboration with the Oprah Winfrey Network: "Oprah's Thank You Game." You can find out more at http://kellymcgonigal.com/tag/gratitude.

7. I learned this practice directly from Dr. Biswas-Diener at his Strengths Intervention for Work and Relationships Workshop at the Second World Congress on Positive Psychology, held in Philadelphia in June 2011. Another resource for strengths-spotting techniques is his manual for psychology coaching: Robert Biswas-Diener, *Practicing Positive Psychology Coaching: Assessment, Activities and Strategies for Success* (Hoboken, NJ: John Wiley and Sons, 2010). See also Ryan M. Niemiec, "VIA Character Strengths: Research and Practice (The First 10 Years)," in Hans Henrik Knoop and Antonella Delle Fave, eds., *Well-Being and Cultures* (Springer Netherlands, 2013); Sandy Gordon and Daniel F. Gucciardi, "A Strengths-Based Approach to Coaching Mental Toughness," *Journal of Sport Psychology in Action* 2, no. 3 (2011): 143–55; and Carmel Proctor et al., "Strengths Gym: The Impact of a Character Strengths-Based Intervention on the Life Satisfaction and Well-Being of Adolescents," *Journal of Positive Psychology* 6, no. 5 (2011): 377–88.

8. Louise C. Hawkley and John T. Cacioppo, "Loneliness Matters: A Theoretical and Empirical Review of Consequences and Mechanisms," *Annals of Behavioral Medicine* 40, no. 2 (2010): 218–27.

9. John T. Cacioppo and William Patrick, *Loneliness: Human Nature and the Need for Social Connection* (New York: W.W. Norton, 2008).

10. Christopher M. Masi et al., "A Meta-Analysis of Interventions to Reduce Loneliness," *Personality and Social Psychology Review* 15, no. 3 (2010).

11. Kristin Neff, *Self-Compassion: Stop Beating Yourself Up and Leave Insecurity Behind* (New York: William Morrow, 2011).

12. Christopher K. Germer, *The Mindful Path to Self-Compassion: Freeing Yourself from Destructive Thoughts and Emotions* (New York: Guilford Press, 2009).

## *Adventure 2: Ninja Body Transformation*

1. Traci Mann et al., "Medicare's Search for Effective Obesity Treatments: Diets Are Not the Answer," *American Psychologist* 62, no. 3 (2007): 220.

2. Linda Bacon and Lucy Aphramor, "Weight Science: Evaluating the Evidence for a Paradigm Shift," *Nutrition Journal* 10, no. 9 (2011): 2–13.

3. Nancy C. Howarth, Edward Saltzman, and Susan B. Roberts, "Dietary Fiber and Weight Regulation," *Nutrition Reviews* 59, no. 5 (2001): 129–39.

4. Michael Pollan, *In Defense of Food: An Eater's Manifesto* (New York: Penguin, 2008).

5. Susmita Kaushik et al., "Autophagy in Hypothalamic AgRP Neurons Regulates Food Intake and Energy Balance," *Cell Metabolism* 14, no. 2 (2011): 173–83.

6.   Musashi Miyamoto, *A Book of Five Rings*, trans. Victor Harris (London: Allison and Busby; Woodstock, NY: Overlook Press, 1974).

7.   Donn F. Draeger and Robert W. Smith, *Comprehensive Asian Fighting Arts* (New York: Kodansha, 1981).

8.   Ferris Jabr, "Let's Get Physical: The Psychology of Effective Workout Music," *Scientific American*, March 20, 2013.

9.   Mona Lisa Chanda and Daniel J. Levitin, "The Neurochemistry of Music," *Trends in Cognitive Sciences* 17, no. 4 (2013): 179–93.

10.  Yuko Tsunetsugu, Bum-Jin Park, and Yoshifumi Miyazaki, "Trends in Research Related to 'Shinrin-Yoku' (Taking in the Forest Atmosphere or Forest Bathing) in Japan," *Environmental Health and Preventive Medicine* 15, no. 1 (2010): 27–37; J. Lee et al., "Effect of Forest Bathing on Physiological and Psychological Responses in Young Japanese Male Subjects," *Public Health* 125, no. 2 (2011): 93–100; and Bum Jin Park et al., "The Physiological Effects of Shinrin-Yoku (Taking in the Forest Atmosphere or Forest Bathing): Evidence from Field Experiments in 24 Forests Across Japan," *Environmental Health and Preventive Medicine* 15, no. 1 (2010): 18–26.

11.  Stephen Turnbull, *Ninja AD 1460–1650* (Oxford: Osprey, 2003).

## Adventure 3: Time Rich

1.   Tim Kasser and Kennon M. Sheldon, "Time Affluence as a Path Toward Personal Happiness and Ethical Business Practice: Empirical Evidence from Four Studies," *Journal of Business Ethics* 84, no. 2 (2009): 243–55.

2.   Susan Roxburgh, "'There Just Aren't Enough Hours in the Day': The Mental Health Consequences of Time Pressure," *Journal of Health and Social Behavior* 45, no. 2 (2004): 115–31; Alex Szollos, "Toward a Psychology of Chronic Time Pressure Conceptual and Methodological Review," *Time and Society* 18, no. 2–3 (2009): 332–50; and Tim Kasser, "Psychological Need Satisfaction, Personal Well-Being, and Ecological Sustainability," *Ecopsychology* 1, no. 4 (2009): 175–80.

3.   Juliet Schor, *Plenitude: The New Economics of True Wealth* (New York: Penguin Press, 2010).

4.   John De Graaf, ed., *Take Back Your Time: Fighting Overwork and Time Poverty in America* (San Francisco: Berrett-Koehler, 2003).

5.   Dana R. Carney, Amy J. C. Cuddy, and Andy J. Yap, "Power Posing: Brief Nonverbal Displays Affect Neuroendocrine Levels and Risk Tolerance," *Psychological Science* 21, no. 10 (2010): 1363–68.

6.   Alice Moon and Serena Chen, "The Power to Control Time: Power Influences How Much Time (You Think) You Have," *Journal of Experimental Social Psychology* 54 (2014): 97–101.

7.   Cassie Mogilner, Zoë Chance, and Michael I. Norton, "Giving Time Gives You Time," *Psychological Science* 23, no. 10 (2012): 1233–38.

8.   Melanie Rudd, Kathleen D. Vohs, and Jennifer Aaker, "Awe Expands People's Perception of Time, Alters Decision Making, and Enhances Well-Being," *Psychological Science* 23, no. 10 (2012): 1130–36.

9.   Marc Wittmann et al., "Social Jetlag: Misalignment of Biological and Social Time," *Chronobiology International* 23, nos. 1–2 (2006): 497–509.

10.  Till Roenneberg et al., "Social Jetlag and Obesity," *Current Biology* 22, no. 10 (2012): 939–43; Christoph Randler, "Differences Between Smokers and Nonsmokers in Morningness-Eveningness," *Social Behavior and Personality: An International Journal* 36, no. 5 (2008): 673–80.

11.  Russell G. Foster et al., "Sleep and Circadian Rhythm Disruption in Social Jetlag and Mental Illness," *Progress in Molecular Biology and Translational Science* 119 (2012): 325–46; and Rosa Levandovski et al., "Depression Scores Associate with Chronotype and Social Jetlag in a Rural Population," *Chronobiology International* 28, no. 9 (2011): 771–78.

12.  Stefan Klein, *The Secret Pulse of Time: Making Sense of Life's Scarcest Commodity* (Cambridge, MA: Da Capo Press, 2008).

13.  Vani Pariyadath and David Eagleman, "The Effect of Predictability on Subjective Duration," *PLOS ONE* 2, no. 11 (2007): e1264.

14.  David M. Eagleman et al., "Time and the Brain: How Subjective Time Relates to Neural Time," *Journal of Neuroscience* 25, no. 45 (2005): 10369–71.
15.  Jennifer L. Aaker, Melanie Rudd, and Cassie Mogilner, "If Money Does Not Make You Happy, Consider Time," *Journal of Consumer Psychology* 21, no. 2 (2011): 126–30.
16.  Seth Lajeunesse and Daniel A. Rodríguez, "Mindfulness, Time Affluence, and Journey-Based Affect: Exploring Relationships," *Transportation Research Part F: Traffic Psychology and Behaviour* 15, no. 2 (2012): 196–205.
17.  Bodhipaksa, "10 Tips for Mindful Driving," http://www.wildmind.org/applied/daily-life/mindful-driving. For more tips, see Michele McDonald, *Awake at the Wheel: Mindful Driving* (audiobook; More Than Sound Productions, 2011).
18.  Mihaly Csikszentmihalyi and Jeremy Hunter, "Happiness in Everyday Life: The Uses of Experience Sampling," *Journal of Happiness Studies* 4, no. 2 (2003): 185–99.

### *About the Science*

1.  Ann Marie Roepke et al., "Randomized Controlled Trial of SuperBetter, a Smartphone-Based/Internet-Based Self-Help Tool to Reduce Depressive Symptoms," *Games for Health Journal* 4, no. 3 (2015): 235–46.

# Index

curiosity (*cont.*)
  and game playing, 2
  increasing of, 338
  and quests, 214
  as top strength, 269, 328
Curwin, Joyce, 127

DePaul University, 234
depression, 2–3, 5, 29, 86–87, 127, 153, 167, 186,
  215, 221
  alleviation of, 4, 12, 19–20, 23, 35, 46–47,
    51, 105–6, 126, 134–35, 152, 327, 339,
    351, 418, 424
  and allies, 254, 256
  and attention control, 50–51
  and bad guys, 200, 417–18
  and challenge mindset, 138, 142, 158
  and epic wins, 292, 306, 312
  and escapist mindset, 116
  and game playing, 4, 19–20, 29, 46–47, 51,
    239, 424
  increase in, 116
  measuring of, 326–27
  and physical activity, 312
  and positive emotions, 168
  and power-ups, 170, 173, 181, 417–18
  and quests, 214, 230–31, 417–18
  and self-compassion, 362
  and signature strengths, 278
  tests/trials for, 416–20
  and vagal tone, 163
determination, 91, 97, 388–89, 392
  benefits of, 313
  down side of, 87
  and epic wins, 302, 310–11
  and game playing, 2–3, 78, 94, 119, 131
  increasing of, 85–86, 88, 96, 103, 152,
    328, 338
  natural capacity for, 1, 78
  and secret identities, 261, 263
  and self-efficacy, 96, 103
  supercharging of, 24, 82, 104, 121, 125, 340
  and tackling challenges, 19
  as top strength, 324
diabetes, 11, 139, 163, 241, 312, 370
dieting, 171–72, 347, 369–71, 375–76, 390
digital games. *See* games; specific titles
domestic violence, 202–3
dopamine, 85–93, 96, 103, 162
dreams, 6–7, 112, 120, 203–4, 211–12
drugs, 30, 42, 78–79, 85, 87, 105, 107, 138, 384

Eagleman, Dr. David, 406
East Carolina University (ECU), 45–47
eating habits, 133, 161, 222
  to feel stronger, 369–70, 390–91
  and game playing, 19
  healthy, 39, 135, 147, 171–72, 396
  and physical activity, 233
  power-foods for, 347, 372–73, 385–86, 391
  power-ups for, 171–72
  unhealthy, 107, 185, 278, 380, 383, 394, 404
  *See also* cravings; dieting; weight issues

echocardiogram (ECG), 163–64
economic hardship, 141, 150, 192
electroencephalographic (EEG) changes, 46–48
Eliot, T. S., 184–85
embodied cognition, 211
emotional
  benefits, 111–12, 121, 251, 284, 422
  challenges, 255, 302
  distress, 36, 116, 215
  experiences, 166–69
  habits, 397
  passion, 379–80, 392–93
  power-ups, 144, 172–74, 183
  strength, 12–13, 50, 153–54, 313, 318
  support, 68
emotional resilience, 293, 341
  and bad guys, 186, 189–90
  building of, 18, 20, 35, 155, 178
  and game playing, 217
  increasing of, 29
  and longevity, 336
  power-ups for, 161, 178
  quests for, 16–18
  strategies for, 152
  *See also* positive emotion ratio
emotions, 48, 85
  avoidance of, 116
  controlling of, 50–51, 104, 125, 128, 163, 165,
    286, 340
  and game playing, 51, 58, 131
  and health, 46, 164–65, 247
  managing of, 111–12, 142
  and mirror/mimic activity, 55–56, 58
  paying attention to, 408
  power-ups for, 160–61, 165
  and stress, 168, 286
  and vagus nerve, 162
  and vagal tone, 163–64
empathy, 53–56, 62, 64–65, 74–76, 244, 339
energy, 135–36, 221
  and allies, 253
  and bad guys, 186, 197, 202
  and epic wins, 305
  and game playing, 46, 114, 121
  and health, 284, 371, 394
  improvement in, 14, 46, 114, 121, 253, 305, 389
  music's impact on, 383–84, 391
  and power foods, 373, 385–86
  power-ups for, 160–61, 176
  and quests, 166, 214, 225, 231, 236, 289, 380
environment, the, 222, 376
Epic Win Possibility Scale, 313–15
epic wins, 144, 228, 281, 332, 338, 341
  and allies, 241, 245–47, 298, 300, 304–5,
    315–16
  benefits of, 294, 421
  breakthrough moments, 297–300, 303, 309,
    311–13, 316
  examples of, 292–93, 295, 298, 300–313, 316
  explanation of, 8–9, 292–95, 316
  and gameful mindset, 315–16
  and GSI inventory, 328
  and life expectancy, 337

neural
circuitry, 91, 284
coupling/connection, 53–54, 56, 58
networks, 89, 96, 115
processing, 110
reorganization, 88–89
neurological
benefits, 152, 386
changes, 74
circuits, 89
disorder, 134
links, 53, 59, 61–62, 65, 75
neurophysiologic state, 163
neuroplasticity, 88–89
neuroscience, 10, 12, 20, 77–78, 84–90, 163, 415
New Jersey Medical School, 43
New Mexico State University, 232–33
New York University's Stern School of Business, 99–101
Nike, 83, 332, 345
Nintendo. *See Wii Bowling* game

obstacles, unnecessary ones, 144–50, 158. *See also* bad guys
Ohio State University Wexner Medical Center, 10, 126, 189, 319, 326–27, 415–16, 421–25
online games, 40, 66–71, 73, 75–76, 80, 119, 256–57, 260, 317. *See also* specific titles
optimism, 88, 137, 166, 362
and allies, 254
and bad guys, 185
and cancer patients, 78, 80
and challenge mindset, 149, 284
in daily life, 132
definition of, 216
down side of, 87
and epic wins, 311
and game playing, 2–3, 78, 80, 94, 131, 225
and gratitude, 354
increasing of, 20, 86, 126, 136, 152, 216–19, 424
and life expectancy, 337
measuring of, 326–28
and quests, 18, 217, 229, 236
Oxford University study, 36–38

*Pac-Man*, 159, 179, 336
pain, 43, 134, 215, 221
and attention control, 30–32, 50–51
avoidance of, 193, 199
and bad guys, 186, 197, 208
blocking of, 19, 23, 30, 32, 51, 108, 186, 286
and breathing techniques, 82–83, 322–23
facing challenge of, 19, 133–34
fear of, 192–93
and game playing, 29–32, 50–51
and heart rate, 83
less vulnerable to, 312–13, 323
lessening of, 30–32, 82, 135
mindfulness of, 191
music's impact on, 383–84
and power-ups, 177
prevention of, 12, 29, 37
and psychological flexibility, 192–93

and quests, 236
and self-efficacy, 84
and signature strengths, 278
and traditional medicines, 19, 23, 30
and vagal tone, 163
*See also* chronic: pain
"palms up" quest, 26–27
panic attacks, 36, 43, 82, 144, 201
pattern-matching games, 37, 39–40, 67, 120
Patterson, Dr. David, 31
Pediatric Oncology Support Team, 290
*Peggle*, 47
perseverance, 25, 77, 87, 91, 97, 310
persistence, 87, 269, 340
Petersen, Dr. Christopher, 268
Pew Internet Life study, 24
physical
activity, 115, 192–93, 214, 233, 332, 336, 415, 418
benefits, 96, 283
challenges, 220, 302
energy, 253, 279, 404
fitness, 262, 292, 305, 308, 338, 370, 389
health, 45, 64, 109, 119, 128, 139, 142, 158, 163–65, 222, 377, 396–97
power-ups, 144, 170–71, 174, 181, 183
sensations, 43, 48, 50, 136
strength, 12–13, 20, 212, 313, 318, 347
triumphs, 135, 312–13, 316, 374–75
physical resilience, 238, 293, 341
and bad guys, 186, 188
building of, 18, 20, 139, 155, 178
and longevity, 336
measuring of, 51
power-ups for, 161, 178
quests for, 14, 230–31
strategies for, 152
and vagal tone, 165
physiological
benefits, 48, 152
changes, 43, 46–48, 74
links, 53, 59
sensations, 43
stress markers, 163, 183
Pollan, Michael, 373
PopCap Games, 46
Porges, Dr. Stephen, 163
*Portal*, 111–12
positive emotion ratio, 164, 166–69, 175, 181, 183
positive emotions, 178, 192, 278, 366, 415
access to, 8, 16–17
and athletic epic win, 313
and battling bad guys, 208
benefits of, 16–17, 164–65, 168–69, 337
building of, 239
and competence/control, 217
and game playing, 111, 121, 239
and gratitude, 354
and hope, 216–17
and life expectancy, 337
list of, 166
power-ups for, 160, 174–75, 182–83